Evidence-Based Practice of Anesthesiology

Evidence-Based Practice of Anesthesiology

Editor: Tiffany Johnson

FOSTER ACADEMICS

www.fosteracademics.com

www.fosteracademics.com

FOSTER ACADEMICS

Cataloging-in-Publication Data

Evidence-based practice of anesthesiology / edited by Tiffany Johnson.
p. cm.
Includes bibliographical references and index.
ISBN 978-1-64646-580-4
1. Anesthesiology. 2. Evidence-based medicine. 3. Anesthesia. 4. Anesthesia services.
5. Anesthesia--Complications. I. Johnson, Tiffany.
RD81 .A54 2023
617.96--dc23

Foster Academics,
118-35 Queens Blvd., Suite 400,
Forest Hills, NY 11375, USA

ISBN 978-1-64646-580-4 (Hardback)

Contents

Preface

This book aims to highlight the current researches and provides a platform to further the scope of innovations in this area. This book is a product of the combined efforts of many researchers and scientists, after going through thorough studies and analysis from different parts of the world. The objective of this book is to provide the readers with the latest information of the field.

Anesthesiology refers to the perioperative care of patients before, during and after the surgery. It also includes intensive care medicine, pain medicine and critical emergency medicine. Its primary principle includes the use of anesthesia and anesthetics for safely supporting a patient's vital functions during a surgery. An understanding of operative risk and complications, the methods to mitigate such risks, and the management of the illness is crucial to the practice of anesthesiology. Active airway management, ultrasonography, echocardiography imaging and hemodynamic monitoring are also performed within this discipline. In recent years, the scope of anesthesiology has extended to the identification of high-risk patients and optimization of their fitness, improvement of safety during the surgery and promotion of recovery. The topics covered in this book offer the readers new insights in the field of anesthesiology. It traces the progress of this field and highlights some of its key concepts and applications. The book is appropriate for students seeking detailed information in this area of medicine as well as for experts.

I would like to express my sincere thanks to the authors for their dedicated efforts in the completion of this book. I acknowledge the efforts of the publisher for providing constant support. Lastly, I would like to thank my family for their support in all academic endeavors.

Editor

1

Effect of PEEP and I:E ratio on cerebral oxygenation in ARDS: An experimental study in anesthetized rabbit

Federica Lovisari[1,2], Gergely H. Fodor[1], Ferenc Peták[3], Walid Habre[1,4] and Sam Bayat[1,5,6*]

Abstract

Background: Although PEEP and inversed I:E ratio have been shown to improve gas exchange in ARDS, both can adversely affect systemic hemodynamics and cerebral perfusion. The goal of this study was to assess how changes in PEEP and I:E ratio affect systemic and cerebral oxygenation and perfusion in normal and injured lung.

Methods: Eight anesthetized Chinchilla-Bastard rabbits were ventilated at baseline with pressure-regulated volume control mode, $V_T = 6$ ml/kg, PEEP = 6 cmH_2O, $FIO_2 = 0.4$; respiratory rate set for $ETCO_2 = 5.5\%$, and I:E = 1:2, 1:1 or 2:1 in random order. Ultrasonic carotid artery flow (CF), arterial (PaO_2), jugular venous blood gases and near infrared spectroscopic cerebral oxygenation (ΔHBO_2) were recorded for each experimental condition. After induced lung injury, the animals were ventilated with PEEP = 9 followed by 6 cmH_2O.

Results: At baseline, inverse-ratio ventilation (IRV) significantly reduced cerebral oxygenation (ΔO_2HB; − 27 at 1:2; − 15 at 1:1 vs. 0.27 μmol/L at 2:1; $p < 0.05$), due to a significant reduction in mean arterial pressure and CF without modifying gas exchange. In injured lung, IRV improved gas exchange but decreased cerebral perfusion without affecting brain oxygenation. The higher PEEP level, however, improved PaO_2 (67.5 ± 19.3 vs. 42.2 ± 8.4, $p < 0.05$), resulting in an improved ΔHBO_2 (− 13.8 ± 14.7 vs. −43.5 ± 21.3, $p < 0.05$), despite a drop in CF.

Conclusions: Our data suggest that unlike moderate PEEP, IRV is not effective in improving brain oxygenation in ARDS. In normal lung, IRV had a deleterious effect on brain oxygenation, which is relevant in anesthetized patients.

Keywords: Mechanical ventilation, Near-infrared spectrometry, Blood flow/regional, Acute respiratory distress syndrome, Lung function, Hemodynamics

Background

Positive-pressure mechanical ventilation is the mainstay of respiratory supportive therapy in patients with acute respiratory distress syndrome (ARDS) [1, 2]. The goal of mechanical ventilation in this setting is to open the alveoli and maintain lung aeration throughout the respiratory cycle, while avoiding excessive mechanical stretch on the lung tissue, and cyclic opening and closing of small airways and alveoli [3, 4], which can both lead to ventilator-induced lung injury. Application of positive end-expiratory pressure (PEEP) is one of the main strategies for maintaining lung aeration following alveolar recruitment [5, 6]. Another proposed approach is to increase the time during which positive pressure is applied at the airway opening, through inverse-ratio ventilation (IRV) [7–9]. This prolonged inspiratory time has been demonstrated to reduce alveolar collapse and to improve oxygenation in patients with ARDS [10, 11].

The beneficial effects of both PEEP and IRV, however, come at the potential cost of detrimental hemodynamic consequences, as the increase in intra-thoracic pressure reduces cardiac output, compromising peripheral tissue perfusion, and ultimately oxygenation [12]. Brain tissue oxygenation is directly affected by the changes in both systemic hemodynamics and blood oxygenation. It closely depends on blood perfusion and cellular metabolism in the brain, which are intricately and continuously

* Correspondence: sbayat@chu-grenoble.fr
[1]Unit for Anesthesiological Investigations Department of Anesthesiology Pharmacology and Intensive Care, University of Geneva, Geneva, Switzerland
[5]Inserm UA7 STROBE Laboratory, University of Grenoble, Grenoble, France

coupled [13]. Moreover, cerebral blood flow is locally autoregulated within physiological limits of cerebral perfusion pressure [14, 15]. Available data suggest that cerebrovascular autoregulation may be impaired in a significant number of patients with ARDS [16]. Currently, it is not well understood how the potentially conflicting effects of positive pressure ventilation settings, namely PEEP and ratio of inspiratory to expiratory time (I:E), on cerebral perfusion and blood oxygenation affect brain tissue oxygenation. The importance of understanding the impact of ventilator settings on brain oxygenation is further underscored by the high prevalence of cognitive impairment in ARDS survivors [17], where both mechanical ventilation [18] and brain tissue hypoxia [19] may play a causative role.

The aim of this study was to characterize how changes in PEEP and I:E ratio affect cerebral perfusion and brain tissue oxygenation in an experimental model of ARDS in anesthetized rabbits. We hypothesized that the improvements in gas exchange by either strategy could potentially improve brain oxygenation in the presence of lung injury.

Methods

Ethics approval

All experiments and procedures were conducted under approval from the Swiss Animal Welfare Committee (Geneva Cantonal Veterinary Office, registration number GE/164/15).

Animal preparation

Eight male pathogen-free Chinchilla-Bastard rabbits (3.5 ± 0.3 kg), purchased from the University of Geneva (Animalerie d'Arare, Plan-les-Ouates, Switzerland), were sedated with intramuscular Xylazine (Provet SA, Lyssach, Switzerland; 5.0 mg/kg). Following the insertion of a 22G catheter in a marginal ear vein, general anesthesia was initiated and maintained by a continuous infusion of propofol (B. Braun Medical AG, Sempach, Switzerland, 15–20 mg/kg/h) and fentanyl (Sintetica SA, Mendrisio, Switzerland; 5 μg/kg/h). All animals were intubated using a 3.0 mm cuffed endotracheal tube. Mechanical ventilation was initiated with the pressure-controlled mode using a pediatric respirator (SERVO-i, Maquet Critical Care, Solna Sweden), with, at baseline: a fraction of inspired oxygen (FiO_2) of 0.4, a PEEP of 3 cmH_2O and an inspiratory pressure of 6 cmH_2O above PEEP. Tidal volume (VT) was approximately 6 ml/kg and respiratory rate (RR) was adjusted to maintain end-tidal CO_2 ($ETCO_2$) between 5.5 and 6%.

After ensuring proper depth of anesthesia, muscle relaxation was induced by a continuous infusion of atracurium (Tracrium, Labatec Pharma SA, Meyrin, Switzerland; 0.6 mg/kg/h). Fluid status was maintained by an IV infusion of lactated Ringer's solution (Fresenius Kabi AG, Oberdorf, Switzerland; 4 ml/kg/h) after an initial bolus of 0.5 to 1.0 ml per kg of hydroxyethyl starch at the time of anesthesia induction.

The right internal jugular vein was cannulated with a 16G catheter for monitoring central venous pressure (CVP; Arrow, Teleflex Medical Europe, Westmeath, Ireland). A second 20G catheter was inserted in the left internal jugular vein cranially to allow cerebral venous blood sampling for blood gas analysis (Abbott i-Stat Handheld, Abbott Medical, Baar/Zug, Switzerland). A Doppler ring probe was positioned around the left internal carotid artery for continuous carotid blood flow (CF) measurement (Transonic Systems, Ithaca, NY). The left femoral artery was cannulated (22 G, Abbocath, Abbott Medical) for invasive blood pressure monitoring and arterial blood gas analysis. The electrocardiogram (ECG) was continuously monitored (Bio Amp, ADInstruments, Dunedin, New Zealand). The animals were placed on a thermostatic heating pad and internal body temperature was maintained at 38–39 °C (Harvard Apparatus, South Natick, MA, USA). An alveolar recruitment maneuver was then performed by inflating the lungs twice to 25 cmH_2O for 15 s to standardize volume history. Arterial, central venous and respiratory pressure, ECG and CF signals were digitized and recorded at 1 kHz using an analog/digital interface (Powerlab model 8/35, ADInstruments). Physiological parameters were allowed to stabilize for 15 min before starting the experimental protocol.

Brain oxygenation monitoring by near-infrared spectroscopy

Brain and muscle oxygenation was measured concomitantly to determine whether the observed changes in brain oxygenation result from local or systemic processes. Following appropriate skin shaving and cleaning, probes were placed on the head and the mid-dorsal region of the animal to monitor brain and muscle tissue oxygenation, using a NIRS monitor (NIRO-200NX, Hamamatsu, Solothurn, Switzerland). The device provides the following indices: the change in oxygenated hemoglobin (ΔHbO_2), the change in deoxygenated hemoglobin (ΔHHO_2), and the tissue oxygenation index (TOI), which is defined as the ratio of oxygenated to total tissue hemoglobin [20].

Measurement of respiratory mechanics

Mechanics of airways and respiratory tissue were measured using the forced oscillation technique, as detailed previously [21]. Briefly, a loudspeaker-in-box system was used to generate a small-amplitude (1 cmH_2O peak to peak) composite pressure forcing signal in a frequency range of 0.5–21 Hz through the tracheal cannula during short (10 s) pauses interposed with mechanical ventilation. A model including frequency-independent airway resistance (Raw) and inertance (Iaw), in series with a constant-phase tissue model [22], including damping (G) and elastance (H) was fit to the respiratory impedance (Zrs) spectra. As previously established, Raw mainly reflects the flow resistance of the airways, Iaw is related to the cyclic acceleration and deceleration of the intra-thoracic gas, G describes the energy loss within the respiratory tissues (resistance), and H characterizes the the respiratory tissues elastance. Raw and Iaw values were corrected by removing the instrumental components of the ET-cannula and the connecting tubing.

Study protocol

The study was performed in a single group ($n = 8$), each animal serving as its own control. The experiments were carried out at an academic laboratory between approximately 8 AM and 4 PM. Fifteen minutes before baseline measurements, the ventilation mode was switched to pressure-regulated volume control mode, with a VT of 6 ml/kg, FiO_2 of 0.4, PEEP of 6 cmH_2O and RR set to maintain $ETCO_2$ between 5.5 and 6%. The animals were then randomized to one of three different I:E ratios (1:2, 1:1 or 2:1). After 10 min with the initial I:E ratio, arterial and jugular venous blood gases and respiratory mechanics data were collected, and the I:E ratio was changed in random order following a recruitment maneuver to reset lung volume history.

ARDS was subsequently induced by a bolus intravenous lipopolysaccharide injection (from *Escherichia coli* O111:B4, 300 μg/kg, Sigma, Saint Louis, Missouri, USA) and whole lung lavage by instillation and recovery of 60 ml of 30 °C normal saline 5 times through the tracheal cannula. This was followed by injurious ventilation using volume-controlled ventilation with a VT of 10 ml/kg, a PEEP of 0, a FiO_2 of 1.0 and I:E ratio of 1:2, until an arterial oxygen tension (PaO_2)/fractional inspired oxygen (FiO_2) ratio between 100 and 200 was reached (in approximately 20 to 30 min) which corresponds to moderate ARDS according to the Berlin definition [1]. Following the induction of ARDS, the same procedures performed at baseline were repeated, first at a PEEP of 9 cmH_2O and again at PEEP of 6 cmH_2O, and an FIO_2 of 0.9. At the end of the study, the animal was euthanized by intravenous injection of sodium pentobarbital (120 mg/kg).

Statistical analysis

Data are presented as mean ± standard error (SEM). Brain oxygenation indices were considered as the main outcome of the study. A formal sample size estimate could not be performed a priori since the variability of the main outcome parameter in rabbit was not known. Three-way repeated measures analysis of variance (ANOVA) with Dunnett's post hoc tests were used to assess the effects of lung injury (control vs. injured), PEEP level (6 vs. 9 cmH2O) and I:E ratio (1:2, 1:1 and 2:1) on parameters reflecting ventilation, brain and muscle oxygenation, hemodynamics, and respiratory mechanics. The associations between hemodynamic and brain oxygenation indices were assessed with Pearson product-moment correlation tests. The statistical tests were performed within the R core package with the lme4 [23] and lsmeans [24] packages and SigmaPlot (version 12.5, Systat Software, Inc., Chicago, IL, USA) with a significance level of $p < 0.05$, and all p values were two-sided.

Results

The changes in airway pressures following the application of the different I:E ratios are shown in Fig. 1. Increasing I:E from 1:2 to 1:1 and 2:1 led to significant elevations in mean airway pressure regardless of the presence of injury ($p < 0.001$). In normal lungs, IRV resulted in both an increase in peak airway pressure (PIP, $p < 0.05$) and the appearance of a slight but significant

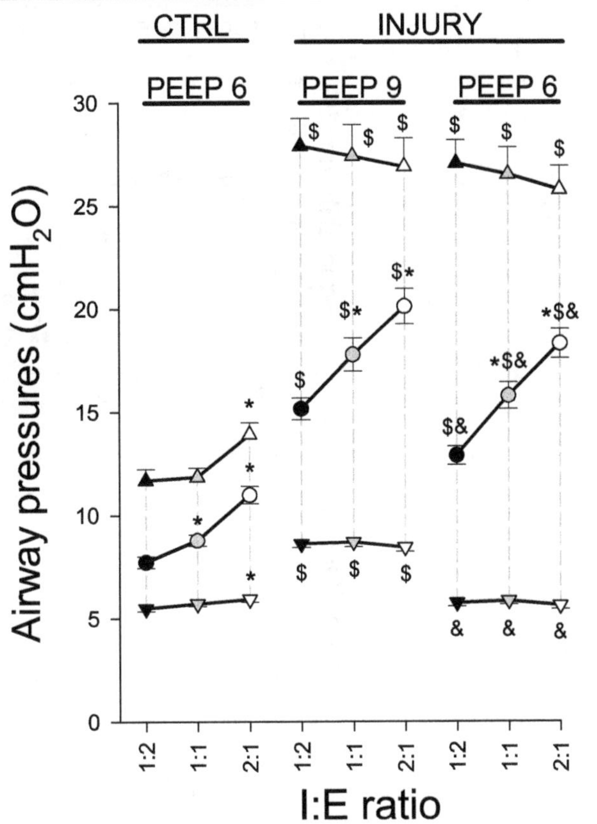

Fig. 1 Airway pressures. CTRL: control; *triangles*: peak airway pressure; *circles*: mean airway pressure; *inverted triangles*: end-expiratory pressure (PEEP); *: vs. 1:2; $: vs. control; &: vs. injury at PEEP 9 cmH_2O

intrinsic PEEP ($p < 0.05$). Conversely, no change in PIP and PEEP was evident in injured lungs.

Figure 2 summarizes the effects of lung injury and the changes in I:E ratio on brain and peripheral muscle tissue oxygenation as measured by NIRS. Under the control conditions, IRV led to a significant decrease in ΔO_2Hb ($p < 0.05$), whereas all other brain and muscle oxygenation indices remained constant. Induction of lung injury resulted in significant deterioration in these indices at the lower PEEP level ($p < 0.05$). These detrimental changes were effectively counteracted at the higher PEEP level in injured lungs ($p < 0.05$).

Changes in systemic hemodynamics are depicted in Fig. 3. Under control conditions, increasing the I:E ratio decreased venous return as suggested by the decrease in CVP ($p < 0.005$). The MAP ($p < 0.02$) and CF ($p < 0.001$) were also decreased significantly. Following the induction of lung injury, the observed hemodynamic changes were variable and influenced by both the PEEP level and the I:E ratio. IRV in the injured lungs led to significant changes in CVP ($p < 0.05$), HR ($p < 0.002$) and CF ($p < 0.02$).

Figure 4 shows the main gas exchange parameters, and a complete picture of changes in blood gas parameters and brain oxygen uptake are shown in Table 1. Lung injury compromised gas exchange significantly, which was manifested in the drop in both arterial and jugular venous blood oxygen partial pressures ($p < 0.05$). Arterial and jugular venous O_2 ($p < 0.001$ and $p < 0.005$, respectively), CO_2 partial pressures ($p < 0.001$ and $p < 0.01$, respectively) and O_2 saturation ($p < 0.001$ for both) were significantly higher at the higher PEEP level of 9 cmH_2O. Ventilation with IRV had no significant effect on arterial blood gas parameters in normal lungs. In the injured lungs however, applying an I:E ratio of 2:1 led to an improvement in PaO_2 at both PEEP levels ($p < 0.005$).

Figure 5 presents the airway and respiratory tissue mechanical parameters. In the presence of the lower PEEP and a normal I:E ratio (1:2), lung injury resulted in marked and statistically significant increases in Raw ($p < 0.002$) and decreases in Iaw ($p < 0.02$). At the lower PEEP level, significant deteriorations in respiratory tissue mechanics were present in the injured lung independently of the I:E ratio applied ($p < 0.05$ for all). The Raw ($p < 0.05$), G

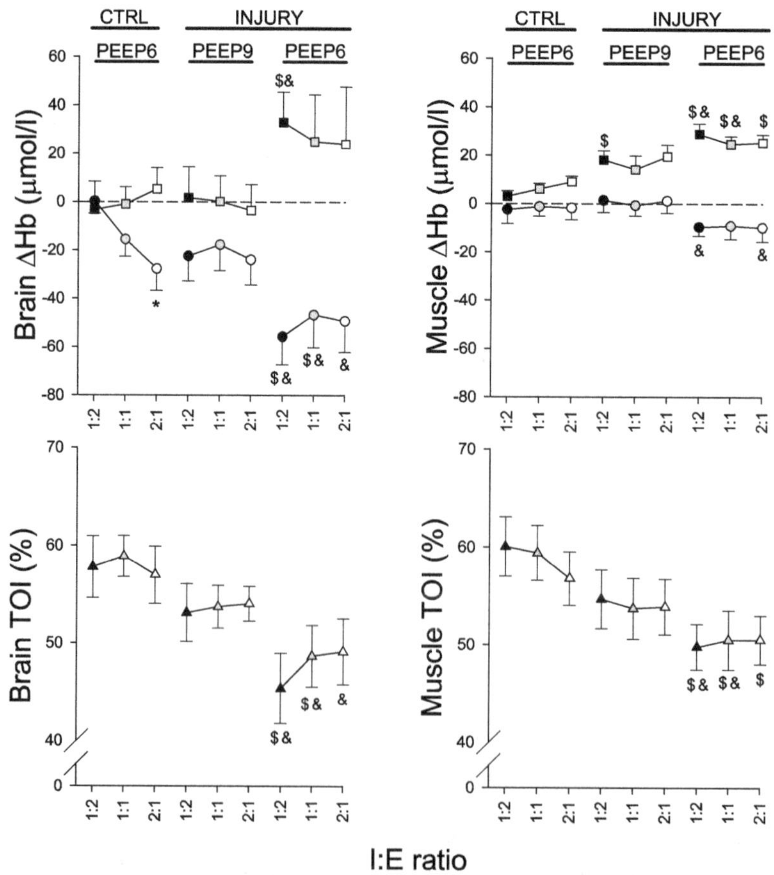

Fig. 2 Oxygenation indices for brain and spinal muscle; ΔHb: change in hemoglobin; *circles*: change in oxygenated hemoglobin (ΔO_2Hb); *squares*: change in deoxygenated hemoglobin (ΔHHb); *triangles*: tissue oxygenation index (TOI); *: vs. 1:2; $: vs. control; &: vs. injury at PEEP 9 cmH_2O

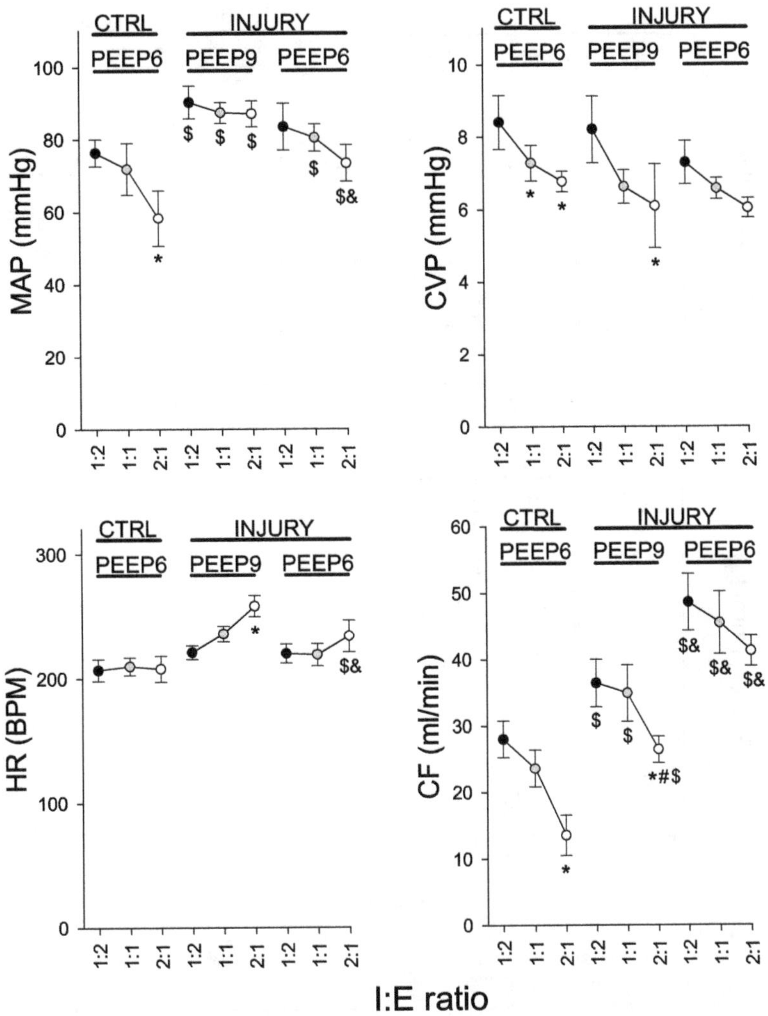

Fig. 3 Hemodynamic parameters. CTRL: control; MAP: mean arterial pressure; CVP: central venous pressure; HR: heart rate; CF: carotid artery flow; *: vs. 1:2; #: vs. 1:1; \$: vs. control; &: vs. injury at PEEP 9 cmH_2O

($p < 0.05$) and H ($p < 0.03$) were all significantly lower at the higher PEEP level of 9 cmH_2O in injured lungs.

Discussion

The main findings of this study were that in injured lungs, there was no evidence for an effect of IRV on brain oxygenation despite a positive effect on gas exchange. Conversely, in normal lungs, IRV led to a deterioration of brain oxygenation with a decrease in ΔO_2Hb. This effect was consequent to the significant drop in both mean systemic arterial pressure (MAP) and CF. Unlike with IRV, brain oxygenation was significantly better with a moderate PEEP of 9 cmH_2O as compared to a lower PEEP level of 6 cmH_2O, in injured lungs. Overall, our data suggest that the beneficial effect of a moderate level of PEEP was more prominent than that observed with IRV.

One of the most challenging aspects of ventilating patients with ARDS is the tradeoff between maintaining optimal gas exchange with appropriate systemic hemodynamic parameters and regional tissue oxygenation. In this study, we applied a model of lung injury which reproduces the cardinal features of ARDS, with a $PaO_2/FiO_2 < 200$ [1] and a major reduction in respiratory tissue compliance. To our knowledge, despite extensive studies of the cardiorespiratory effects of IRV [25–30] no data are available on the effects of PEEP and IRV on brain oxygenation in the presence of ARDS, without concomitant brain injury.

The rationale behind the use of IRV is to improve alveolar recruitment by prolonging the time during which positive pressure is applied at the airway opening during inspiration. Lengthening inspiratory time leads to an increase in mean airway pressure, without increasing peak pressures. Therefore, increasing I:E ratio has the

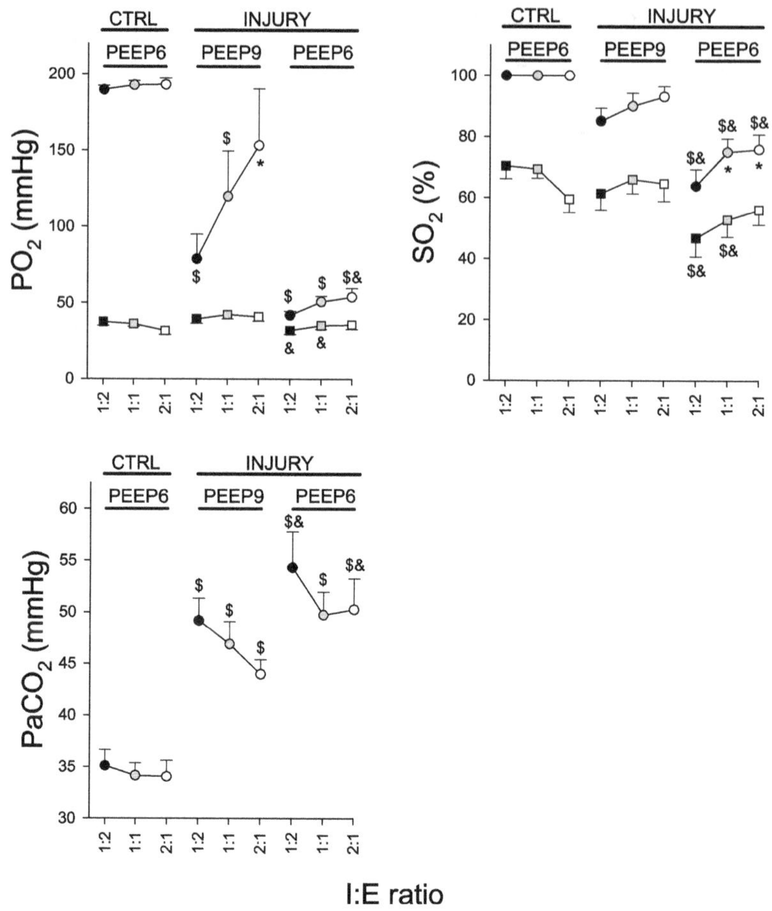

Fig. 4 Gas exchange parameters. CTRL: control; PO_2: oxygen partial pressure in arterial and jugular venous blood; $PaCO_2$: arterial carbon dioxide partial pressure; SO_2: oxygen saturation in arterial and jugular venous blood; *circles*: values obtained from arterial blood; *squares*: values obtained from arterial blood; *: vs. 1:2; $: vs. control; &: vs. injury at PEEP 9 cmH_2O

potential to improve the mechanical properties of the airways and respiratory tissues and gas exchange [25, 26, 28]. However, both PEEP and IRV can potentially reduce venous return due to an increase in intrathoracic pressure, thereby decreasing cardiac output [27, 28]. Both could contribute to a decrease in CF due to a reduction in effective cerebral perfusion pressure, and in cerebral oxygenation. Examination of the physiological consequences of these modes on cerebral oxygenation are therefore important and relevant. Although IRV is not widely used in clinical practice, recent studies in the literature suggest that it might be used to maintain end-expiratory recruitment without the adverse effects of PEEP [29]. Other ventilation modes have been proposed such as airway pressure-release ventilation (APRV), which is an inverse-ratio pressure controlled, intermittent mandatory ventilation, that is intensely used in some centers and used as the primary mode in ARDS [31, 32]. This mode bears similarities with IRV in that mean airway pressure is increased through a prolonged inspiratory time, without increasing peak airway pressure [33].

Inverse-ratio ventilation resulted in a net decrease in ΔO_2Hb at baseline. In injured lung however, the effect of IRV on brain oxygenation was not significant. These changes may be attributed to the concomitant changes in gas exchange and brain perfusion as measured by CF. In turn, CF depended on MAP and was significantly influenced by $PaCO_2$ (Additional file 1: Figure S1). At baseline, the drop in ΔO_2Hb with IRV may be attributed to a decreased carotid flow, while the gas exchange parameters were unchanged. The decrease in CF under IRV in this case, may have resulted from a decreased cardiac output. This is in line with the decrease in MAP. Moreover, the decrease in CVP suggests a reduced venous return with IRV (Fig. 3). Additionally, the decrease in CF was correlated to Paw_m (Additional file 1: Figure S1). On the other hand, the lack of a significant effect of IRV on ΔO_2Hb in ARDS may be due to a concomitant increase in PaO_2 and a drop in CF (Figs. 3 and 4) at the higher PEEP level of 9 cmH_2O.

In normal lung, the correlations between CF and brain oxygenation indices (Additional file 1: Figure S1) were

Table 1 Gas exchange data

		CTRL			INJURED					
		PEEP6			PEEP9			PEEP6		
	I:E ratio	1:2	1:1	2:1	1:2	1:1	2:1	1:2	1:1	2:1
Artery	pH	7.459 ±0.02	7.467 ±0.03	7.454 ±0.02	7.244$^{\$}$ ±0.03	7.253$^{\$}$ ±0.04	7.269$^{\$}$ ±0.04	7.202$^{\$}$ ±0.04	7.221$^{\$}$ ±0.02	7.218$^{\$}$ ±0.02
	$PaCO_2$ (mmHg)	35.1 ±1.54	34.1 ±1.24	34.0 ±1.60	49.2$^{\$}$ ±2.15	46.9$^{\$}$ ±2.18	44.0$^{*\$}$ ±1.39	54.3$^{\$\&}$ ±3.47	49.7$^{\$\&}$ ±2.21	50.3$^{\$\&}$ ±2.99
	PaO_2 (mmHg)	189.6 ±2.78	192.6 ±2.93	193 ±4.21	78.8$^{\$}$ ±16.1	119.9$^{\$}$ ±29.7	153.1$^{*\$}$ ±37.0	42.0$^{\$\&}$ ±2.67	50.9$^{\$\&}$ ±3.51	53.9$^{*\$\&}$ ±5.82
	PaO_2/FIO_2	474.1 ±6.96	481.6 ±7.32	482.5 ±10.5	87.5$^{\$}$ ±17.9	133.2$^{\$}$ ±33.0	170.1$^{*\$}$ ±41.1	46.7$^{\$\&}$ ±2.96	56.5$^{\$\&}$ ±3.91	59.9$^{\$\&}$ ±6.47
	HCO_3^-(mmol/l)	24.9 ±0.68	24.7 ±1.04	23.8 ±0.80	21.2$^{\$}$ ±0.54	20.8$^{\$}$ ±1.2	20.4$^{\$}$ ±1.2	21.2$^{\$}$ ±1.0	20.3$^{\$}$ ±0.5	20.3$^{\$}$ ±0.6
	BE (mmol/l)	1.0 ±0.93	0.89 ±1.42	−0.13 ±1.10	−6.4$^{\$}$ ±0.98	−6.4$^{\$}$ ±1.7	− 6.5$^{\$}$ ±1.8	−6.9$^{\$}$ ±1.6	− 7.3$^{\$}$ ±0.75	−7.5$^{\$}$ ±0.50
	SaO_2 (%)	100.0 ±0.0	100 ±0.0	100 ±0.0	85.1$^{\$}$ ±4.2	90.0$^{\$}$ ±4.3	93.1$^{\$}$ ±3.4	63.9$^{\$\&}$ ±5.4	75.0$^{\$\&}$ ±4.4	75.9$^{\$\&}$ ±4.8
	Lac (mmol/l)	2.67 ±0.44	2.61 ±0.43	3.07 ±0.50	4.98 ±1.0	5.03 ±1.1	5.71 ±1.1	6.36$^{\$}$ ±1.2	5.9$^{\$}$ ±0.80	5.9$^{\$}$ ±0.45
Vein	pH	7.406 ±0.016	7.412 ±0.02	7.400 ±0.02	7.227$^{\$}$ ±0.03	7.232$^{\$}$ ±0.04	7.238$^{\$}$ ±0.03	7.191$^{\$}$ ±0.04	7.197$^{\$}$ ±0.02	7.225$^{\$}$ ±0.01
	$PvCO_2$ (mmHg)	38.5 ±2.0	38.2 ±1.83	39.9 ±1.85	53.7$^{\$}$ ±2.80	47.7$^{\$}$ ±2.8	49.5$^{\$}$ ±2.9	56.0$^{\$}$ ±4.7	54.8$^{\$\&}$ ±2.3	52.1$^{\$}$ ±2.6
	PvO_2 (mmHg)	37.5 ±2.3	36.3 ±1.86	31.8* ±2.49	39.4 ±2.71	42.3 ±2.79	40.9$^{\$}$ ±2.92	32.0$^{\$}$ ±2.5	35.3$^{\&}$ ± 2.5	35.7$^{\&}$ ± 2.8
	HCO_3^-(mmol/l)	24.09 ±1.0	24.38 ±1.3	24.5 ±1.1	22.2$^{\$}$ ±0.5	20.3$^{\$}$ ±1.5	21.0$^{\$}$ ±0.96	21.1$^{\$}$ ±1.0	21.2$^{\$}$ ±0.61	21.5$^{\$}$ ±1.0
	BE (mmol/l)	−0.50 ±1.0	−0.25 ±1.5	−0.5 ±1.3	−5.5$^{\$}$ ±0.8	−7.1$^{\$}$ ±2.1	−6.4$^{\$}$ ±5.8	−7.1$^{\$}$ ±1.5	−7.0$^{\$}$ ±0.9	−6.1$^{\$}$ ±1.1
	SvO_2 (%)	70.4 ±4.2	69.4 ±2.9	59.5* ±4.3	61.4 ±5.4	66.0 ±4.7	64.6 ±5.8	46.8$^{\$\&}$ ±6.1	52.8$^{\$\&}$ ±5.6	56.0$^{\$\&}$ ±4.8
	Lac (mmol/l)	8.41 ±0.31	8.37 ±0.33	8.19 ±0.28	8.16 ±0.28	7.63 ±0.64	7.93 ±0.31	7.71 ±0.33	8.16 ±0.31	8.27 ±0.56
	$C(a\text{-}v)O_2$ (ml/dl)	3.82 ±0.57	3.91 ±0.22	4.98* ±0.50	2.79$^{\$}$ ±0.31	2.66$^{\$}$ ±0.33	3.49$^{*\$}$ ±0.31	1.84$^{\$\&}$ ±0.25	2.53$^{\$}$ ±0.27	2.73$^{*\$}$ ±0.48
	Brain $\dot{Q}\,O_2$ (ml/min)	2.05 ±0.24	1.82 ±0.19	1.22* ±0.24	1.95 ±0.17	1.82 ±0.25	1.84$^{\$}$ ±0.22	1.71 ±0.21	2.36* ±0.31	2.28$^{*\$}$ ±0.40

Gas exchange and brain metabolic parameters; *BE*: base excess; *SaO_2, SvO_2*: arterial and venous hemoglobin oxygen saturation, respectivley; *Lac*: blood lactate; *$C(a\text{-}v)O_2$*: difference in arterio-venous oxygen content; $\dot{Q}\,O_2$:brain O_2 uptake; *: vs. 1:2, $: vs. CTRL, &: vs. injury at PEEP 9 cmH_2O; by 3-way repeated measures ANOVA

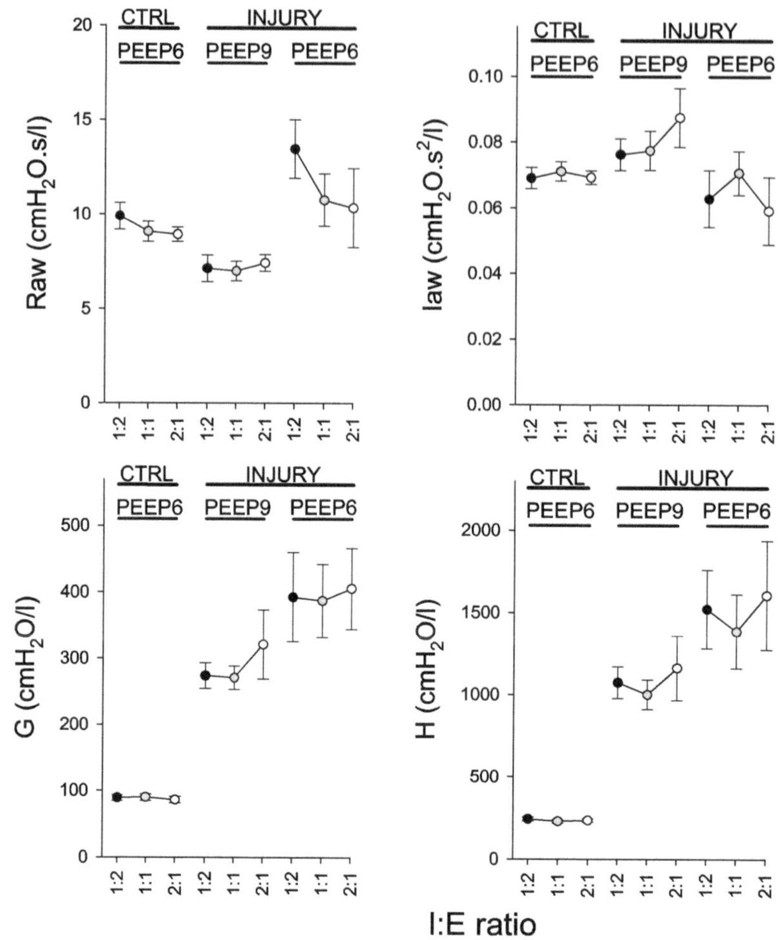

Fig. 5 Forced oscillatory respiratory mechanical parameters; Raw: airway resistance; Iaw: airway inertance; H: respiratory tissue elastance; G: respiratory tissue damping; CTRL: control; *: vs. 1:2; #: vs. 1:1; $: vs. control; &: vs. injury at PEEP 9 cmH_2O

opposite to those observed in moderate ARDS. This is explained by the fact that the predominant effect of an increase in Paw_m was a drop in CF, while gas exchange was not significantly affected (Fig. 4). Under this condition, brain oxygenation indices were primarily determined by brain perfusion, which was itself dependent upon the MAP, which is illustrated by a strong correlation between MAP and CF.

In injured lung, IRV significantly increased PaO_2 and reduced $PaCO_2$, although this effect was highly dependent on PEEP: a much larger improvement in PaO_2 and a reduction in $PaCO_2$ was observed at the higher PEEP level of 9 cmH_2O. The lower PEEP level of 6 cmH_2O resulted in a severe hypoxemia and hypercapnia. Despite a higher carotid flow promoted by hypercapnic cerebral vasodilation, brain oxygenation was significantly decreased as a consequence of severe hypoxemia. Under this condition, IRV had no significant effect on brain oxygenation.

A potential mechanism for the improved gas exchange on PEEP 9 cmH_2O, may be that small increments in Paw_m under IRV, resulted in lung recruitment. However, although a modest increase in PEEP improved respiratory tissue elastance suggesting recruitment, no additional decreases in H were observed by increasing I:E (Fig. 5). It should be noted that IRV did not produce any intrinsic PEEP at either PEEP levels in injured lung, although a slight intrinsic PEEP was observed at baseline (Fig. 1). Nevertheless, poorly compliant alveoli with faster emptying time constants, that derecruit upon end-expiration are likely to be aerated for longer periods of time during IRV. This mechanism would contribute to gas exchange [34], but would not be measured by respiratory elastance, which is measured upon expiration. However, in injured lung IRV did not significantly increase the dynamic compliance either, despite a significant improvement with the PEEP increment from 6 to 9 cmH2O (Additional file 1: Figure S1). Our data therefore, do not demonstrate a better alveolar recruitment under IRV.

Another possible mechanism for the observed improvement in gas exchange is that the prolonged inspiration lengthens the time for admixture of alveolar and dead space gas, thereby reducing physiologic dead space [25, 27, 34]. This effect may have been more prominent in the presence of a larger alveolar gas compartment due to the recruitment induced by the slightly higher PEEP level.

Ventilating the lung with a slightly higher PEEP (9 vs. 6 cmH_2O) with an I:E of 0.5, improved tissue oxygenation markedly in the brain and, to a lesser degree, in peripheral muscle. This effect on brain oxygenation occurred despite a significant decrease in CF (Fig. 3) that occurred in parallel to a reduction in $PaCO_2$, while MAP and CVP were unchanged. This suggests that increased brain oxygenation in this case, was mainly due to improved gas exchange (Fig. 4). This interpretation is further illustrated by the negative correlation between CF and brain oxygenation indices (TOI, ΔHbO_2) in injured lung (Additional file 1: Figure S1).

Our study had several methodological limitations. Only a single PEEP level was tested at baseline. This was because higher PEEP levels are seldom applied in normal lung, and our data show that higher airway pressures in healthy lungs can indeed compromise cerebral perfusion and systemic hemodynamics without improving gas exchange. To avoid the confounding effects of evolving lung injury and limited time, only one PEEP increment was assessed in injured lung. However, the single PEEP increment was sufficient to characterize the effect of elevated PEEP on the brain oxygenation indices; further PEEP elevations would likely produce similar trends with changes of larger magnitude. In this study, we did not alter respiratory rate in order to adjust $PaCO_2$ between the various ventilatory conditions; we rather maintained the same level of external PEEP and minute ventilation, and modified the I:E ratio. While this resulted in changes in physiologic parameters with significant colinearity amongst themselves, this is inherent to in-vivo studies in general and similar to the comparison of standard I:E and IRV in the clinical setting [27]. Moreover, manipulating the respiratory rate would have modified Paw_m raising further issues. We therefore maintained a study design that allows assessing the integral effect of manipulating I:E on cerebral oxygenation. We did not measure cardiac output, and it should be noted that CVP may be a weak indicator of volume status [35], although it has been shown to decrease with hypovolemia and rise with resuscitation in rabbits [36]. However, the drop in MAP is highly suggestive of a drop in cardiac output under IRV at baseline. Finally, as in any study using animal models, extrapolation to human subjects should be made with appropriate caution. However, cerebrovascular autoregulation in rabbit has been widely used as a consistent model of human physiology [37, 38].

Conclusions

We found that the mechanical ventilation strategy in the presence of lung injury significantly impacted brain oxygenation. In normal lung, IRV had a deleterious effect on brain oxygenation, and clinicians should be aware of the potential adverse effect of this ventilation mode. Moreover, we observed no effect of IRV on brain oxygenation in moderate ARDS, as the beneficial effects of IRV on gas exchange were counteracted by decreases in cerebral perfusion. In contrast, a modest PEEP significantly improved brain oxygenation in injured lung, since the substantial improvement in gas exchange overcame the concomitant decrease in brain perfusion. Overall, our data suggest that unlike moderate PEEP, IRV is not effective in improving brain oxygenation in ARDS.

Abbreviations

APRV: Airway pressure-release ventilation; ARDS: Acute respiratory distress syndrome; CF: Carotid flow; ECG: Electrocardiogram; ET-cannula: Endotracheal cannula; $ETCO_2$: End-tidal CO_2; FiO_2: Fraction of inspired O_2; G: respiratory tissue damping; H: respiratory tissue elastance; I:E: Ratio of inspirartory/expiratory time; Iaw: Respiratory inertance; IRV: Inverse-ration ventilation; MAP: Mean arterial pressure; NIRS: Near-infrared spectroscopy; PaO_2: arterial O_2 partial pressure; PEEP: Positive end-expiratory pressure; PIP: Peak inspiratory pressure; Raw: Airway resistance; RR: Respiratory rate; TOI: Tissue oxygenation index; VT: tidal volume; Zrs: respiratory impedance; ΔHbO_2: change in oxygenated hemoglobin; ΔHHO_2: change in deoxygenated hemoglobin

Acknowledgements

The authors thank Xavier Belin and Sylvie Roulet for their technical assistance.

Authors' contributions

SB, FL, FP, and WH designed the study; SB and FL acquired the data; SB, FL, GHF and FP carried out the data analysis; SB, FL, FP and WH drafted the manuscript. All authors read, edited and approved the final version of the article.

Author details

[1]Unit for Anesthesiological Investigations Department of Anesthesiology Pharmacology and Intensive Care, University of Geneva, Geneva, Switzerland. [2]University of Milano-Bicocca, Milan, Italy. [3]Department of Medical Physics and Informatics, University of Szeged, Szeged, Hungary. [4]Pediatric Anesthesia Unit, Geneva Children's Hospital, Geneva, Switzerland. [5]Inserm UA7 STROBE Laboratory, University of Grenoble, Grenoble, France. [6]Department of Clinical Physiology, Sleep and Exercise, Grenoble University Hospital, Grenoble, France.

References

1. Ranieri VM, Rubenfeld GD, Thompson BT, Ferguson ND, Caldwell E, Fan E, et al. Acute respiratory distress syndrome: the Berlin definition. JAMA. 2012;307(23):2526–33.
2. Wang C, Wang X, Chi C, Guo L, Zhao N, Wang W, et al. Lung ventilation strategies for acute respiratory distress syndrome: a systematic review and network meta-analysis. Sci Rep. 2016;6:22855.
3. Gattinoni L, Carlesso E, Caironi P. Stress and strain within the lung. Curr Opin Crit Care. 2012;18(1):42–7.
4. Protti A, Cressoni M, Santini A, Langer T, Mietto C, Febres D, et al. Lung stress and strain during mechanical ventilation: any safe threshold? Am J Respir Crit Care Med. 2011;183(10):1354–62.
5. Briel M, Meade M, Mercat A, Brower RG, Talmor D, Walter SD, et al. Higher vs lower positive end-expiratory pressure in patients with acute lung injury and acute respiratory distress syndrome: systematic review and meta-analysis. JAMA. 2010;303(9):865–73.

6. Brower RG, Lanken PN, MacIntyre N, Matthay MA, Morris A, Ancukiewicz M, et al. Higher versus lower positive end-expiratory pressures in patients with the acute respiratory distress syndrome. N Engl J Med. 2004;351(4):327–36.
7. Zhang WP, Zhu SM. The effects of inverse ratio ventilation on cardiopulmonary function and inflammatory cytokine of bronchoaveolar lavage in obese patients undergoing gynecological laparoscopy. Acta Anaesthesiol Taiwanica : Off J Taiwan Soc Anesthesiol. 2016;54(1):1–5.
8. Armstrong BW Jr, MacIntyre NR. Pressure-controlled, inverse ratio ventilation that avoids air trapping in the adult respiratory distress syndrome. Crit Care Med. 1995;23(2):279–85.
9. Wang X, Wang P, Wang K, Jiang T, Xu Z. Pressure-controlled inverse ratio ventilation during general anesthesia for open abdominal surgery improves postoperative pulmonary function. J Biomed Sci Eng. 2016;9(01):17.
10. Lessard MR, Guerot E, Lorino H, Lemaire F, Brochard L. Effects of pressure-controlled with different I:E ratios versus volume-controlled ventilation on respiratory mechanics, gas exchange, and hemodynamics in patients with adult respiratory distress syndrome. Anesthesiology. 1994;80(5):983–91.
11. Gore DC. Hemodynamic and ventilatory effects associated with increasing inverse inspiratory-expiratory ventilation. J Trauma. 1998;45(2):268–72.
12. Michard F, Teboul JL. Using heart-lung interactions to assess fluid responsiveness during mechanical ventilation. Crit Care. 2000;4(5):282–9.
13. Yarowsky PJ, Ingvar DH. Symposium summary. Neuronal activity and energy metabolism. Fed Proc. 1981;40(9):2353–62.
14. Lassen NA. Cerebral blood flow and oxygen consumption in man. Physiol Rev. 1959;39(2):183–238.
15. Joshi B, Ono M, Brown C, Brady K, Easley RB, Yenokyan G, et al. Predicting the limits of cerebral autoregulation during cardiopulmonary bypass. Anesth Analg. 2012;114(3):503–10.
16. Schramm P, Closhen D, Felkel M, Berres M, Klein KU, David M, et al. Influence of PEEP on cerebral blood flow and cerebrovascular autoregulation in patients with acute respiratory distress syndrome. J Neurosurg Anesthesiol. 2013;25(2):162–7.
17. Hopkins RO, Jackson JC. Long-term neurocognitive function after critical illness. Chest. 2006;130(3):869–78.
18. Pelosi P, Rocco PR. The lung and the brain: a dangerous cross-talk. Crit Care. 2011;15(3):168.
19. Hopkins RO, Myers CE, Shohamy D, Grossman S, Gluck M. Impaired probabilistic category learning in hypoxic subjects with hippocampal damage. Neuropsychologia. 2004;42(4):524–35.
20. Suzuki S, Takasaki S, Ozaki T, et al. A tissue oxygenation monitor using NIR spatially resolved spectroscopy, vol. 11. Bellingham, WA, ETATS-UNIS: Society of Photo-Optical Instrumentation Engineers; 1999.
21. Bayat S, Strengell S, Porra L, Janosi TZ, Petak F, Suhonen H, et al. Methacholine and ovalbumin challenges assessed by forced oscillations and synchrotron lung imaging. Am J Respir Crit Care Med. 2009;180(4):296–303.
22. Hantos Z, Daroczy B, Suki B, Nagy S, Fredberg JJ. Input impedance and peripheral inhomogeneity of dog lungs. J Appl Physiol. 1992;72(1):168–78.
23. Bates D, Mächler M, Bolker B. Walker S. fitting linear mixed-effects models using lme4. 2015. 2015;67(1):48.
24. Lenth RV. Least-squares means. The R Package lsmeans 2016. 2016;69(1):33.
25. Cole AG, Weller SF, Sykes MK. Inverse ratio ventilation compared with PEEP in adult respiratory failure. Intensive Care Med. 1984;10(5):227–32.
26. Yanos J, Watling SM, Verhey J. The physiologic effects of inverse ratio ventilation. Chest. 1998;114(3):834–8.
27. Mercat A, Titiriga M, Anguel N, Richard C, Teboul JL. Inverse ratio ventilation (I/E = 2/1) in acute respiratory distress syndrome: a six-hour controlled study. Am J Respir Crit Care Med. 1997;155(5):1637–42.
28. Neumann P, Berglund JE, Andersson LG, Maripu E, Magnusson A, Hedenstierna G. Effects of inverse ratio ventilation and positive end-expiratory pressure in oleic acid-induced lung injury. Am J Respir Crit Care Med. 2000;161(5):1537–45.
29. Boehme S, Bentley AH, Hartmann EK, Chang S, Erdoes G, Prinzing A, et al. Influence of inspiration to expiration ratio on cyclic recruitment and derecruitment of atelectasis in a saline lavage model of acute respiratory distress syndrome. Crit Care Med. 2015;43(3):e65–74.
30. Muller-Redetzky HC, Felten M, Hellwig K, Wienhold SM, Naujoks J, Opitz B, et al. Increasing the inspiratory time and I:E ratio during mechanical ventilation aggravates ventilator-induced lung injury in mice. Crit Care. 2015;19:23.
31. Habashi NM. Other approaches to open-lung ventilation: airway pressure release ventilation. Crit Care Med. 2005;33(3 Suppl):S228–40.
32. Jain SV, Kollisch-Singule M, Sadowitz B, Dombert L, Satalin J, Andrews P, et al. The 30-year evolution of airway pressure release ventilation (APRV). Intensive Care Med Exp. 2016;4(1):11.
33. Mireles-Cabodevila E, Kacmarek RM. Should airway pressure release ventilation be the primary mode in ARDS? Respir Care. 2016;61(6):761–73.
34. Knelson JH, Howatt WF, DeMuth GR. Effect of respiratory pattern on alveolar gas exchange. J Appl Physiol. 1970;29(3):328–31.
35. Kumar A, Anel R, Bunnell E, Habet K, Zanotti S, Marshall S, et al. Pulmonary artery occlusion pressure and central venous pressure fail to predict ventricular filling volume, cardiac performance, or the response to volume infusion in normal subjects. Crit Care Med. 2004;32(3):691–9.
36. Chen S, Zhu X, Wang Q, Li W, Cheng D, Lei C, et al. The early effect of Voluven, a novel hydroxyethyl starch (130/0.4), on cerebral oxygen supply and consumption in resuscitation of rabbit with acute hemorrhagic shock. J Trauma. 2009;66(3):676–82.
37. Aksenov D, Eassa JE, Lakhoo J, Wyrwicz A, Linsenmeier RA. Effect of isoflurane on brain tissue oxygen tension and cerebral autoregulation in rabbits. Neurosci Lett. 2012;524(2):116–8.
38. Tureen JH, Dworkin RJ, Kennedy SL, Sachdeva M, Sande MA. Loss of cerebrovascular autoregulation in experimental meningitis in rabbits. J Clin Invest. 1990;85(2):577–81.

2

Pleth variability index versus pulse pressure variation for intraoperative goal-directed fluid therapy in patients undergoing low-to-moderate risk abdominal surgery

Sean Coeckelenbergh[1,2*†], Amélie Delaporte[1,2†], Djamal Ghoundiwal[1,2], Javad Bidgoli[1,2], Jean-François Fils[1,3], Denis Schmartz[1,2] and Philippe Van der Linden[1,2]

Abstract

Background: Goal-directed fluid therapy (GDFT) based on dynamic indicators of fluid responsiveness has been shown to decrease postoperative complications and hospital length of stay (LOS) in patients undergoing major abdominal surgery. The usefulness of this approach still needs to be clarified in low-to-moderate risk abdominal surgery. Both pulse-pressure variation (PPV) and pleth variability index (PVI) can be used to guide GDFT strategies. The objective of this prospective randomized controlled trial was to determine if the use of PVI guided GDFT, when compared to PPV guided GDFT, would lead to similar hospital LOS in patients undergoing low-to-moderate risk surgery. Secondary outcomes included amount of fluid administered and incidence of postoperative complications.

Methods: Patients were randomized into either PVI or PPV guided GDFT groups. Both received a baseline 2 ml kg^{-1} h^{-1} Lactated Ringer infusion. Additional fluid boluses consisted of 250 mL of colloid that was infused over a 10 min period if PVI was > 15% or PPV was > 13% for at least five minutes. The primary outcome was to determine if hospital LOS, which was defined as the number of days from surgery up to the day the surgeon authorized hospital discharge, was equivalent between the two groups.

Results: A total of 76 patients were included and they were randomized into two groups of 38 patients. Baseline characteristics were similar in both groups. Both PVI and PPV guided GDFT strategies were equivalent for the primary outcome of LOS (median [interquartile range]) (days) 2.5 [2.0–3.3] vs. 3.0 [2.0–5.0], $p = 0.230$, respectively. Fluids infused, postoperative complications, and all other outcomes were not different between groups.

Conclusion: In patients undergoing low-to-moderate risk abdominal surgery, PVI seems to guide GDFT similarly to PPV in regards to hospital LOS, amount of fluid, and incidence of postoperative complications. However, in low-risk patients undergoing these surgical procedures optimizing stroke volume may have limited impact on outcome.

Keywords: Anesthesia, Anesthesiology, Goal-directed therapy, Colloids, Crystalloids, Fluid responsiveness, Hemodynamics

* Correspondence: secoecke@ulb.ac.be
†Sean Coeckelenbergh and Amélie Delaporte contributed equally to this work.
[1]Department of Anesthesiology, CHU Brugmann, 4, Place Van Gehuchten, 1020 Bruxelles, Belgium
[2]Université Libre de Bruxelles, Brussels, Belgium

Background

Goal-directed fluid therapy (GDFT), guided by dynamic indicators of fluid responsiveness, (e.g. pulse pressure variation (PPV)) has been shown to decrease postoperative complications and to shorten length of stay (LOS) during major abdominal surgery [1–3]. Dynamic indicators are based on cardiopulmonary interactions during mechanical ventilation and predict fluid responsiveness better than static indicators (e.g. central venous pressure and non-invasive blood pressure) [4–8].

Pulse pressure variation can guide GDFT [9], but it requires the insertion of an arterial catheter and its inherent risks [10]. This is not always desirable, especially for low-to-moderate risk surgeries where blood loss and fluid shifts are minimal. In cases where the risks of an invasive catheter outweigh its potential benefits, pleth variability index (PVI) may be a valuable alternative. PVI is a totally non-invasive monitor which only requires a pulse oximeter [11]. PVI-based GDFT has been shown to reduce postoperative lactate levels and improve postoperative outcome in patients undergoing high-risk abdominal surgery [12–14]. It is safe, easily implemented, and non-invasive. Nevertheless, PVI's correlation to PPV has been shown to be weak during major abdominal surgery and cardiac surgery, which may be due to intraoperative or chronic changes in arteriolar compliance, sympathetic tone, and heart rate variability [15, 16]. In low-to-moderate risk abdominal surgery, however, such effects on arteriolar and sympathetic tone are probably less frequent and the clinical impact of PVI remains to be determined. PVI may thus be useful in guiding GDFT in this population where these hemodynamic alterations are scarce.

The primary objective of this prospective randomized controlled trial was to demonstrate that the use of PVI guided GDFT and PPV guided GDFT would lead to equivalent hospital LOS in patients undergoing low-to-moderate risk abdominal surgery. Secondary objectives included the amount of fluid administered and the incidence of postoperative complications associated to each GDFT strategy.

Methods

This single center prospective parallel group randomized controlled trial was performed at the CHU-Brugmann Hospital after ethical committee approval (Brussels, Belgium) (N°CE/201134 and B077201112471) and was registered on clinicaltrials.gov (NCT02908256). Patients gave written informed consent, were adults scheduled for elective low-to-moderate risk abdominal surgery lasting at least one hour, and were allocated into each group after randomization with a ratio of 1:1. Patients were randomized with internet-based software (http://www.randomization.com) and the determined groups were placed in numbered sealed envelopes. AD and DG generated the randomization sequence, enrolled patients, and assigned patients to the interventions. Exclusion criteria consisted of patients younger than 18 years, American Society of Anesthesiologist physical status score greater than III, a body mass index $> 35\ \text{kg m}^{-2}$, chronic cardiac arrhythmias, altered myocardial function (left ventricular ejection fraction < 25%), peripheral vascular disease, severe respiratory disease, gelatin allergy, and end stage renal failure (creatinine clearance $< 30\ \text{ml min}^{-1}$).

Anesthesia protocol

Patients fasted at least 6 h for solids and 2 h for clear liquids preoperatively and received oral alprazolam 0.5mg one hour before induction of general anesthesia. Patient monitoring included 5 lead electrocardiogram, non-invasive blood pressure, and peripheral pulse oximetry. The Masimo Radical 7 Set pulse oximeter (Masimo Corp, Irvine, CA, USA) was applied on the index finger, contralateral to the blood pressure cuff, and covered from ambient light for the continuous monitoring of the PVI. A 20-G radial artery catheter was placed ipsilateral to the pulse oximeter after induction of anesthesia. PPV were displayed on the IntelliVue MP5 monitor (Philips Healthcare, Best, Netherlands). Investigators were blinded to the values not pertaining to the allocated GDFT protocol. Entropy sensors (GE Healthcare, Chalfont St Giles, United Kingdom) monitored anesthesia depth and values were kept between 40 and 60 for all patients. Anesthetists induced anesthesia with a propofol bolus of $1–2\ \text{mg kg}^{-1}$ and a sufentanil $0.3\ \text{ng ml}^{-1}$ target controlled infusion Gepts model [17] (Alaris PK syringe pump, CardinalHealth, Rolle, Switzerland). Rocuronium $0.5\ \text{mg kg}^{-1}$ facilitated oral tracheal intubation and muscle paralysis was maintained with additional doses of $0.1\ \text{mg kg}^{-1}$ to maintain a train of four ratio of 0:4 (TOF Watch, Alsevia Pharma, France). Anesthesia was maintained with sevoflurane and sufentanil with a target concentration of $0.2\ \text{ng ml}^{-1}$. Rectal temperature was measured continuously and a forced-air warming blanket was added to maintain normothermia. Tidal volume was maintained at of $8\ \text{ml kg}^{-1}$ of ideal body weight and the respiratory frequency was set to maintain expiratory carbon dioxide between 30 and 35 mmHg. Positive end-expiratory pressure was set to 5 cm H_2O in all patients. Trendelenburg was set at 10° using a goniometer (iPhone, Apple, Cupertino, CA, USA) that was placed lateral to each patient's head. Postoperative pain control was achieved with the following analgesics (if not contraindicated): paracetamol, diclofenac, tramadol, and patient controlled intravenous morphine. Use of nitrous oxide, ketamine, or clonidine was prohibited intraoperatively.

GDFT protocol

Patients were randomized into either PPV GDFT or PVI GDFT groups. Anesthetists were blinded to the monitor not corresponding to their allocated group while patients and postoperative care givers were blinded to the intervention. All patients received a baseline 2 ml $kg^{-1} h^{-1}$ Lactated Ringer infusion. The fluid challenge consisted of a 250 ml bolus of colloid (Geloplasma, Fresenius Kabi SA, Belgium) that was infused over a 10 min period. Patients in the PVI GDFT group received a fluid challenge if PVI was higher than 15% for more than 5 min while patients in the PPV GDFT group received a fluid challenge if PPV was higher than 13% for more than 5 min [11, 18, 19]. Boluses were repeated until patients were no longer over the PVI or PPV fluid challenge thresholds. Phenylephrine was titrated if mean arterial blood pressure remained below 65 mmHg despite preload optimization (i.e. PVI or PPV values were below the predetermined fluid responsiveness threshold) (Fig. 1). Additional crystalloids infused for antibiotic and analgesic administration were recorded and added to the total infused volume. Management of acute hemodynamic instability associated with hemorrhage was left at the attending anesthesiologist's discretion. There was no change in threshold values during pneumoperitoneum and the GDFT protocols were the same regardless of the use of laparoscopy.

Outcomes variables

The primary outcome was hospital the LOS, which was defined as the number of days from surgery up to the day the surgeon authorized hospital discharge. If patients remained hospitalized longer than the date decided by the surgeon, the surgical discharge date noted in the medical record was still used to calculate hospital LOS. Other outcomes included total infused colloid, total infused crystalloid, estimated blood loss, diuresis, intraoperative use of phenylephrine (i.e., mean arterial blood pressure remained below 65 mmHg despite preload optimization), post-anesthesia care unit (PACU) LOS, number of anti-emetics administered at the PACU, post-operative complications (Additional file 1), time to first ambulation, and postoperative day 1 pain evaluation using visual analogue scale score.

Statistical analysis

The primary objective of the study was to demonstrate that hospital LOS was equivalent between the two groups. For a difference of one day and equivalence margin of two days a study with a power of 90% and an alpha of 0.01 would require 30 patients per group. Since we estimated a drop-out rate of about 20%, we elected to recruit 38 patients per group. The R package TrialSize was used based on the work of Chow et al. [20]. We planned to determine if groups had comparable variances with Bartlett's test for homogeneity of variance and if the residuals of the t-test were normally distributed. In the case of non-normal distribution, a non-parametric approach would be used with the R package nparcomp [21] to take into account the non-parametric Behrens-Fisher problem [22]. This package tests whether the observations in one group tend to be different than those of another. If the 95% confidence

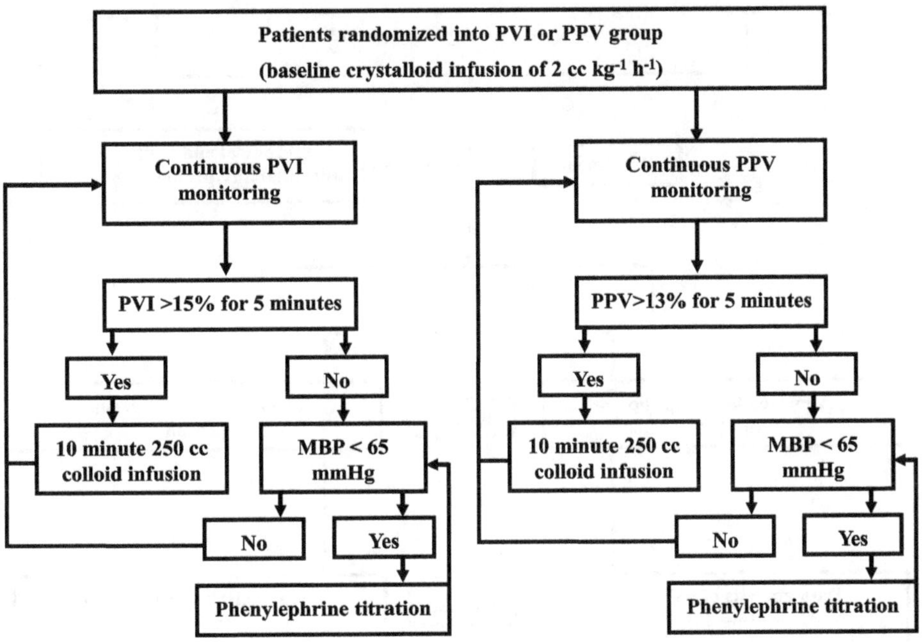

Fig. 1 Goal-directed fluid therapy protocols. Patients were randomized into either PVI or PPV guided groups. *PPV pulse pressure variation, PVI Pleth variability index*

interval does not contain 0.5 the two groups are significantly different.

The Schapiro-Wilk test determined normality for continuous variables. Normally distributed variables were analyzed with student-t test and non-normal variables were analyzed with Mann-Whitney U test. Categorical variables were analyzed with Chi-square. Statistics were carried out using Minitab statistical software (Paris, France). Group allocation was revealed after data analysis.

Results

A total of 76 patients of the initially 129 screened patients were included from July 2011 to October 2013 (Fig. 2). Baseline characteristics were similar in both groups (Table 1). Anesthesia and surgical times were similar between groups. Patients remained in their pre-assigned group throughout the study period. Bartlett's test of homogeneity of variance ($Chi^2 = 19.69$, $df = 1$, p-value < 0.001) indicated that variances were not equal between groups and the Shapiro-Wilk normality test indicated that the residuals were not normally distributed for LOS. Therefore, the non-parametric approach was applied, and no difference was observed for the primary outcome of LOS (median [interquartile range]) 2.5 [2.0–3.3] vs. 3.0 [2.0–5.0] days, $p = 0.230$, for PVI and PPV, respectively (Fig. 3). The 95% confidence interval equals [0.291–0.549]. Since it contains the 0.5 value, the two groups are equivalent for LOS.

Infused crystalloid volume, infused colloid volumes, estimated blood loss, diuresis, time to first ambulation, and pain evaluation at post-operative day 1 were not different between groups (Table 2). The use of phenylephrine to correct hypotension in preload optimized patients was not different between groups. There was no difference in individual postoperative complications or composite postoperative complications. None of the patients required supplementary fluids due to hemorrhage associated hemodynamic instability. No harm was caused by the intervention and no patient died during the study period. No correction was done for missing data.

Discussion

In patients undergoing low-to-moderate risk abdominal surgery PVI and PPV guided GDFT are considered equivalent for the primary outcome of hospital LOS and no difference was found between the secondary outcomes. Both strategies seem to optimize preload equally and lead to similar outcome. PVI nonetheless has the distinct advantages of being totally non-invasive. Although PPV can be displayed continuously with certain monitors, it is invasive and does not improve outcome when compared to PVI in this population.

Several studies have shown that PVI guided GDFT, when compared to fluid therapy guided by static parameters of fluid responsiveness, can lead to decreased infused fluid volume, decreased time to first stool, and decreased perioperative lactate levels [12, 13, 23, 24]. Trials comparing different GDFT strategies to PVI, such as esophageal Doppler, have however resulted in conflicting results. For

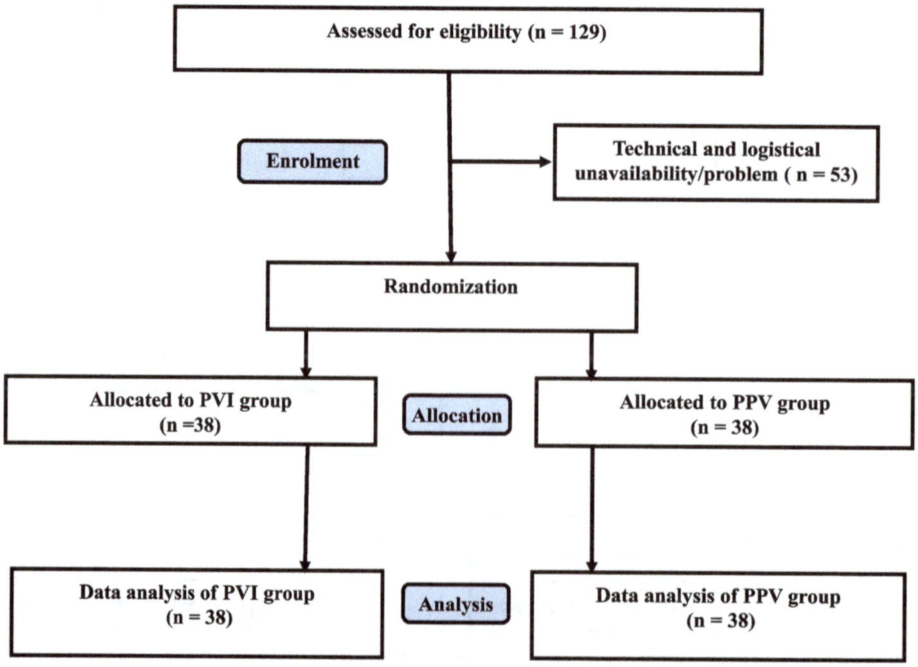

Fig. 2 Flow chart of enrolment, allocation, and analysis

Table 1 Baseline characteristics, expressed as % (number), mean (+/−SD), or median [IRQ]

	PVI ($n = 38$)	PPV ($n = 38$)	p-value
Age (year)	45 (+/−13)	50 (+/− 13)	0.124
Female gender	92.1 (35)	94.7 (36)	0.644
Weight (kg)	72 (+/−15)	66 (+/− 15)	0.096
ASA Score			0.154
ASA physical status 1	29.0 (11)	44.7 (17)	
ASA physical status 2	71.1 (27)	55.3 (21)	
Medications %			
Aspirin	2.6 (1)	10.5 (4)	0.165
Beta-blocker	13.2 (5)	10.5 (4)	0.723
ACEI	7.9 (3)	2.6 (1)	0.304
ARB	5.3 (2)	5.3 (2)	1.00
Calcium channel blocker	5.3 (2)	2.6 (1)	0.556
SSRI	5.3 (2)	5.3 (2)	1.000
Antidepressant other	15.8 (6)	7.9 (3)	0.287
Benzodiazepine	13.2 (5)	15.8 (6)	0.744
Hypertension	31.6 (12)	15.8 (6)	0.105
Diabetes	5.3 (2)	2.6 (1)	0.556
Obstructive pulmonary	5.3 (2)	13.2 (5)	0.234
Previous major surgery	21.1 (8)	23.7 (9)	0.783
Type of surgery			0.312
Laparoscopy (%)	65.8 (25)	76.3 (29)	
Laparotomy (%)	34.2 (13)	23.7 (9)	
Surgery Duration (min)	130 (+/− 75)	122 (+/−47)	0.599
Anesthesia Time (min)	180 [136–215]	183 [142–229]	0.670

ASA American Society of Anesthesiology, *ACEI* angiotensin converting enzyme inhibitor, *ARB* aldosterone receptor blocker, *SSRI* selective serotonin reuptake inhibitor

example, when compared to esophageal Doppler in patients requiring renal transplantation, PVI was shown to detect fluid responsiveness less consistently [25]. These patients may have pathological endothelial changes affecting arterial compliance that lead to poor capillary distribution. Since PVI is a direct measure of arterial compliance [26], these effects may alter the fluid response threshold. However, when compared to esophageal Doppler GDFT in patients requiring colorectal resection, a population more comparable to ours, fluid administration and outcome was not different [27]. Bahlmann et al. also showed that PVI and stroke volume optimization assessed by esophageal Doppler during open abdominal surgery had similar outcome [28]. Our results parallel the latter studies and indicate that in low-to-moderate risk abdominal surgery, PVI seems to be an adequate guide for GDFT.

It is important to consider, nevertheless, that low-to-moderate risk abdominal surgery may itself explain the lack of difference between groups. Two recent studies on the impact of non-invasively guided GDFT (Clearsight/ccNexfin) in patients undergoing moderate risk abdominal surgery, when compared to restrictive fluid therapy, were unable to demonstrate any difference between groups [29, 30]. Two possible reasons for these findings are that the non-invasive monitor did not adequately optimize cardiac output or that preload optimization has little impact on outcome in low-to-moderate risk abdominal surgery. However, other studies focusing on low-to-moderate risk abdominal surgery reported that perioperative fluid management could still have an impact on postoperative outcome in this particular population indicating that fluid administration should be individualized and goal directed [31].

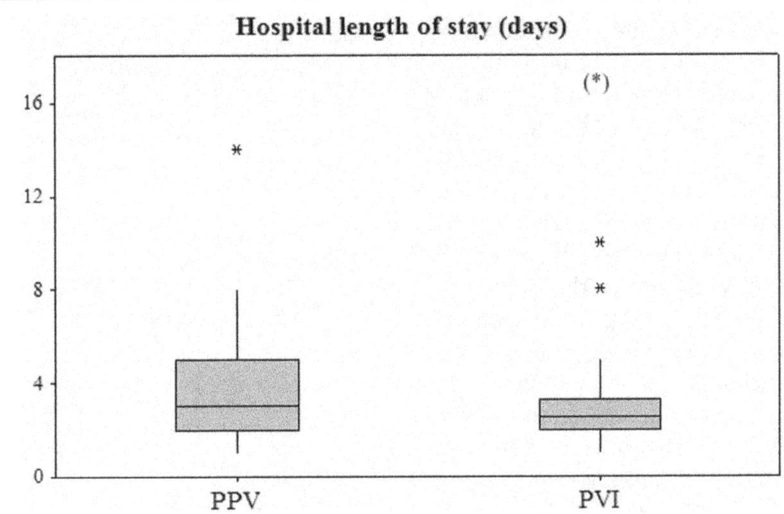

Fig. 3 Box-plot comparison of the primary outcome, length of stay (LOS). (*) In order to improve readability, one outlier (LOS = 35 days) is not represented in this figure

Table 2 Study outcomes, expressed as % (number), mean (+/−SD), or median [IRQ]

	PVI	PPV	*p*-value
Intraoperative data			
Total colloid (ml)	500 [0–750]	250 [0–500]	0.275
Total crystalloid (ml)	500 [350–740]	550 [450–663]	0.458
Estimated blood loss (ml)	100 [50–300]	100 [50–163]	0.445
Urine output (ml)	150 [79–250]	150 [100–250]	0.803
Intraoperative phenylephrine	26.3 (10)	21.1 (8)	0.589
Postoperative data			
LOS PACU (min)	105 [90–135]	90 [45–135]	0.382
PACU PONV	10.5 (4)	7.9 (3)	0.692
Number of antiemetics PACU			0.330
0	89 (34)	92 (35)	
1	5.3 (2)	7.9 (3)	
2	5.3 (2)	0 (0)	
Hypotension PACU	5.3 (2)	7.9 (3)	0.644
VAS Day 1 score	1 [0–2]	2 [0–2]	0.925
Ward PONV	7.9 (3)	7.9 (3)	1.000
Fever	7.9 (3)	2.6 (1)	0.304
Post-operative complications	4 (10.5)	2 (5.3)	0.395
Time to first ambulation	1 [1–2]	2 [1–2]	0.231

LOS length of stay, *PONV* postoperative nausea or vomiting, *PACU* post anesthesia care unit, *VAS* visual analogue scale

This randomized controlled trial had several limitations. In addition to the limitations intrinsic to a single center study, we did not measure protocol compliance, which is a key predictor of GDFT impact [3]. However, since both interventions required similar workloads, compliance should have been similar in both groups. In addition, this study was performed according to an intention to treat analysis and our results consequently reflect clinical practice. The vast majority of patients were women undergoing laparoscopic surgery and this should be noted when applying our GDFT strategies to patients. Another limitation inherent to PVI is its dependence on perfusion index, which varies depending on vascular tone [32]. This limitation nonetheless does not seem to have had an impact on our results since no difference was found between PVI and PPV groups in the amount of fluids administered or on outcome in this overwhelmingly healthy population. Another important point to consider is that this lack of difference between groups may be due to the low impact of GDFT on outcome in the studied population which ultimately consisted of low-risk patients undergoing low-to-moderate risk surgery. Nevertheless, physicians who still wish to implement a GDFT strategy for these patients should prefer a non-invasive monitor, such as PVI, to a more invasive monitor.

Conclusion

In patients undergoing low-to-moderate risk abdominal surgery, PVI seems to guide GDFT similarly to PPV in regards to hospital LOS, amount of fluid, and incidence of postoperative complications. However, in low-risk patients undergoing these surgical procedures optimizing stroke volume may have limited impact on outcome.

Abbreviations

ACEI: Angiotensin converting enzyme inhibitor; ARB: Aldosterone receptor blocker; ASA: American Society of Anesthesiology; GDFT: Goal-directed fluid therapy; LOS: Length of stay; PACU: Post anesthesia care unit; PPV: Pulse pressure variation; PVI: Pleth variability index; SSRI: Selective serotonin reuptake inhibitor; VAS: Visual analogue scale

Acknowledgements

The authors would like to acknowledge the medical and nursing staff of Brugmann CHU for their help in assuring the highest quality of care to all patients.

Authors' contributions

SC: Study design, data collection, data analysis, initial draft, approval of manuscript. AD: Study design, patient recruitment, data collection, critical revision and approval of manuscript. DG: Study design, patient recruitment, data collection, critical revision and approval of manuscript. JB: Study design, patient recruitment, data collection, critical revision and approval of manuscript. JFF: data analysis, critical revision and approval of manuscript. DS: data analysis, critical revision and approval of manuscript. PVdL: Study design, data collection, data analysis, initial draft, approval of manuscript. All authors have read and approved the manuscript.

Author details

[1]Department of Anesthesiology, CHU Brugmann, 4, Place Van Gehuchten, 1020 Bruxelles, Belgium. [2]Université Libre de Bruxelles, Brussels, Belgium. [3]Ars Statistica SPRL, Nivelles, Belgium.

References

1. Salzwedel C, Puig J, Carstens A, Bein B, Molnar Z, Kiss K, Hussain A, Belda J, Kirov MY, Sakka SG, Reuter DA. Perioperative goal-directed hemodynamic therapy based on radial arterial pulse pressure variation and continuous cardiac index trending reduces postoperative complications after major abdominal surgery: a multi-center, prospective, randomized study. Crit Care. 2013;17(5):R191.
2. Joosten A, Coeckelenbergh S, Delaporte A, Ickx B, Closset J, Roumeguere T, Barvais L, Van Obbergh L, Cannesson M, Rinehart J, Van der Linden P. Implementation of closed-loop-assisted intra-operative goal-directed fluid therapy during major abdominal surgery: a case-control study with propensity matching. Eur J Anaesthesiol. 2018;35(9):650–8.
3. Pearse RM, Harrison DA, MacDonald N, Gillies MA, et al. Effect of a perioperative, cardiac output-guided hemodynamic therapy algorithm on outcomes following major gastrointestinal surgery: a randomized clinical trial and systematic review. JAMA. 2014;311(21):2181–90.
4. Lee S, Chun Y, Oh Y, Shin S, Park S, Kim S, Choi Y. Prediction of fluid responsiveness in the beach chair position using dynamic preload indices. J Clin Monit Comput. 2016;30(6):995–1002.
5. Wu C, Cheng Y, Liu Y, Wu T, Chien C, Chan K. Predicting stroke volume and arterial pressure fluid responsiveness in liver cirrhosis patients using dynamic preload variables: a prospective study of diagnostic accuracy. Eur J Anaesthesiol. 2016;33(9):645–52.
6. Vos JJ, Kalmar AF, Struys MM, Wietasch JK, Hendriks HG, Scheeren TW. Comparison of arterial pressure and plethysmographic waveform-based dynamic preload variables in assessing fluid responsiveness and dynamic arterial tone in patients undergoing major hepatic resection. Br J Anaesth. 2013;110(6):940–6.
7. Lu W, Dong J, Xu Z, Shen H, Zheng J. The pleth variability index as an indicator of the central extracellular fluid volume in mechanically ventilated patients after anesthesia induction: comparison with initial distribution volume of glucose. Med Sci Monit. 2014;20:386–92.

8. van der Zee EN, Egal M, Gommers D, Groeneveld AB. Targeting urine output and 30-day mortality in goal-directed therapy: a systematic review with meta-analysis and meta-regression. BMC Anesthesiol. 2017;17(1):22.
9. Benes J, Giglio M, Brienza N, Michard F. The effects of goal-directed fluid therapy based on dynamic parameters on post-surgical outcome: a meta-analysis of randomized controlled trials. Crit Care. 2014;18(5):584.
10. Scheer B, Perel A, Pfeiffer UJ. Clinical review: complications and risk factors of peripheral arterial catheters used for haemodynamic monitoring in anaesthesia and intensive care medicine. Crit Care. 2002;6(3):199–204.
11. Cannesson M, Desebbe O, Rosamel P, Delannoy B, et al. Pleth variability index to monitor the respiratory variations in the pulse oximeter plethysmographic waveform amplitude and predict fluid responsiveness in the operating theatre. Br J Anaesth. 2008;101(2):200–6.
12. Forget P, Lois F, de Kock M. Goal-directed fluid management based on the pulse oximeter-derived pleth variability index reduces lactate levels and improve fluid management. Anesth Analg. 2010;111(4):910–4.
13. Cesur S, Çardaközü T, Kuş A, Türkyılmaz N, Yavuz Ö. Comparison of conventional fluid management with PVI-based goal directed fluid management in elective colorectal surgery. J Clin Monit Comput. 2018; [Epub ahead of print].
14. Thiele RH, Rea KM, Turrentine FE, Friel CM, Hassinger TE, McMurry TL, Goudreau BJ, Umapathi BA, Kron IL, Sawyer RG, et al. Standardization of care: impact of an enhanced recovery protocol on length of stay, complications, and direct 30 costs after colorectal surgery. J Am Coll Surg. 2015;220:430–43.
15. Hengy B, Gazon M, Schmitt Z, Benyoub K, et al. Comparison between respiratory variations in pulse oximetry plethysmographic waveform amplitude and arterial pulse pressure during major abdominal surgery. Anesthesiology. 2012;117(5):973–80.
16. Ganter MT, Geisen M, Hartnack S, Dzemali O, Hofer CK. Prediction of fluid responsiveness in mechanically ventilated cardiac surgical patients: the performance of seven different functional hemodynamic parameters. BMC Anesthesiol. 2018;18(1):55.
17. Gepts E, Shafer S, Camu F, Stanski D, Woestenborghs R, Van Peer A, Heykants J. Linearity of pharmacokinetics and model estimation of Sufentanil. Anesthesiology. 1995;83(6):1194–204.
18. Cai QF, Mi WD, Yuan WX. The ability of pleth variability index to predict fluid responsiveness in mechanically ventilated patients under general anaesthesia. Zhonghua Wai Ke Za Zhi. 2010;48(21):1628–32.
19. Benes J, Haidingerova L, Pouska J, Stepanik J, Stenglova A, Zatloukal J, Pradl R, Chytra I, Kasal E. Fluid management guided by a continuous non-invasive arterial pressure device is associated with decreased postoperative morbidity after total knee and hip replacement. BMC Anesthesiol. 2015;15:148.
20. Chow S, Shao J, Wang H. Sample Size Calculations in Clinical Research. 2nd ed. New York: Marcel Dekker; 2008.
21. Konietschke F, Placzek M, Schaarschmidt F, et al. Nparcomp:an R software package for nonparametric multiple comparisons and simultaneous confidence intervals. J Stat Softw. 2015;64:1–17.
22. Brunner E, Munzel U. The nonparametric Behrens-fisher problem: asymptotic theory and a small-sample approximation. Biom J. 2000;1(1):17–21.
23. Demirel İ, Bolat E, Altun AY, Özdemir M, Beştaş A. Efficacy of goal-directed fluid therapy via Pleth variability index during laparoscopic roux-en-Y gastric bypass surgery in morbidly obese patients. Obes Surg. 2018;28(2):358–63.
24. Yu Y, Dong J, Xu Z, Shen H, Zheng J. Pleth variability index-directed fluid management in abdominal surgery under combined general and epidural anesthesia. J Clin Monit Comput. 2015;29:47–52.
25. Le Guen M, MD FA, Gayat E, Fischler M. The plethysmographic variability index does not predict fluid responsiveness estimated by esophageal Doppler during kidney transplantation a controlled study. Medicine. 2018;97:20.
26. Shelley KH, Murray WB, Chang D. Arterial-pulse oximetry loops: a new method of monitoring vascular tone. J Clin Monit. 1997;13:223–8.
27. Warnakulasuriya S, Davies S, Wilson R, Yates D. Comparison of esophageal Doppler and plethysmographic variability index to guide intraoperative fluid therapy for low-risk patients undergoing colorectal surgery. J Clin Anesth. 2016;34:600–8.
28. Bahlmann H, Hahn RG, Nilsson L. Pleth variability index or stroke volume optimization during open abdominal surgery: a randomized controlled trial. BMC Anesthesiol. 2018;18(1):115.
29. Joosten A, Raj Lawrence S, Colesnicenco A, Coeckelenbergh S, Vincent JL, Van der Linden P, Cannesson M, Rinehart J. Personalized versus Protocolized fluid management using noninvasive hemodynamic monitoring (Clearsight system) in patients undergoing moderate-risk abdominal surgery. Anesth Analg. 2018; [Epub ahead of print].
30. Stens J, Hering JP, van der Hoeven CWP, Boom A, et al. The added value of cardiac index and pulse pressure variation monitoring to mean arterial pressure-guided volume therapy in moderate-risk abdominal surgery (COGUIDE): a pragmatic multicentre randomised controlled trial. Anaesthesia. 2017;72(9):1078–87.
31. Holte K, Foss NB, Andersen J, Valentiner L, et al. Liberal or restrictive fluid administration in fast-track colonic surgery: a randomized, double-blind study. Br J Anaesth. 2007;99(4):500–8.
32. Broch O, Bein B, Gruenewald M, Höcker J, Schöttler J, Meybohm P, Steinfath M, Renner J. Accuracy of the pleth variability index to predict fluid responsiveness depends on the perfusion index. Acta Anaesthesiol Scand. 2011;55:686–93.

3

Abnormal cisatracurium pharmacodynamics and pharmacokinetics among patients with severe aortic regurgitation during anesthetic induction

Xiaocong Huang[1], Lei Chen[2], Yujing Cai[3], Jinfeng Wei[4], Lina Lin[5], Jie Sun[5], Xuemei Peng[2] and Sheng Wang[1,6*]

Abstract

Background: This study was designed to examine whether severe aortic regurgitation will affect the pharmacodynamics (PD) and pharmacokinetics (PK) of cisatracurium during anesthetic induction.

Methods: A total of 32 patients were divided into two groups: the AR group ($n = 16$) and the control group (n = 16). Arterial blood samples were drawn before and at 1, 2, 4, 6, 8, 10, 16 and 20 min after intravenous injection of 0.15 mg/kg cisatracurium. TOF tests were applied to determine the onset time of maximal muscle relaxation. The concentration of cisatracurium in plasma was determined by high-performance liquid chromatography.

Results: The onset time to maximal neuromuscular block was prolonged from 2.07 ± 0.08 min to 4.03 ± 0.14 min, which indicated that the PD responses to cisatracurium were significantly delayed in the AR group ($P < 0.05$) compared to the control group.
A conventional two-compartment PK model showed a higher plasma concentration of cisatracurium among the AR group with markedly reduced intercompartment transfer rate ($K_{12} = 0.19 \pm 0.02$ and $K_{21} = 0.11 \pm 0.01$ in the AR group vs. $K_{12=}0.26 \pm 0.01$ and $K_{21} = 0.19 \pm 0.01$ in the control group, $P < 0.01$) compared to the control group.

Conclusion: Backward blood flow during diastole in severe AR impaired distribution of cisatracurium from the central compartment to the peripheral compartment, which accounted for the lagged PD responses.
Findings in this study underlie the importance of muscular blockade monitoring among patients with severe aortic regurgitation during anesthetic induction.

Registration: Name of the registry: Abnormal Cisatracurium Pharmacodynamics and Pharmacokinetics among Patients with Severe Aortic Regurgitation during Anesthetic Induction.

Keywords: Cisatracurium, Severe aortic regurgitation, Neuromuscular blockade, Intercompartment transfer rate

* Correspondence: shengwang_gz@163.com
[1]Department of Anesthesiology, Guangdong Provincial Cardiovascular Institute, Guangdong Provincial People's Hospital (previously called Guangdong General Hospital), Guangdong Academy of Medical Sciences, Guangzhou 510630, China
[6]Department of Anesthesiology, Linzhi People's Hospital, Xizang 860000, China

Background

Cisatracurium besilate (NIBEX, 51 W89) is a nondepolarizing neuromuscular blocking agent widely used in anesthesia and ICU [1, 2]. About 77% of total clearance of cisatracurium undergoes Hoffmann degradation, which is characterized by spontaneous temperature- and pH-dependent chemical degradation in plasma and tissues [3]. Tetrahydropapaverine, the major metabolite of cisatracurium, has no neuromuscular blocking effect. In addition, histamine release reports are less seen in cistracurium than in other muscle relaxants [4].

Aortic regurgitation (AR) is a disorder in which the aortic valve fails to close properly and some blood flows back into the left ventricle during diastole [5]. According to the American Heart Association and the American College of Cardiology, severe aortic regurgitation is diagnosed in patients with ≥0.3cm^2 regurgitant orifice area or ≥ 50% regurgitant fraction [6, 7]. The LV systolic function begins to aggravate if the disease developes naturally. Prognosis depends on the severity of regurgitation [6]. Surgery is proved to be the optimal treatment to protect left ventricle function and extend life expectancy for patients with severe AR [8, 9].

Compared with other muscle relaxants, cisatracurium is more favorable during anesthetic induction among patients with severe AR because of its low propensity to cause adverse cardiovascular effect [10]. Previous studies proved that the drug effect of cisatracurium would be compromised by some types of heart diseases with abnormal hemodynamics [11, 12]. The abnormal hemodynamics of aortic regurgitation, which is characterized by regurgitation into the left ventricle during diastole, may cause pharmacological change of cisatracurium in severe AR pateints. Thus it's necessary to determine the pharmacodynamics (PD) and pharmacokinetics (PK) of cisatracurium in severe AR patients and this study was aimed to provide evidence to decide whether the common administration method should be modified in consideration of clinical efficacy and safety for the severe AR population.

Methods

Subjects

This clinical trial (No. GDREC2015297H) was approved by the Guangdong Provincial People's Hospital Ethics Committee. The online registration number was ChiCTR1800019654. Patients were informed the objectives and risks of this trial before the operations. Written informed consents were obtained from all individual participants. From December 2018 to April 2019, 32 patients were enrolled in this study and divided into 2 groups: the AR group ($n = 16$) and the control group (n = 16). Patients in the AR group suffered from severe AR according to the diagnostic criteria published by AHA and ACC [5, 7]. And they were going to undergo elective aortic valve replacement. Patients in the control group suffered from breast fibroadenoma or thyroid adenoma, and their heart structure and function were proved to be intact by clinical examination, electrocardiography and echocardiography. And they underwent elective excision of breast fibroadenoma or thyroid adenoma.

Inclusion criteria for both groups are as follows:

(1) age 20–60 years old;
(2) BMI 20–24 kg/m^2;
(3) American Society of Anesthesiologists grade I or II.

Patients were excluded if they show any signs below:

(1) history of allergy to cisatracurium or other anesthetics in this trial's protocol;
(2) compromised renal, liver or neuromuscular function.

Preparation before anesthesia

Demographic information was collected and routine laboratory tests were applied in each case. Patients were prohibited from eating for 8 h and drinking for 4 h before elective surgeries. No preoperative anesthetic was administered before anesthesia.

Anesthetic induction

Anesthetic induction was conducted intravenously in every subject through a peripheral catheter in the median cubital vein. 0.05 mg/kg midazolam, 1.5–2.5 mg/kg propofol and 5 μg/kg fentanyl were administered by bolus. After loss of eyelash reflex and unresponsiveness to oral instructions in the subject, a bolus of 0.15 mg/kg cisatracurium was injected. 4-6 mg/kg/h propofol and 0.05–0.1 μg/kg/min remifentanyl were infused to maintain stable hemodynamics and sufficient anesthesia.

Neuromuscular monitoring

Pharmacodynamics was assessed by the Train-of-Four (TOF) tests. The negative and positive electrodes of TOF-Watch SX (Organon, Ireland) were placed on the ulnar side of the left forearm after skin cleaning. Calibration is carried out by single stimuli at 1 Hz upon the adductor pollicis muscles for 3 min in a row before the administration of cisatracurium and the start of TOF stimulation at 2 Hz every 15 s. TOF-Watch SX Monitor (version 2.2 int) was a software used to record the values of T_1, T_2, T_3, T_4 every 15 s. The values of T_4, T_3, T_2 and T_1 will decrease after muscle relaxants begin to take effect. T_4, T_3, T_2 and T_1 will become zero in turn as neuromuscular blockade increase. Finally T_1 equals zero when skeletal muscles reach maximal blockade. Therefore, the onset time is defined as the interval between the moment cisatracurium is adminstered and the moment T_1 first reaches zero.

Blood sampling

Arterial blood samples (about 5 ml in each) were collected before (time 0) and at 1, 2, 4, 8, 12, 16, 20 min after cisatracurium administration. Blood samples were transferred to heparin-primed centrifuge tubes and centrifuged at 9000 *g* for 3 min (4 °C). Then the supernatant was mixed with 100 μl H_2SO_4 immediately and stored at − 80 °C until analysis.

Acetonitrile (800 μl) was used to deproteinize plasma samples (200 μl). The mixture was vortexed for 3 min and centrifuged at 15,000 *g* for 15 min. The resulting supernatant was obtained and dried using Eppendorf Concentrator Plus (Hamburg, Germany). The residue was reconstituted in a solution of water/acetonitrile [50: 50(v/v);200 μl] before being centrifuged at 15,000 *g* for 15 min (4 °C). An aliquot of supernatant (5 μl) was injected into the UPLC-QTOF/MS system for quantification analysis.

Quantification of plasma cisactracurium by UPLC-QTOF/MS system

An UPLC-QTOF/MS system equipped with an Acquity UPLC device and a Xevo G2 QTOF mass spectrometer (Waters, Milford, MA) was used to quantify the concentration of cisatracurum. A BEH column (2.1x50mm, 1.7 μm; Waters) was used to perform chromatographic separation. Formic acid (0.1%) in water (mobile phase A) and acetonitrile (mobile phase B) at a flow rate of 0.45 ml/min were used perform the gradient elution, which was 5% B at 0 to 1 min, 5 to 85% B at 1 to 3 min, 85% B at 3 to 3.5 min, and 85 to 5% B at 3.5 to 4 min. Cisatracurium concentration was quantified by full scan analysis and extracted ion chromatograms reported by MassLynx software (version 4.1; Waters).

Limit of quantification and precision

The limit of quantification was defined as the final compound concentration with a signal-to-noise ratio larger than 10. Precision equals standard deviation of measured concentration divided by mean of measured concentration. A 1/× 2 weighted linear least-squares regression method was used to determine the linearity of the standard curve.

PK analysis

A conventional two-compartment model was constructed by WinNonlin software (Pharmsight, Mountain View, CA, USA) to analyze the PK data for cisatracurium (Fig. 1) [13].

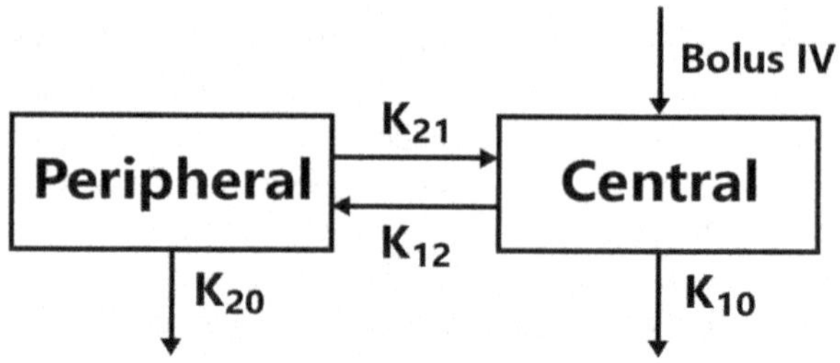

Fig. 1 Schematic diagram of a conventional two-compartment model. IV, intravenous; K_{12}, transfer rate constant from central compartment to peripheral compartment; K_{21}, transfer rate constant from peripheral compartment to central compartment; K_{10}, elimination rate constant for central compartment; K_{20}, elimination rate constant for peripheral compartment

Statistical analysis

Categorical variables were represented as percentage and were tested by Pearson chi-squared analysis. Data of continuous variables were presented as mean ± standard deviation (SD). The unpaired Student's t-test was performed to analyze the differences in PK and PD parameters between AR and control groups. The level of significance was set at $P < 0.05$. IBM SPSS Statistics 22.0 was used to conduct statistical calculation.

Results

Baseline data

Between the AR and control groups, there was no significant difference in demographic profile including age, gender, BMI and comorbid diseases (Table 1). In addition, no statistical difference was found between the two groups in parameters derived from blood gas analysis (Table 2).

Abnormal cisatracurium PK in patients with severe AR

Figure 2 is a diagram presenting plasma concentration vs. time curves for both groups. Mean plasma cisatracurium concentration was significantly higher ($P < 0.05$) at early time points (1,2 and 4 min after cisatracurium injection) in the severe AR group than in the control group.

The mean values for the PK parameters derived from the conventional two-compartment model for both groups were presented in Table 3. A significant decrease in the intercompartmental transfer rate K_{12}, K_{21} and $T_{1/2\alpha}$($P < 0.01$) was seen in the AR group compared with

Table 1 Demographic Profile

Parameter	Control (*n* = 16)	AR (*n* = 16)
Male/Female (n)	8/8	8/8
Age (years)	54.54 ± 9.07	52.88 ± 10.03
BMI (kg/m^2)	21.74 ± 1.14	21.64 ± 1.22
Comorbid diseases	no	no

Table 2 Parameters Derived from Blood Gas Analysis

Parameter	Control ($n = 16$)	AR ($n = 16$)
Body Temperature (°C)	36.37 ± 0.10	36.35 ± 0.15
Blood pH	7.40 ± 0.03	7.39 ± 0.03
Hemoglobin (g/L)	137.88 ± 4.86	140.13 ± 6.54
Hematocrit (%)	40.17 ± 2.44	41.92 ± 3.28

the control group. Meanwhile, This finding is consistent with higher plasma concentrations of cisatracurium (at 1,2 and 4 min) in the AR group than in the control group. PK parameters evaluating drug elimination such as K_{10},K_{20} and $T_{1/2\beta}$ were unaltered statistically in the AR group.

Abnormal cisatracurium PD in patients with severe AR

A column diagram depicting the onset time of two groups was shown in Fig. 3. The onset time of the control group and AR group were 2.07 ± 0.08 min and 4.03 ± 0.14 min respectively. The onset time of cisatracurium was significantly prolonged in severe AR patients compared with control patients ($P < 0.05$).

Discussion

This is the first study examining the PK and PD of cisatracurium in patients with severe AR.

Cisatracurium mainly metabolizes by Hoffmann degradation, which is a spontaneous temperature- and pH-dependent chemical degradation in plasma and tissues [2, 3]. Thus, cisatracurium is barely affected by differences of liver and kidney function among patients so it helps us focus on the drug distribution difference between the two groups and make it easier to find the link between delayed drug distribution and lagged PD response.

The conventional two-compartment model was proved to precisely depict the PK profile of cisatracurium in previous studies [11, 12]. An elevation in plasma concentration of cisatracurium and slower transfer rate between the central and peripheral compartments were observed in the AR group. These PK characteristics are consistent with severe AR patients' prolonged onset time (4.03 ± 0.14 min in AR group vs. 2.07 ± 0.08 min in control group). On the contrary, PK parameters evaluating drug elimination such as K_{10},K_{20} and $T_{1/2\beta}$ were unaltered statistically in the AR group. This finding is consistent with the fact that cisatracurium metabolizes mainly by pH- and temperature-dependent Hoffmann reaction [4, 14] since no statistical difference was found in the blood gas analysis. Abnormal hemodynamics in severe AR patients could contribute to markedly altered distribution of cisatracurium but could not affect its elimination condition. Thus it's reasonable to infer that the higher plasma concentration of cisatracurium resulted from impaired drug distribution instead of altered drug elimination [15]. Slower distribution of cisatracurium caused by severe AR's abnormal hemodynamics underlies the lagged onset of maximal neuromuscular blockade.

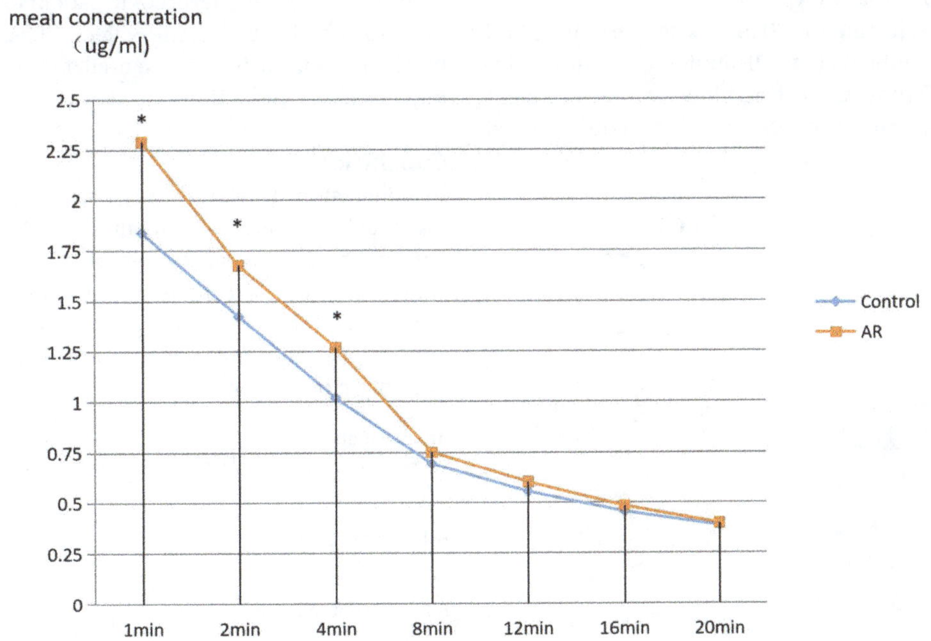

Fig. 2 Mean plasma concentration vs time curves between the control and AR groupswere shown in this figure. The 1, 2, 4-min time points were marked with asteriks, indicating statistical differences in the mean plasma concentration between two groups ($P < 0.05$)

Table 3 Pharmacokinetic Parameters Derived from the Conventional Two-compartment Model after Administration of Cisatracurium

Parameter	Control	AR
K_{10} (1/min)	0.06 ± 0.01	0.07 ± 0.01
K_{20} (1/min)	0.04 ± 0.01	0.04 ± 0.01
K_{12} (1/min)	0.26 ± 0.02	0.19 ± 0.01*
K_{21} (1/min)	0.19 ± 0.01	0.11 ± 0.01*
V_1 (ml/kg)	56.68 ± 7.79	52.34 ± 5.67
V_2 (ml/kg)	41.31 ± 6.26	38.90 ± 5.48
$T_{1/2\alpha}$ (min)	1.52 ± 0.12	2.56 ± 0.16*
$T_{1/2\beta}$ (min)	21.82 ± 3.02	23.76 ± 3.34
CL (ml/min/kg)	6.76 ± 1.36	7.06 ± 1.51
AUC (min*μg/ml)	23.81 ± 5.14	28.79 ± 6.25*

The mean values of PK parameters for both groups were shown here. All data were presented as means±SD. Statistcal differences between the two groups were indicated by asteriks (**$P < 0.01$). K_{10}, elimination rate constant for central compartment; K_{20}, elimination rate constant for peripheral compartment; K_{12}, transfer rate constant from central compartment to peripheral compartment; K_{21}, transfer rate constant from peripheral compartment to central compartment; V_1, volume of the central compartment; V_2, volume of the peripheral compartment; $T_{1/2\alpha}$, distribution half-life; $T_{1/2\beta}$, elimination half-life; *CL* clearance; *AUC* area under the curve

The cause for the impaired transfer rate between the central and peripheral compartments in severe AR patients was not clearly elucidated before. But according to the typical abnormal pathology and pathophysiology of severe aortic regurgitation, it is reasonable to infer that the abnormal diastolic regurgitation primarily leads to reduction of forward blood flow and slower distribution of cisatracurium. And this study provided PD and PK evidence to suppor that viewpoint.

The sampling schedule (0–20 min) seems be short and could raise the doubt that if it'll limit the scientific significance of this study. Collecting blood samples at eight time points during the 20-min sampling schedule proved sufficient to elaborate on the PK profile of cisatracurium due to two reasons. Firstly, the marked differences in plasma concentration of cisatracurium between the two groups were observed in the early 4 min after administration of cisatracurium. Secondly, the onset time to maximal neuromuscular blockade for both groups were both within the early 4 min though they were statistically different. Hence, it is assuring to say that the 20-min sampling schedule is long enough to examine the PK and PD characteristics in this trial.

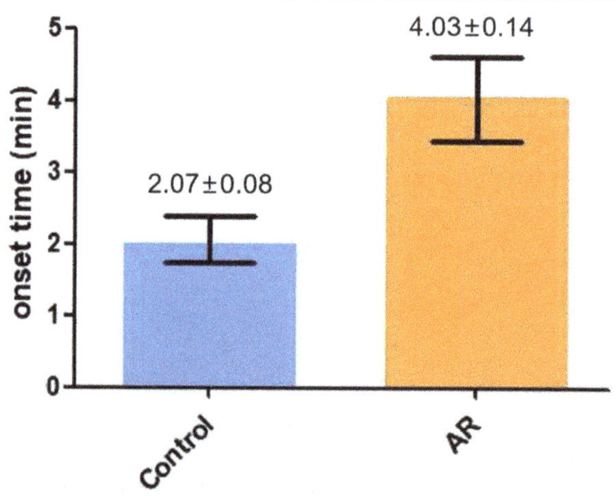

Fig. 3 A comparison of onset time of the control and AR group

A potential limitation of this study is that we do not have the post-operative PK and PD parameters of intravenous bolus of cisatracurium because it is against ethical code and clinical practice protocol to repeat the test after surgeries with the only purpose of collecting data. Our inferences of the impact of severe AR on PK and PD will be proved if pre-operative and post-opeartive parameters of PK and PD are found to be statistically different. Therefore, it's worth to investigate in the future whether patients who have intact prosthetic aortic valves will present normal cisatracurium PK and PD characteristics when they undergo non-cardiac surgeries.

Out of clinical safety concern, anesthesiologists should be aware of the changes in PK and PD properties resulting from diseases and pathophysiological conditions. In clinical practices, it's common for them to perform endotracheal entubation 2 minutes after the intravenous injection of 0.15 mg/kg cisatracurium without TOF monitoring [16]. Based on the findings in this study, 2 minutes are sufficient for patients with intact cardiac structure and function to obtain perfect neuromuscular blockade. However, severe AR patients require at least 4 min to obtain the same effect. Therefore, muscular blockade monitoring is essential for these patients during anesthetic induction.

Conclusions

In conclusion, this study demonstrated that by PD and PK anaylsis severe AR impaired distribution of cisatracurium from central to peripheral compartment and caused lagged PD responses. These findings underlie the importance of neuromuscular blockade monitoring among patients with severe aortic regurgitation during anesthetic induction.

Abbreviations

AR: Aortic Regurgitation; PD: Pharmacodynamics; PK: Pharmacokinetics; TOF: Train of Four

Acknowledgements

Not applicable.

Authors' contributions

SW conceived of the study, designed the study protocol and reviewed the manuscript. XH designed the study procotol, performed anesthesia, collected blood samples and wrote the manuscript. YC performed anesthesia, collected blood samples and wrote the manuscript. LC determined the cisatracurium concentration, analyzed data and performed statistics. JW performed anesthesia and collected blood samples. JS and LL collected blood samples and determined the cisatracurium concentration. XP analyzed data and performed statistics. All authors read and approved the final manuscript. XH, LC and YC made equal contributions to this study and should be considered co-first authors.

Author details
[1]Department of Anesthesiology, Guangdong Provincial Cardiovascular Institute, Guangdong Provincial People's Hospital (previously called Guangdong General Hospital), Guangdong Academy of Medical Sciences, Guangzhou 510630, China. [2]Department of Anesthesiology, the First Affiliated Hospital of Jinan University, Guangzhou 510632, China. [3]Department of Anesthesiology, Guangdong Provincial People's Hospital (previously called Guangdong General Hospital), Guangdong Academy of Medical Sciences, Guangzhou 510630, China. [4]Department of Anesthesiology, Guangdong Provincial People's Hospital (previously called Guangdong General Hospital), Guangzhou 510630, China. [5]College of Pharmacy, Jinan University, Guangzhou 510632, China. [6]Department of Anesthesiology, Linzhi People's Hospital, Xizang 860000, China.

References

1. Bryson HM, Faulds D. Cisatracurium besilate. A review of its pharmacology and clinical potential in anaesthetic practice. Drugs. 1997;53(5):848–66.
2. Liu X, Kruger PS, Weiss M, Roberts MS. The pharmacokinetics and pharmacodynamics of cisatracurium in critically ill patients with severe sepsis. Br J Clin Pharmacol. 2012;73(5):741–9.
3. Welch RM, Brown A, Ravitch J, Dahl R. The in vitro degradation of cisatracurium, the r, cis-r'-isomer of atracurium, in human and rat plasma. Clin Pharmacol Ther. 1995;58(2):132–42.
4. Welch RM, Brown A, Dahl R. The degradation and metabolism of 51w89, the r,cis-r1,cis isomer of atracurium, in human and rat plasma. Anesthesiology. 1994;81(SUPPLEMENT):A1092.
5. Akinseye OA, Pathak A, Ibebuogu UN. Aortic valve regurgitation: a comprehensive review. Curr Probl Cardiol. 2017.
6. Goldbarg SH, Halperin JL. Aortic regurgitation: disease progression and management. Nat Clin Pract Cardiovasc Med. 2008;5(5):269–79.
7. Yeung AC, Plappert T, Sutton MGSJ. Calculation of aortic regurgitation orifice area by doppler echocardiography: an application of the continuity equation. Br Heart J. 1992;68(2):236.
8. Mentias A, Feng K, Alashi A, Rodriguez LL, Gillinov AM, Johnston DR, et al. Long-term outcomes in patients with?Aortic regurgitation and preserved?Left ventricular ejection fraction. J Am Coll Cardiol. 2016;68(20): 2144–53.
9. Nkomo VT. Indications for surgery for aortic regurgitation. Curr Cardiol Rep. 2003;5(2):105–9.
10. Vanderweide L, Abdel-Rasoul M, Gerlach AT. The incidence of hypotension with continuous infusion atracurium compared to cisatracurium in the intensive care unit. Int J Crit Illn Inj Sci. 2017;7(2):113–8.
11. Wu Z, Wang S, Peng X, Lu C, Ye X, Wu B. Altered cisatracurium pharmacokinetics and pharmacodynamics in patients with congenital heart defects. Drug Metab Dispos. 2015;44(1):75–82.
12. Liu J, Lu C, Zou Q, Wang S, Peng X. Altered pharmacodynamics and pharmacokinetics of cisatracurium in patients with severe mitral valve regurgitation during anaesthetic induction period. Brit J Clin Pharm. 2017; 83(2):363–9.
13. Kisor DDF, Schmith VD. Clinical pharmacokinetics of cisatracurium besilate. Clin Pharmacokinet. 1999;36(1):27–40.
14. Kim JH, Lee YC, Lee SI, Park SY, Choi SR, Lee JH, et al. Effective doses of cisatracurium in the adult and the elderly. Korean J Anesthesiol. 2016;69(5): 453–9.
15. Bergeron L, Bevan DR, Berrill A, Kahwaji R, Varin F. Concentration–effect relationship of cisatracurium at three different dose levels in the anesthetized patient. Anesthesiology. 2001;95(2):314–23.
16. Mellinghoff H, Diefenbach C. the clinical pharmacology of cisatracurium. Der Anaesthesist. 1997;46(6):481.

4

Usefulness of intra-operative neuromuscular blockade monitoring and reversal agents for postoperative residual neuromuscular blockade

Gonzalo Domenech[1*], Matías A. Kampel[1], María E. García Guzzo[1], Delfina Sánchez Novas[1], Sergio A. Terrasa[2] and Gustavo Garcia Fornari[1]

Abstract

Background: Complete avoidance of residual neuromuscular blockade (RNMB) during the postoperative period has not yet been achieved in current anesthesia practice. Evidently, compliance with NMB monitoring is persistently low, and the risk of RNMB during the perioperative period remains underestimated. To our knowledge, no publications have reported the incidence of RNMB in a university hospital where access to quantitative NMB monitoring and sugammadex is unlimited and where NMB management is not protocolised. The primary aim of this study was to estimate the incidence of RNMB in patients managed with or without sugammadex or neostigmine as antagonists and quantitative NMB monitoring in the operating room. The secondary aim was to explore the associations between RNMB and potentially related variables.

Methods: This retrospective observational cohort study was conducted at a tertiary referral university hospital in Buenos Aires, Argentina. Records created between June 2015 and December 2015 were reviewed. In total, 240 consecutive patients who had undergone elective surgical procedures requiring NMB were included. All patients were monitored via acceleromyography at the adductor pollicis muscle within 5 min of arrival in the postanaesthesia care unit (PACU). Scheduled recovery in the intensive care unit was the only exclusion criterion.

Results: RNMB was present in 1.6% patients who received intra-operative quantitative NMB monitoring and 32% patients whose NMB was not monitored ($P < 0.01$). Multivariable analysis revealed that the use of intra-operative quantitative NMB monitoring and sugammadex were associated with a lower incidence of RNMB, with calculated odds ratios of 0.04 (95% confidence interval [CI]: 0.005 to 0.401) and 0.18 (95% CI: 0.046 to 0.727), respectively.

Conclusions: The results of the present study suggest that intra-operative quantitative NMB monitoring and use of sugammadex are associated with a decreased incidence of RNMB in the PACU, reinforcing the contention that the optimal strategy for RNMB avoidance is the use of quantitative NMB monitoring and eventual use of reversal agents, if needed, prior to emergence from anaesthesia.

Keywords: Neuromuscular blockade, Residual neuromuscular blockade, Neuromuscular blockade monitoring

* Correspondence: gonzalo.domenech@hospitalitaliano.org.ar
[1]Department of Anesthesiology, Italiano de Buenos Aires Hospital, Presidente Teniente General Juan Domingo Perón 4190, Postal Code, 1199 Buenos Aires, Argentina

Background

Complete avoidance of residual neuromuscular blockade (RNMB) during the postoperative period has not yet been achieved. The clinical implications of RNMB are not clearly defined, but several studies suggest that it can prolong postoperative recovery, adversely affect respiratory function, impair airway-protective reflexes, and induce unpleasant symptoms associated with muscle weakness [1]. RNMB is currently defined as the presence of a train-of-four (TOF) ratio (TOFR; ratio of the fourth to the first twitch height) of < 0.9 (90%) [2]. The reported incidence varies from 20 to 50% in the postanaesthesia care unit (PACU), depending on the TOFR threshold (0.7 or 0.9) used to define RNMB in each study, type of neuromuscular blocking drugs (NMBDs) used, and the use of objective or intra-operative quantitative monitoring of neuromuscular function [3].

Despite the high incidence of RNMB reported in modern PACUs, reported as high as 45% [4], awareness of its clinical implications remains limited. In an online survey, 15% of anaesthesiologists in the United States and Europe reported that they had never observed an episode of RNMB in their patients [5]. Recently, a consensus statement on the perioperative use of NMB monitoring strongly recommended the use of quantitative NMB monitoring whenever a nondepolarising NMBD is administered [6]. Also, several reports suggest that clinical evaluation and qualitative neuromuscular monitoring approaches are not sensitive enough to detect the presence of RNMB [7–9].

In 2 previous studies, the selective agent γ-cyclodextrin sugammadex was proven to eliminate RNMB in the PACU among patients receiving intra-operative quantitative NMB monitoring and to accelerate reversal times when compared with neostigmine [10, 11]. In another study, however, sugammadex reportedly failed to prevent postoperative TOFR values of < 0.9 without the concomitant use of intra-operative NMB monitoring [12].

To date, no publications have reported the incidence of RNMB in a hospital where access to quantitative NMB monitoring and sugammadex is unlimited and where NMB management is not protocolised. Regarding this matter, our hypothesis was that our PACU would have an incidence of RNMB as high as 45%, as reported by Debaene B, et al. [13] and that both intra-operative quantitative NMB monitoring and the use of reversal agents would be associated with a lower incidence of RNMB.

Objectives

Primary aim

To estimate the incidence of RNMB in patients managed with or without sugammadex and neostigmine as antagonists, and quantitative NMB monitoring in the operating room.

Secondary aim

To explore the associations between RNMB and potentially related variables such as the use of NMB monitoring, duration of surgery, type of NMBD, type of reversal agent, and time between the last NMBD administration and TOFR in the PACU.

Methods

Ethical approval for this retrospective cohort study was provided by the Ethical Committee of the Hospital Italiano de Buenos Aires in Buenos Aires, Argentina (Chairperson: Dr. Augusto Pérez, Ethical Committee N° 2832) on June 10, 2016. This study was conducted at the Italiano de Buenos Aires Hospital, a tertiary referral university hospital in Buenos Aires, Argentina. A medical record review of 240 consecutive patients who had undergone elective surgical procedures requiring NMB was performed. Scheduled recovery in the intensive care unit was the only exclusion criterion. Acceleromyography (AMG) in the PACU was routine clinical practice during 2015 as part of a clinical audit to improve patient care. Cases between June 2015 and December 2015 were reviewed. The jurisdictional Institutional Review Board that approved the study waived the need for informed consent from the patients due to the retrospective nature of the study.

The patient variables recorded included sex, age, the American Society of Anesthesiologists (ASA) physical status classification score, weight, height, and body mass index. The surgery-related data assessment included duration of surgery, NMBD used (compound, total dose, and time from last dose to TOFR in the PACU), antagonist for NMBD (sugammadex or neostigmine), and the use of quantitative neuromuscular function monitoring. All data were obtained via electronic medical records.

Two different types of NMB monitoring were used due to limited availability of monitors. Intra-operative TOFR measurements were determined via a Philips IntelliVue NMT Module 865,383 (Phillips Healthcare, Amsterdam, the Netherlands), attached to multiparameter monitors in every operating room as it is not portable. A different monitor, TOF-Watch® SX (Organon Ireland Ltd., a division of MSD, Dublin, Ireland), was available as a portable device for PACU measurements. Although both monitors use the same measuring principle (AMG), there is no published evidence on the similarity of measurements between them. No qualitative monitors were used during the study. The site of monitoring as well as the results of quantitative monitoring (depth of block and TOFR prior to tracheal extubation) were not manually recorded nor automatically transferred to the electronic anaesthesia record. The retrospective nature of the study precluded possible methods for obtaining this information. Results from TOFRs before tracheal extubation were verbally communicated to the physician performing TOF monitoring in the PACU in cases in which NMB monitoring or reversal agents had been used. Results from TOFRs in the PACU were added manually in the postanaesthetic subsection of the electronic anaesthesia record.

Within 5 min of arriving in the PACU, all patients were monitored via AMG of the adductor pollicis muscle (TOF-Watch® SX). TOFR measurements were performed by anaesthesia trainees who had previous training in NMB monitoring. Surface electrodes were placed 3 cm apart over the ulnar nerve as routine practice. The skin was prepared using alcohol cleansing pads to decrease resistance to stimulation. Uncalibrated TOF stimulation was applied and free movement of the thumb was ensured in the monitored extremity. Electrode placement for TOF monitoring was standardised, and it was not manually recorded. Nonetheless, it is highly likely that NMB monitors were applied to the thumb opposite existing peripheral venous or arterial catheters in both the operating room and the PACU.

The stimulation current was set at 50 mA (4 pulses of 0.2 ms duration at a frequency of 2 Hz) and 3 consecutive stimuli were applied to each patient, separated by 15 s. Baseline settings of the TOF Watch SX monitor include a stimulating current of 50 mA. The mean of the 3 resulting TOFRs was used for decision making. An NMBD antagonist (sugammadex or neostigmine) was administered if the TOFR was < 0.9.

The primary outcome was the presence of RNMB, defined as a TOFR of < 0.9. The secondary outcomes were the associations between RNMB and potentially related variables as per a multivariable regression model.

Statistical analysis

We assumed a 45% incidence of RNMB [13] and calculated a required sample size of 222 patient records. This sample size allowed an incidence estimation with a 95% confidence interval (CI) margin of error that did not exceed 7%. Eventually, 240 electronic medical records were analysed after considering a missing data rate of 10%.

Descriptive analyses were performed using the mean ± standard deviation for continuous variables and numbers and percentages for categorical variables. Qualitative variables derived from each group were compared using the chi-square test or Fisher's exact test in cases involving low expected counts. The Student's t-test was used to analyse normally distributed quantitative data, while the nonparametric Wilcoxon rank-sum test was used to analyse non-normally distributed quantitative data.

In the first step, we evaluated the association between the different potentially predictive variables and the outcome (RNMB) through a bivariate analysis. Since we had a total of 58 outcomes, we predicted that we could build a multivariable model with a maximum of 5 potential predictors as recommended by Norman et al. [14]

The multivariable model was built using the 4 variables (use of monitoring, type of reversal agent, duration of surgery, and the time between the last administration of NMBD and the presence of a TOFR in the PACU) that had shown a statistically significant association ($P < 0.1$) in the bivariate analysis. In addition, we forced the entry of the NMBD type as a variable for clinical reasons.

Once the model was built, we tested whether the elimination of those variables with no statistical significance ($P > 0.05$) modified the odds ratio (OR) of the other variables in the model in a substantial way (more than 10%). For this reason, the duration of surgery was retained as a variable in the model.

The final model was established using the following variables: use of NMB monitoring, type of reversal agent used, duration of surgery, time between the last administration of NMBD and TOFR in the PACU, and type of NMBD used.

Results

A total of 240 patients were included in this retrospective observational study. The overall incidence of RNMB was 24% (58/240). One of 63 patients (1.6%) who received intra-operative quantitative NMB monitoring and 57 of 177 (32%) patients who were not monitored exhibited RNMB ($P < 0.01$; Table 1). The mean TOFR in patients who exhibited RNMB (TOFR < 0.9) was 0.68 ± 0.20, while that in patients without RNMB was 0.94 ± 0.03. The incidence of a TOFR of < 0.7 was 10%.

Demographic patient characteristics are presented in Table 1. Intra-operative quantitative NMB monitoring was used in 63 of 240 patients (26%). There were no significant differences pertaining to age, sex, body mass index, ASA physical status, or type of NMBD used in both groups. The mean duration of surgery was 142.3 ± 67.20 min in the nonmonitored group and 154.8 ± 65.69 min in the monitored group ($P = 0.204$).

Rocuronium, vecuronium, and atracurium were administered to 73, 23, and 3% patients with mean doses of 54.15 ± 29.06, 8.23 ± 6.52, and 41.87 ± 16.89 mg, respectively (Table 2). All patients who received atracurium as an NMBD were reversed with neostigmine and all patients who received sugammadex were under NMB after rocuronium or vecuronium administration.

Among the 63 monitored patients, 9 received neostigmine and 42 received sugammadex prior to tracheal extubation (51/63, 81%). Five and 19 of the 177

Table 1 Patient demographics and anaesthetic variables

	Nonmonitored group (n = 177)	Monitored group (n = 63)	P value
Age (years)	53.3 ± 17.82	57 ± 16.66	0.15⊥
Sex (male/female)	60/117	29/34	0.087*
Body mass index	26.4 ± 5.16	28.1 ± 5.97	0.029⊥
ASA physical status (I/II/III/IV)	17/123/37/0	6/36/19/2	0.05#
Duration of surgery (min)	142.3 ± 67.20	154.8 ± 65.69	0.204⊥
NMBD used			
Vecuronium	7	1	0.804#
Atracurium	42	14	
Rocuronium	128	48	
Interval between last NMBD administration and TOFR measurement (min)	134.43 ± 61.66	105.33 ± 61.08	0.014⊥
NMB antagonist, n/total (%)	24/177 (13.5)	51/63 (81)	< 0.01*
Neostigmine	5/24	9/63	< 0.01*
Sugammadex	19/24	42/63	
Dose of NMB antagonist			
Neostigmine (μg kg^{-1})	29.51 ± 9.83	29.64 ± 1.06	0.98⊥
Sugammadex (mg kg^{-1})	3.22 ± 1.23	3.90 ± 2.66	0.29⊥
RNMB, n/total (%)	57/177 (32%)	1/63 (1.6%)	< 0.001

Data are expressed as the mean ± standard deviation or numbers
ASA American Society of Anesthesiologists, *NMB* Neuromuscular blockade, *NMBD* Neuromuscular blocking drug, *RNMB* Residual neuromuscular blockade, *TOFR* Train-of-four ratio
⊥Student's t-test
*Chi-square test
#Fisher's exact test

nonmonitored patients received neostigmine and sugammadex (24/177, 13.5%), respectively. Postoperative RNMB was present in 2 of the 5 patients (40%) who received neostigmine without quantitative NMB monitoring and none of the patients who received neostigmine with quantitative NMB monitoring (P = 0.11). Sugammadex failed to reverse the blockade in 3 of 19 patients (16%) in the nonmonitored group and none of the patients in the monitored group (P = 0.028; Table 3).

Multivariable analysis revealed that the use of intra-operative quantitative NMB monitoring and the use of sugammadex were associated with a lower incidence of RNMB, with calculated ORs of 0.04 (95% CI: 0.005 to 0.401) and 0.18 (95% CI: 0.046 to 0.727), respectively. A longer period since last NMBD administration and the presence of a TOFR at the PACU was also associated with a lower incidence of RNMB (OR, 0.98; 95% CI: 0.977 to 0.995; Table 4).

Discussion

The incidence of RNMB in patients without NMB monitoring in the present study (32%) is similar to the incidence reported in previous studies [15–17]. Moreover, the incidence of RNMB in monitored patients was significantly lower (1.6%; $P < 0.01$) than in non-monitored patients. These results are corroborated by substantial evidence suggesting that the use of intra-operative quantitative NMB monitoring is associated with a decreased incidence of RNMB in the PACU [18, 19].

The rate of quantitative NMB monitoring in the current study was 26%, which is very low considering the availability of monitoring equipment in every operating room. As Todd et al. [20] described, we believe the low NMB monitoring rates could be related to a poor understanding of the pharmacology of nondepolarising NMBDs. Additionally, very few adverse respiratory events in the PACU are confirmed to be a consequence

Table 2 Nondepolarising neuromuscular blockade management

	Agent	n/total (%)	Total dose (mg)	Total dose (mg kg^{-1})
Nondepolarising neuromuscular blockade	Rocuronium	176/240 (73%)	54.15 ± 29.06	0.61 ± 0.18
	Vecuronium	56/240 (23.3%)	8.23 ± 6.52	0.08 ± 0.025
	Atracurium	8/240 (3.3%)	41.87 ± 16.89	0.42 ± 0.067

n Number of patients
Data are presented as the mean ± standard deviation or numbers

Table 3 Neuromuscular blockade (NMB) monitoring and the use of NMB antagonists

	Intra-operative NMB monitoring (n = 63)		No intra-operative NMB monitoring (n = 177)		P value
	TOFR > 0.9	RNMB	TOFR > 0.9	RNMB	
Non-reversed (n = 165)	11/12	1/12	101/153	52/153	0.106#
Neostigmine (n = 14)	9/9	0/9	3/5	2/5	0.11#
Sugammadex (n = 61)	42/42	0/42	16/19	3/19	0.028#

RNMB Residual neuromuscular blockade
#Fisher's exact test

of RNMB; hence, it is often not considered a clinically relevant problem and anaesthesiologists remain reluctant to use NMB monitoring.

Fifty-one of the 63 monitored patients (81%) received a reversal agent, while only 24 of the 177 nonmonitored patients (14%) received such an agent in our study. This shows that anaesthesiologists who do not use monitoring despite its availability probably do not consider the need for NMB reversal agents. On the contrary, anaesthesiologists who apply NMB monitoring routinely are more likely to consider peri-operative NMB management as an important aspect of patient safety and quality of care. These physicians likely administer reversal agents, whenever needed, following NMB monitoring results.

It is established that the spontaneous recovery of neuromuscular function (at least 4 responses measured by TOF) is crucial for successful antagonism with neostigmine [21]. As this is a retrospective study, we did not have access to data about the depth of paralysis at which neostigmine was administered. The incidence of RNMB in patients who received neostigmine in the nonmonitored group was 40 and 0% in the monitored group. A recent study showed a significant decrease in the incidence of severe postoperative RNMB in patients who received neostigmine in adjusted doses 10 min after a TOF count of 4 was confirmed at the thumb. However, RNMB was not completely prevented [22, 23]. Administration of neostigmine at an incorrect depth of paralysis could be a reason for failure to negate RNMB in the absence of NMB monitoring in the current study.

Table 4 Multivariable logistic regression analysis for the association between residual neuromuscular blockade and potentially related factors

	OR	95% CI	P value
Intra-operative NMB monitoring	0.043	0.004 to 0.400	0.006
Sugammadex	0.182	0.045 to 0.727	0.016
Neostigmine	0.798	0.124 to 5.099	0.812
Duration of surgery	1.002	0.995 to 1.009	0.522
Time from last NMBD dose	0.986	0.977 to 0.995	0.002
Rocuronium	0.861	0.174 to 4.247	0.855
Atracurium	1.846	0.349 to 9.751	0.470

OR Odds ratio, *CI* Confidence interval, *NMB* Neuromuscular blockade, *NMBD* Neuromuscular blocking drug

Our results show that sugammadex administration in the absence of NMB monitoring is not an effective strategy to avoid RNMB (16% incidence of RNMB). In these cases, reversal failure was likely due to an insufficient dosage, assuming the anaesthesiologists' underestimation of the NMB depth. Although Kotake et al. [12] reported a lower incidence than noted in the present study for reversal failure with sugammadex in nonmonitored patients (4.3%; interquartile range: 1.7 to 9.4%), they also state that an incidence as high as 9.4% is not acceptable; therefore, sugammadex should not be used in the absence of NMB monitoring.

The current study had some limitations. First, it was an observational single-centre study conducted in a tertiary referral university hospital, rendering it difficult to generalise the applicability of the study results. Second, physicians in charge of TOFR measurements in the PACU were not blinded to the type of NMBD used, use of intra-operative NMB monitoring, or use of reversal agents. Third, 2 different monitors were used for intra-operative and postoperative periods because of limited availability. Fourth, the sample size for patients who received antagonists was not adequate to draw conclusions regarding this aspect. Last, we did not collect patient temperature data during the surgery or in the PACU, which may have affected the TOF measurements. Although the multivariable regression model showed an association between the use of NMB monitoring and the use of sugammadex, and a lower incidence of RNMB, the CIs of both ORs overlap. Consequently, we cannot state whether monitoring or sugammadex has a greater influence on the incidence of RNMB.

One patient in the monitored group exhibited RNMB. The patient presented in the PACU with an average TOFR (3 consecutive stimuli) of 0.87, and before extubation showed no apparent need for reversal. Despite having no electronic data available on TOFR results prior to extubation, it was verbally stated that all monitored patients who were extubated in the operating room had presented acceptable recovery of neuromuscular function, defined as TOFR > 0.9. Although TOFR results in the PACU should not be discordant because different monitors were used, the results could vary because of the patient's wakefulness and responses to noxious stimuli.

All measurements were conducted when patients were conscious. Stimulation currents of ≤50 mA are acceptable in terms of patient comfort [24]. All TOFR measurements made in the PACU were obtained without prior calibration. There have been critical appraisals of the use of the TOF-Watch SX monitor without prior calibration. This monitor's baseline configuration values provide both supramaximal stimulation and appropriate sensitivity for most typical adult patients. Also, this monitor has been used without calibration in several research studies [15, 24, 25]. We believe it is unlikely that calibration prior to our measurements would have modified the results of the present study.

Regarding the accuracy of TOFR measurements in conscious patients, it appears that 2 successive measurements may not be reliable; [26] however, some authors were able to report consecutive, stable, and concordant results using 3 TOFR measurements, similar to the protocol followed at our institution [13].

Conclusions

The results of the present study suggest that intra-operative quantitative NMB monitoring and the use of sugammadex are associated with a decreased incidence of RNMB in the PACU, reinforcing the contention that the optimal strategy for RNMB avoidance is the use of quantitative NMB monitoring and the eventual use of reversal agents, if needed, prior to emergence from anaesthesia. Antagonism with either neostigmine or sugammadex without the use of NMB monitoring fails to prevent RNMB in the PACU. Further efforts should aim towards increasing awareness of RNMB and monitoring rates.

Abbreviations

AMG: Acceleromyography; ASA: American Society of Anesthesiologists; CI: Confidence interval; NMB: Neuromuscular blockade; NMBD: Neuromuscular blocking drug; OR: Odds ratio; PACU: Postanaesthesia care unit; RNMB: Residual neuromuscular blockade; TOF: Train-of-four; TOFR: Train-of-four ratio

Acknowledgements

We would like to thank Editage [http://www.editage.com] for editing and reviewing this manuscript for English language.

Authors' contributions

GD conceived the original idea and collaborated on the design of the study. This author also analysed and interpreted the patient data and participated in writing the manuscript. MK was the main person in charge of collecting the data for the study and participated in the statistical analysis. MGG analysed and interpreted the patient data and was in charge of collecting data and writing the manuscript. DSN analysed and interpreted the patient data and was in charge of writing the manuscript. GGF, as head of the Anesthesiology Department, authorised the present study, was an active mentor throughout its development and substantively revised the final manuscript. ST helped with the study design and statistical analysis. All authors read and approved the final manuscript.

Author details

[1]Department of Anesthesiology, Italiano de Buenos Aires Hospital, Presidente Teniente General Juan Domingo Perón 4190, Postal Code, 1199 Buenos Aires, Argentina. [2]Department of Research, Italiano de Buenos Aires Hospital, Buenos Aires, Argentina.

References

1. Murphy GS, Szokol JW, Marymont JH, Greenberg SB, Avram MJ, Vender JS. Residual neuromuscular blockade and critical respiratory events in the postanesthesia care unit. Anesth Analg. 2008;107:130–7.
2. Brull SJ, Naguib M, Miller RD. Residual neuromuscular block: rediscovering the obvious. Anesth Analg. 2008;107:11–4.
3. Donati F. Residual paralysis: a real problem or did we invent a new disease? Can J Anaesth. 2013;60:714–29.
4. Murphy GS, Brull SJ. Residual neuromuscular block: lessons unlearned. Part I: definitions, incidence, and adverse physiologic effects of residual neuromuscular block. Anesth Analg. 2010;111:120–8.
5. Naguib M, Kopman AF, Lien CA, Hunter JM, Lopez A, Brull SJ. A survey of current management of neuromuscular block in the United States and Europe. Anesth Analg. 2010;111:110–9.
6. Naguib M, Brull SJ, Kopman AF, Hunter JM, Fülesdi B, Arkes HR, et al. Consensus statement on perioperative use of neuromuscular monitoring. Anesth Analg. 2018;127:71–80.
7. Cammu G, De Witte J, De Veylder J, Byttebier G, Vandeput D, Foubert L, et al. Postoperative residual paralysis in outpatients versus inpatients. Anesth Analg. 2006;102:426–9.
8. Nemes R, Fülesdi B, Pongrácz A, Asztalos L, Szabó-Maák Z, Lengyel S, et al. Impact of reversal strategies on the incidence of postoperative residual paralysis after rocuronium relaxation without neuromuscular monitoring: a partially randomised placebo controlled trial. Eur J Anaesthesiol. 2017;34: 609–16.
9. Beemer GH, Rozental P. Postoperative neuromuscular function. Anaesth Intensive Care. 1986;14:41–5.
10. Della Rocca G, Pompei L, Pagan de Paganis C, Tesoro S, Mendola C, Boninsegni P, et al. Reversal of rocuronium induced neuromuscular block with sugammadex or neostigmine: a large observational study. Acta Anaesthesiol Scand. 2013;57:1138–45.
11. Brueckmann B, Sasaki N, Grobara P, Li MK, Woo T, de Bie J, et al. Effects of sugammadex on incidence of postoperative residual neuromuscular blockade: a randomized, controlled study. Br J Anaesth. 2015;115:743–51.
12. Kotake Y, Ochiai R, Suzuki T, Ogawa S, Takagi S, Ozaki M, et al. Reversal with sugammadex in the absence of monitoring did not preclude residual neuromuscular block. Anesth Analg. 2013;117:345–51.
13. Debaene B, Plaud B, Dilly MP, Donati F. Residual paralysis in the PACU after a single intubating dose of nondepolarizing muscle relaxant with an intermediate duration of action. Anesthesiology. 2003;98:1042–8.
14. Norman G, Monteiro S, Salama S. Sample size calculations: should the emperor's clothes be off the peg or made to measure? BMJ. 2012;345: e5278.
15. Esteves S, Martins M, Barros F, Barros F, Canas M, Vitor P, et al. Incidence of postoperative residual neuromuscular blockade in the postanaesthesia care unit: an observational multicentre study in Portugal. Eur J Anaesthesiol. 2013;30:243–9.
16. Yip PC, Hannam JA, Cameron AJ, Campbell D. Incidence of residual neuromuscular blockade in a post-anaesthetic care unit. Anaesth Intensive Care. 2010;38:91–5.
17. Butterly A, Bittner EA, George E, Sandberg WS, Eikermann M, Schmidt U. Postoperative residual curarization from intermediate-acting neuromuscular blocking agents delays recovery room discharge. Br J Anaesth. 2010;105: 304–9.
18. Baillard C, Clec'h C, Catineau J, Salhi F, Gehan G, Cupa M, et al. Postoperative residual neuromuscular block: a survey of management. Br J Anaesth. 2005;95:622–6.
19. Murphy GS, Szokol JW, Avram MJ, Greenberg SB, Marymont JH, Vender JS, et al. Intraoperative acceleromyography monitoring reduces symptoms of muscle weakness and improves quality of recovery in the early postoperative period. Anesthesiology. 2011;115:946–54.
20. Todd MM, Hindman BJ. The implementation of quantitative electromyographic neuromuscular monitoring in an academic anesthesia department: follow-up observations. Anesth Analg. 2015;121:836–8.

21. Fuchs-Buder T, Nemes R, Schmartz D. Residual neuromuscular blockade: management and impact on postoperative pulmonary outcome. Curr Opin Anaesthesiol. 2016;29:662–7.
22. Thilen SR, Ng IC, Cain KC, Treggiari MM, Bhananker SM. Management of rocuronium neuromuscular block using a protocol for qualitative monitoring and reversal with neostigmine. Br J Anaesth. 2018;121:367–77.
23. Murphy GS, Kopman AF. Neostigmine as an antagonist of residual block: best practices do not guarantee predictable results. Br J Anaesth. 2018;121: 335–7.
24. Murphy GS, Szokol JW, Marymont JH, Franklin M, Avram MJ, Vender JS. Residual paralysis at the time of tracheal extubation. Anesth Analg. 2005; 100:1840–5.
25. Thilen SR, Hansen BE, Ramaiah R, Kent CD, Treggiari MM, Bhananker SM. Intraoperative neuromuscular monitoring site and residual paralysis. Anesthesiology. 2012;117:964–72.
26. Baillard C, Bourdiau S, Le Toumelin P, Ait Kaci F, Riou B, Cupa M, et al. Assessing residual neuromuscular blockade using acceleromyography can be deceptive in postoperative awake patients. Anesth Analg. 2004;98:854–7.

5

Population pharmacokinetic-pharmacodynamic model of propofol in adolescents undergoing scoliosis surgery with intraoperative wake-up test: a study using bispectral index and composite auditory evoked potentials as pharmacodynamic endpoints

Heleen J. Blussé van Oud-Alblas[1,2], Margreke J. E. Brill[3,4], Mariska Y. M. Peeters[4], Dick Tibboel[5], Meindert Danhof[3] and Catherijne A. J. Knibbe[3,4*]

Abstract

Background: In adolescents limited data are available on the pharmacokinetics (PK) and pharmacodynamics (PD) of propofol. In this study we derived a PK-PD model for propofol in adolescents undergoing idiopathic scoliosis surgery with an intraoperative wake-up test with reinduction of anesthesia using both Bispectral Index (BIS) and composite A-line ARX index (cAAI) as endpoints.

Methods: Fourteen adolescents (9.8–20.1 years) were evaluated during standardized propofol-remifentanil anesthesia for idiopathic scoliosis surgery with an intraoperative wake-up test with reinduction of anesthesia. BIS and cAAI were continuously measured and blood samples collected. A propofol PKPD model was developed using NONMEM.

Results: The time courses of propofol concentrations, BIS and cAAI values during anesthesia, intra-operative wakeup and reduction of anesthesia were best described by a two-compartment PK model linked to an inhibitory sigmoidal Emax PD model. For the sigmoidal Emax model, the propofol concentration at half maximum effect (EC_{50}) was 3.51 and 2.14 mg/L and Hill coefficient 1.43 and 6.85 for BIS and cAAI, respectively. The delay in PD effect in relation to plasma concentration was best described by a two compartment effect-site model with a ke_o of 0.102 min^{-1}, ke_{12} of 0.121 min^{-1} and ke_{21} of 0.172 min^{-1}.

Conclusions: A population PKPD model for propofol in adolescents was developed that successfully described the time course of propofol concentration, BIS and cAAI in individuals upon undergoing scoliosis surgery with intraoperative wake-up test and reinduction of anesthesia. Large differences were demonstrated between both monitors. This may imply that BIS and cAAI measure fundamentally different endpoints in the brain.

Keywords: Propofol, Pharmacokinetics, Pharmacodynamics, Population PKPD modeling, Bispectral index, Auditory evoked potentials, Adolescents, Anesthetic depth

* Correspondence: c.knibbe@antoniusziekenhuis.nl
[3]Division of Pharmacology, Leiden Academic Center for Drug Research, Leiden University, Leiden, The Netherlands
[4]Department of Clinical Pharmacy, St. Antonius Hospital, P.O. Box 2500, 3430 EM Nieuwegein, The Netherlands

Background

Propofol is frequently used for induction and maintenance of anesthesia in adults and children, as it has desirable pharmacokinetic and pharmacodynamic properties. While propofol pharmacokinetics (PK) are widely studied [1–5], there is a relative paucity of pharmacodynamic data. For adults, population models are available describing propofol PK PD during various types of surgery [6–8], different co-morbidities [9, 10], and for patients admitted to the ICU [7, 8]. To date, also a limited number of PKPD models in children have been published on the propofol dose-response relationship in children undergoing different types of surgery, and on the depth of sedation in non-ventilated children in the ICU [11–16]. However, even though adolescents are known to differ from both children and adults because of physiologic changes due to unique hormonal profiles and changes in body size and composition, only one PKPD model in (obese) adolescents was reported [17]. Moreover, whereas in adults different PD endpoints have been used in PKPD models, in children only Bispectral Index (BIS) and Comfort scores have been used to describe the time course of propofol effects in relation to the dose.

In this study we aimed to derive a population PK-PD model for propofol in adolescents undergoing idiopathic scoliosis surgery using two different PD endpoints. Scoliosis surgery provides a unique setting to study the PK and PD of propofol because during this type of surgery an intraoperative wake-up test is applied to reduce the risk of motor deficit or paraplegia. This wake-up test consists of waking up patients during and immediately after completion of spinal procedures after which anesthesia is reinduced to allow for completion of surgery and therefore allows for a unique combination of both awake and anesthetic observations in the same individual. As pharmacodynamics endpoints both BIS and composite A-line ARX index (cAAI) were used. Both BIS, derived from the EEG, and the cAAI, derived from auditory evoked potentials, have been evaluated as tools to measure depth of anesthesia.

Methods

The study was approved by the Institutional Ethics Committee of the Erasmus University Medical Center, Rotterdam, The Netherlands. Written informed consent of parents and patients was obtained. Inclusion criteria included patients with American Society of Anesthesiologists physical status I or II undergoing correction of idiopathic scoliosis with an intraoperative wake-up test. Exclusion criteria were hypacusis or deafness, any neurological disease, medication affecting the central nervous system, or any contraindication to the anesthesia protocol.

Anesthesia protocol

Patients received a standardized anesthetic regimen without premedication. Anesthesia was induced with remifentanil 1 mcg. kg^{-1}. min^{-1}, followed by a bolus propofol (4 mg/kg), and rocuronium (0.6 mg/kg) to facilitate endotracheal intubation. The propofol bolus dose was administered over 10 s into a fast running saline infusion into an y-site close to the patient. The lungs were mechanically ventilated to normocapnia (end-tidal carbon dioxide 35–40 mmHg). After induction of anesthesia, a central venous catheter and an arterial line were inserted for invasive continuous measurement of central venous pressure, arterial blood pressure and for arterial blood sampling.

Anesthesia was maintained with propofol by continuous infusion (2–10 mg. kg^{-1}. h^{-1}) and remifentanil (0.2–1 mcg. kg^{-1}. min^{-1}). The attending anesthesiologist conducted anesthesia in order to maintain heart rate and mean arterial pressure within 20% of baseline values obtained before induction of anesthesia. This anesthesiologist was blinded to BIS and cAAI values in order to prevent actual BIS or cAAI values to influence infusion rates of propofol, which is in accordance with current practice in our department. During the surgical procedure intrathecal morphine (5 mcg/kg) was administered by the surgeon for both intra- and postoperative pain treatment. For the wake-up test, propofol and remifentanil infusions were stopped. Patients were then repeatedly asked by the anesthesiologist in charge to move their fingers at least every 30 s until they responded, and thereafter to wiggle their toes. After finishing the wake-up test, patients were reanesthetized with an IV bolus of propofol (3–5 mg/kg) and maintenance of anesthesia was continued as previously described. Thirty minutes before the estimated end of surgery, 100 mcg/kg morphine was administered intravenously. At the end of surgery, propofol and remifentanil infusions were discontinued, and patients were extubated when sufficient spontaneous breathing had returned and they responded to verbal commands. Thereafter, patients were transferred to the Pediatric Surgical Intensive Care Unit. In addition to continuous BIS and cAAI monitoring, electrocardiogram, heart rate, noninvasive and invasive arterial blood pressure, central venous pressure, end tidal carbon dioxide, oxygen saturation via pulse oximetry, and rectal temperature were continuously monitored, collected at 5-s. intervals using Rugloop (Demed, Temse, Belgium), and synchronized with Labgrab software (Demed).

Electroencephalographic and auditory evoked potential recording

BIS and cAAI were measured before induction of anesthesia until return of consciousness of the patient, defined as spontaneous eye opening of the patient. In the

Pediatric Surgical Intensive Care only BIS was registered. In accordance with current practice BIS and cAAI values were not used to adjust propofol dosing regimens (see under Anesthesia protocol).

For the BIS, a four sensor BIS probe (BIS Pediatric Sensor, Covidien B.V. Zaltbommel, Netherlands) was attached to the left side of the patient's forehead. Values were recorded with a BIS™ monitor (A-2000, version 3.2; Aspect Medical Systems, Newton, M.A.). The BIS is ranged from 99 to 0. Values above 90 indicate wakefulness and the target range for a patient under general anesthesia is 40 to 60. For the Auditory Evoked Potentials monitor/2 (Danmeter A/S, Odense, Denmark; software version 1.6), a headphone for auditory stimuli and three disposable electrodes (cAAI; Danmeter A/S, Odense, Denmark) were positioned at the mid-forehead (+), right forehead (reference), and right mastoid (–). The cAAI is ranged from 99 to 0. cAAI levels higher than 45 indicate wakefulness, whereas levels between 15 and 25 are considered to reflect surgical anesthesia.

Blood sampling and analysis

Venous samples (1 ml) were taken before induction of anesthesia, and at approximately 15 or 30 min after the start of propofol infusion. After an arterial line was placed, arterial samples (1 ml) were taken at approximately 45 or 60, 120 or 180, 240 or 360 min after the start of the propofol infusion; at 5–10 or 10–15 min after stopping propofol infusion for the wake-up test; at the time of patient movement to a verbal command during the wake-up test; just before and 1 h after each dose adjustment; just before stopping; and 15 or 30, 45 or 60, and 120 min after the end of the infusion after surgery. The maximum amount for blood sampling was 25 ml per patient. Blood samples were collected in oxalate tubes and stored at 4 °C until analysis (within 1 month). Propofol concentrations were measured in whole blood using high-performance liquid chromatography with fluorescence detection [18]. The limit of quantification was 0.005 mg/l. Inter- and intra-assay coefficients of variation were less than 6.7 and 3.3%, over the concentration range 0.5–20 mg/L.

Data analysis

The Non-Linear Mixed effect Modeling (NONMEM) program (Globomax LLC, Hanover, MD, version VI), with Splus (version 6.2; Insightful software, Seattle, WA) for the visualization of the data, was used for sequential population pharmacokinetic and pharmacodynamic analysis [19, 20]. Using population analysis, population mean parameters and inter- and intraindividual variability (i.e. residual error) are estimated, minimizing the objective function (– 2 log likelihood). The NONMEM option of the first-order conditional estimation (Method 1) with η-ε interaction was used. Model development was performed in four steps: (1) choice of structural pharmacokinetic or pharmacodynamic model (including inter-individual variability assessment), (2) choice of residual error model, (3) covariate analysis and (4) internal validation of the model. Discrimination between different models was made by comparison of the objective function. A value of $p < 0.05$, representing a decrease of 3.8 points in the objective function was considered statistically significant. In addition, goodness-of-fit plots, including observations versus individually predicted, observations versus population predicted, time versus weighted residuals, and population predicted versus weighted residuals were used for diagnostic purposes of both pharmacokinetic and pharmacodynamic data. Finally, the confidence interval of the parameter estimates, the correlation matrix and visual improvement of the individual time versus observation plots were used to evaluate the model.

Covariate analysis

Covariates were plotted independently against the individual post-hoc parameter estimates and the weighted residuals of the basic model without covariates, to visualize potential relationships, as previously described [13]. Bodyweight, age, gender, and remifentanil infusion rates were tested as covariates.

Potential covariates were separately incorporated into the model and considered statistically significant if the objective function decreased 7.8 points ($P < 0.005$) and the 95% confidence interval of the additional parameter did not include 0 (assuming normal distribution). In addition, visual inspection of diagnostic plots was performed.

Model evaluation

The internal validity of the population pharmacokinetic and pharmacodynamic models was primarily assessed by the bootstrap resampling method (repeated random sampling to produce another data set of the same size but with a different combination of individuals). Parameters obtained with the bootstrap replicates were compared to the estimates obtained from the original data set. Deviations up to 5–10% in structural parameters were accepted for the pharmacokinetic model and 15–20% for the pharmacodynamic model. Additionally, normalized prediction distribution errors (NPDE) were computed [21, 22].

Pharmacokinetic model

A two-compartment pharmacokinetic model (NONMEM ADVAN 3 TRANS 4) was used to fit the log-transformed data, parameterized in terms of clearance (CL), central volume of distribution (V_1), inter-compartmental clearance (Q) and peripheral volume of distribution (V_2).

The individual value (post hoc value) of each parameter (P) of the ith subject was modeled by

$$P_i = P_{tv} * e^{\eta i} \quad (1)$$

where P_{tv} is the mean estimated of the typical population parameter value and η_i is a random variable with mean zero and variance ω^2, assuming log-normal distribution of the parameter in the population.

The intraindividual variability was best described by a proportional error model. This means for the jth observed log transformed propofol concentration of the ith individual (Y_{ij}) the relation

$$Y_{ij} = \log c_{pred,ij} + \varepsilon_{ij} \quad (2)$$

where c_{pred} predicted log transformed propofol concentration and ε_{ij} is the random variable with mean zero and variance σ^2.

Pharmacodynamic model

The delay in BIS and cAAI values in relation to propofol concentration in the central pharmacokinetic compartment was characterized on the basis of a hypothetical effect compartment [23], which is an approach that has been applied before for propofol induced BIS values [24, 25].

In this effect compartment approach, it is assumed that the rate of onset and offset of effect is governed by the rate of propofol distribution to and from a hypothetical 'effect-site'. Under this interpretation, the effect compartment is linked to the blood compartment by a first order rate constant k_{e1} and with a rate constant for drug loss k_{e0}. Under the assumption that in equilibrium the effect-site concentration equals the blood concentration, the following equation can be used:

$$\frac{dCe}{dt} = ke0 \cdot (Cb\text{-}Ce) \quad (3)$$

where C_b is the blood concentration in the central pharmacokinetic compartment, C_e represents the effect-site concentration and k_{e0} is the first-order equilibration constant. Beside this previously applied one compartment effect-site model for propofol, also a two compartment effect-site model was explored [26], in which distribution of propofol within the brain is represented by definition of a central effect compartment and a peripheral effect compartment (Fig. 1). Similar to the one-compartment effect model, in this two compartment effect site model, the observed effect is dependent upon the concentration in the central effect compartment, however this concentration is in its turn not only governed by the rate of propofol distribution to and from the central pharmacokinetic compartment but also by the rate of propofol distribution to and from the peripheral effect compartment, k_{e12} and k_{e21}, respectively.

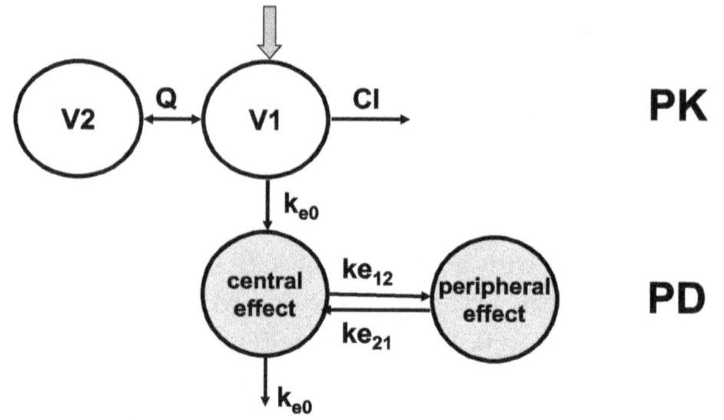

Fig. 1 Schematic representation of the pharmacokinetic (PK) -pharmacodynamic (PD) model for propofol with V1, V2, Q and Cl representing the two compartment pharmacokinetic model and a central and peripheral effect-site compartment characterizing the pharmacodynamics. K_{e0} is the first-order rate constant from central pharmacokinetic compartment to central effect site compartment which equals the rate constant for drug loss of the effect-site compartment, k_{e12} and k_{e21} represent the rate constants from central to peripheral effect site compartment and back. The propofol concentration in the central effect site-compartment is directly responsible for the measured Bispectral Index (BIS) or composite A-Line ARX Index (cAAI) as described using eq. 4

For the pharmacodynamics model, posthoc values of the pharmacokinetic model were used. The full pharmacokinetic-pharmacodynamic model is showed in Fig. 1.

Concentration-effect relationships

For the relation between propofol concentration in central effect compartment and BIS or cAAI values, a sigmoidal E_{max} model was used:

$$PD_{ij} = PD_0 - \frac{\left(E_{\max,\ i} \bullet c_{e,ij}^{\gamma}\right)}{EC_{50,i}{}^{\gamma} + c_{e,ij}{}^{\gamma}} \quad (4)$$

where PD_0 is the baseline BIS or cAAI value, $E_{max,i}$ is the maximum possible effect of propofol on BIS or cAAI in the *i*th subject, $C_{e,ij}$ is the propofol concentration in the central effect compartment in the *i*th subject at the *j*th time point, γ is the Hill coefficient representing the steepness of the concentration versus response relation, and EC_{50} is the propofol concentration (mg/l) at half the maximum score of the BIS or cAAI. Pharmacodynamic parameters were assumed to be log-normally distributed. The interindividual variable (η_i) was assumed to be log-normally distributed with mean zero and variance ω^2. The residual error ε was best characterized by an additive error model.

$$Y_{ij} = PD_{pred,ij} + \varepsilon_{ij} \quad (5)$$

where Y_{ij} represents the observed BIS or cAAI effect in the *i*th subject at the *j*th time point.

Results

Propofol pharmacokinetics

The propofol pharmacokinetic model was based on 225 blood samples from 14 adolescents during propofol-remifentanil anesthesia for scoliosis surgery with an intraoperative wake-up test with reinduction of anesthesia (median duration propofol administration of 410 min). All patient and data characteristics are provided in Table 1. The pharmacokinetics of propofol were adequately described by a two-compartment model. The pharmacokinetic parameter values and their 95% confidence intervals of the final model are shown in Table 2. The fits of 1000 bootstrap replicates of the data set demonstrated the stability of the model. In Fig. 2a and b, the diagnostics of the final pharmacokinetic model is shown. Figure 3a shows the log transformed propofol concentration versus time of a representative individual. None of the explored covariates significantly influence the pharmacokinetic parameters.

Table 2 Pharmacokinetic (PK) model parameter estimates and stability of the parameters using bootstrap validation (BS)

Parameter	PK Model Mean (CV%)	BS PK Model Mean (CV%)
Fixed effects		
CL (l/min)	1.37 (7.0)	1.38 (5.1)
Q (l/min)	1.15 (29.4)	1.16 (44.1)
V_1 (l)	3.6 (10.2)	3.45 (11.3)
V_2 (l)	76.8 (5.0)	77.3 (5.0)
Interindividual variability		
ω^2 of CL in %	22.1 (28.7)	21.4 (25.7)
Residual error		
σ^2	19.0% (11.9)	18.4% (12.5)
Performance measures		
(−2LL)	− 452	− 464.7

BS bootstrap validation, *CL* clearance, *Q* intercompartmental clearance, V_1 central volume, V_2 peripheral volume, ω^2 variance, the square root of the exponential variance of η-1 is the percentage of the interindividual variability in the pharmacokinetic parameters; σ^2 proportional individual variance, *-2LL* objective function. Values in parentheses are coefficient of variation (CV) of the parameter values

Propofol pharmacodynamics

Per patient a median of 113 (66–154) observations for BIS and 100 (60–141) for cAAI were available for the pharmacodynamic analysis. Propofol concentration-effect relationship was described using a sigmoid E_{max} model (eq. 4) for which different parameter values for BIS and cAAI were found.

For BIS, the propofol concentration at half maximum effect (EC_{50}) was 3.51 mg/l with interindividual coefficient of variation of 0.059 which corresponds to a CV of 25% within the context of a two compartment effect site compartment model ($p < 0.001$ compared to one-compartment effect site model). Using BIS, the delay of anesthetic effect with respect to plasma concentrations, was described by a keo of 0.102 min-1, ke12 of 0.121 min-1, ke21 of 0.172 min-1. The T_{max} of the two-compartment biophase distribution model was 2.63 min. The Hill coefficient was 1.43 (CV = 34%).

Table 1 Patients' and data characteristics (*n* = 14)

Gender (M / F)	2 / 12
Age (years)	14.7 (9.8–20.1)
Bodyweight (kg)	51 (36.6–82)
Height (cm)	162.5 (142–183)
Number of blood samples per patient	16 (6–22)
Number of BIS events per patient	113 (66–154)
Number of cAAI events per patient	100 (60–141)
Duration of propofol infusion (minutes)	410.0 (200–460)
Length of wake-up test (minutes)	21.5 (7.6–42.4)
ROC after propofol infusion (minutes)	52.2 (22.6–116.33)

F Female, *M* Male, *BIS* Bispectral Index, *cAAI* composite A-Line ARX Index, *ROC* Return of consciousness. The length of wake-up test is defined as the length of time propofol infusion was stopped during the intraoperative wake-up test during propofol-remifentanil anesthesia. Data are presented as a median (minimum-maximum)

For cAAI EC50 was 2.14 mg/l (CV 42%) within the context of a one compartment effect site model with a keo of 0.067 min-1, as a two-compartment effect-site model was not superior ($P > 0.05$). For cAAI, the baseline value was estimated at 63.4 while the E_{max} was estimated at 49.8, yielding a maximum effect of 14 at the cAAI scale. The Hill coefficient was 6.85 (CV = 126%) (Table 3).

For the pharmacodynamics of propofol no covariates could be identified, though there was a negatively linear trend towards an influence of age on the EC50 ($P > 0.05$) of both BIS and cAAI.

Figure 2 c, d, e, and f show diagnostic plots of the pharmacodynamic models for BIS and cAAI. In Fig. 3 b and c, BIS and cAAI values versus time in a representative adolescent are presented. These plots show that the final pharmacodynamic models describe both BIS and cAAI observations well during induction, wake-up test, reinduction and emergence of anesthesia until return of consciousness, albeit the performance was better for BIS compared to cAAI. The bootstrap validation (250 replications, Table 3) confirmed the stability of the final pharmacodynamic models. Also the results from the computation of the model NPDE demonstrated a normal distribution, with no trend in the output graphs (data not shown)

In Fig. 4 the propofol concentration effect relationships for BIS and cAAI are presented. The figure shows that BIS values gradually change as a result of

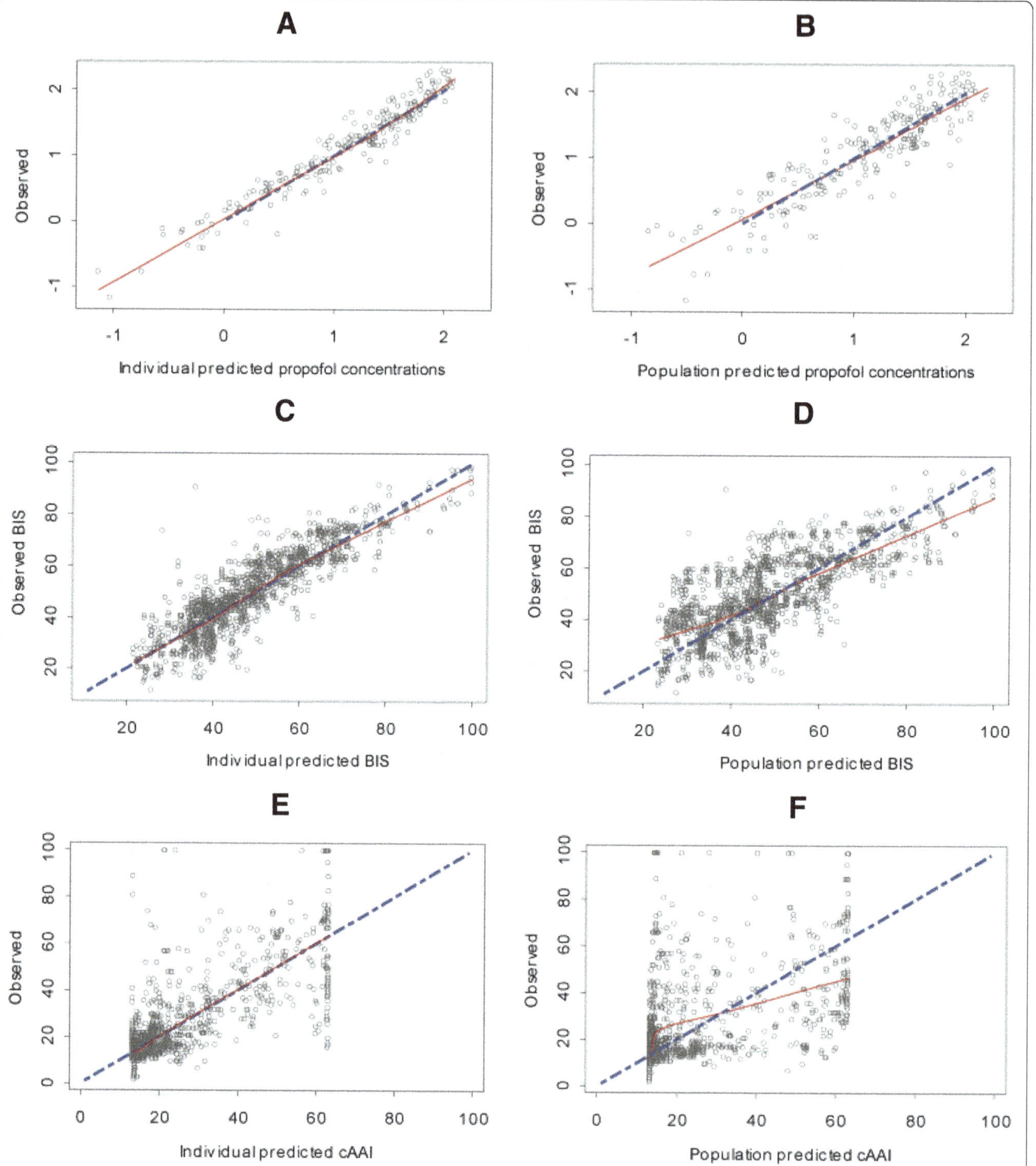

Fig. 2 Diagnostic plots of the final pharmacokinetic (**a** and **b**) and pharmacodynamic models using Bispectral index (BIS) (**c** and **d**) and composite A-Line ARX index (cAAI) (**e** and **f**), including (left) observations versus individual-predicted propofol concentrations or depth of anesthesia, and (right) observations versus population predicted concentrations or depth of anesthesia. The solid line indicates the trend line, the dashed line represents the line of identity, x = y

the propofol concentration, while for cAAI a more rapid change in values are observed as a result of the higher Hilll coefficient.

Discussion

In this study we derived a population PK and PD model for propofol in adolescents undergoing scoliosis surgery

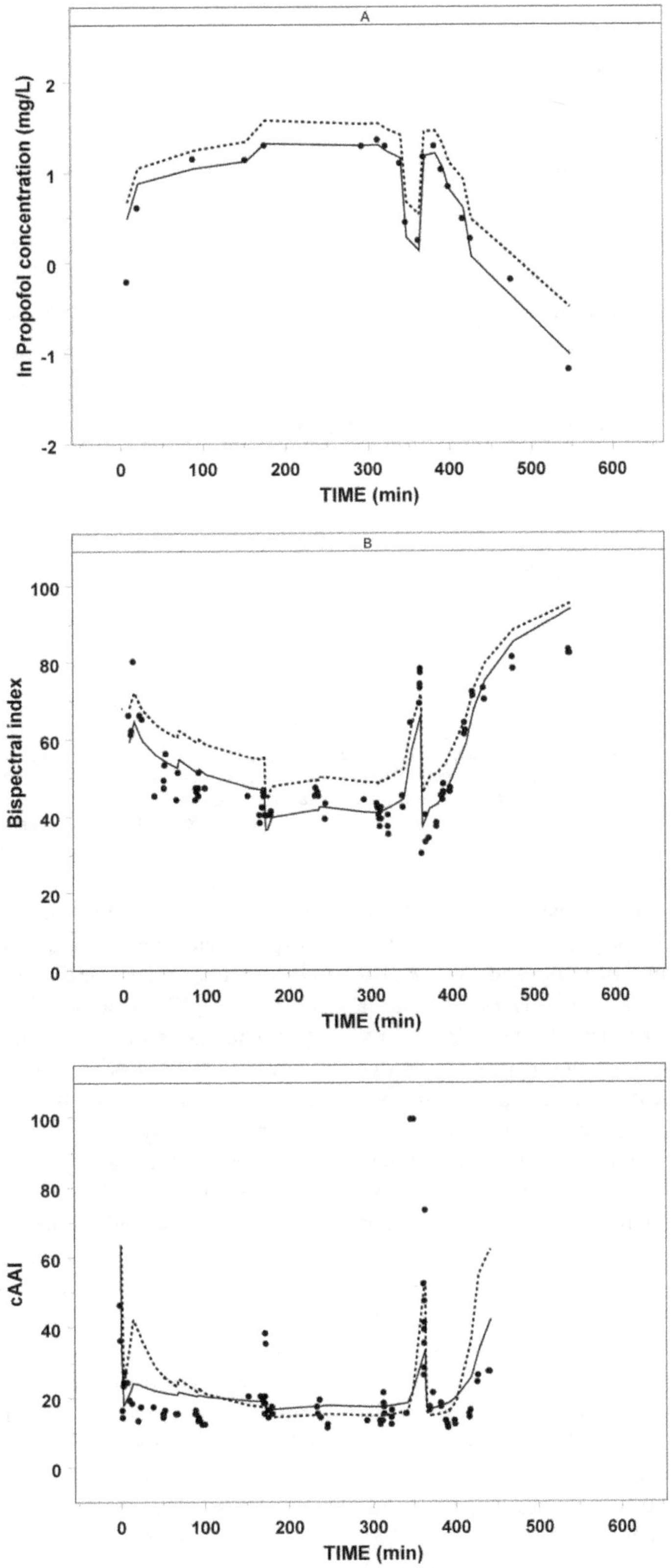

Fig. 3 Log transformed propofol concentrations, Bispectral index and composite A-Line ARX index (cAAI) versus time (minutes) in a representative adolescent. The solid circles represent the observations, the solid lines represent the individual predicted concentration or depth of anesthesia and the dashed line represents the population predicted concentration or depth of anesthesia

Table 3 Population pharmacodynamic parameters for the one-compartment effect model and two compartment effect model for propofol induced changes of the Bispectral index (BIS) and composite A-line ARX index (cAAI)

Parameter	BIS Mean (CV%)	Bs BIS Mean (%)	cAAI Mean (CV%)	Bs cAAI Mean (%)
Fixed effects				
E_0	100 Fixed	100 Fixed	63.4 (14.9)	63.3 (100)
E_{max} (value)	100 Fixed	100 Fixed		
E_{max} (fraction of E_0)			0.786 (6.1)	0.787 (100)
EC_{50} (mg/l)	3.51 (6.61)	3.53 (101)	2.14 (12.4)	2.10 (98)
γ	1.43 (10.1)	1.44 (100)	6.85 (46.4)	7.03 (103)
k_{eo} (min^{-1})	0.102 (20.4)	0.103 (101)	0.067 (14.8)	0.079 (118)
k_{e12}	0.121 (49.3)	0.118 (98)		
k_{e21}	0.172 (35.8)	0.160 (93)		
Interindividual variability				
ω_{EC50}^2	0.059 (48.1)	0.056 (96)	0.159 (33.9)	0.165 (103)
ω_{γ}^2	0.117 (41.0)	0.111 (95)	0.952 (39.3)	1.12 (118)
$\omega_{k_{eo}}^2$	0.192 (49.7)	0.195 (102)	0.498 (38.4)	0.522 (105)
Residual error				
σ^2	59.5 (11.1)	58.4 (98)	133 (18.9)	122 (92)
Performance measures				
-2LL	6.984.424	6972.363 (100)	9354.40	9310.08 (100)

BIS Bispectral index, *cAAI* composite A-Line ARX index, *Bs* bootstrap validation (250 times), *E0* baseline, *Emax* maximum possible effect expressed as absolute value or fraction of E0, *EC50* propofol concentration at half maximum effect, *γ* Hill coefficient, *keO* first-order equilibration constant, *ke12* rate constant from central to peripheral effect site, *ke21* rate constant from peripheral to central effect site, *ω2* variance, the square root of the exponential variance of η minus 1 is the percentage of interindividual variability in the pharmacodynamic parameters, *σ2* additive intraindividual variance, values in parentheses are *CV* coefficient of variation of the parameter values, *-2LL* objective function

with an intraoperative wake-up test using BIS and cAAI as pharmacodynamic endpoints. The data used in this analysis covered a broad range of sleep and awake propofol plasma concentrations and depths of anesthesia endpoints. The time courses of propofol concentrations, BIS and cAAI values during anesthesia, intra-operative wakeup and reduction of anesthesia were best described by a two-compartment PK model linked to an inhibitory sigmoidal Emax PD model. For the sigmoidal Emax model, the propofol concentration at half maximum effect (EC50) was 3.51 and 2.14 mg/L and Hill coefficient 1.43 and 6.85 for BIS and cAAI, respectively. The delay in PD effect in relation to plasma concentration was best described by a two compartment effect-site model with a keo of 0.102 min-1, ke12 of 0.121 min-1 and ke21 of 0.172 min-1.

For the pharmacokinetics of propofol, clearance observed in this study where the median bodyweight was 51 kg, was 1.37 L/min. This result seems in accordance with the results of a recent study in (morbidly) obese adolescents and children (mean total body weight 125 kg), which demonstrated a clearance of 1.72 L/min for a 70 kg standardized individual [27]. The slightly lower propofol clearance in our (non obese) adolescents compared to that of the obese adolescents and children, may be explained by the increased blood volume and cardiac output that may be expected leading to an increased clearance in obese individuals for this high extraction ratio drug [27]. A population pharmacokinetic meta-analysis showed a clearance of 2.37 L/min with a combination of total body weight and age being the best covariates to capture changes in propofol clearance as a result of obesity and ageing which are known to influence both influence hepatic blood flow [28]. Next to this, the central volume in our study (3.6 L) is consistent with previously reported findings in adults during propofol-remifentanil anesthesia, while our estimation of the peripheral volume of distribution (76.8 L) seems very much in accordance with the earlier reported volume of 31.7 L [29].

In target-controlled-infusion (TCI) systems PK and PD models are used to determine the dose required to achieve a desired target concentration in a central or effect-site compartment. In many hospitals, propofol is administered with a target-controlled infusion (TCI) pump. Of the currently available models, the Schnider [30] and Marsh [1] pharmacokinetic models are commonly used, even though they were developed from studies in healthy subjects. Understanding the pharmacokinetics allows clinicians to adjust the delivered dose

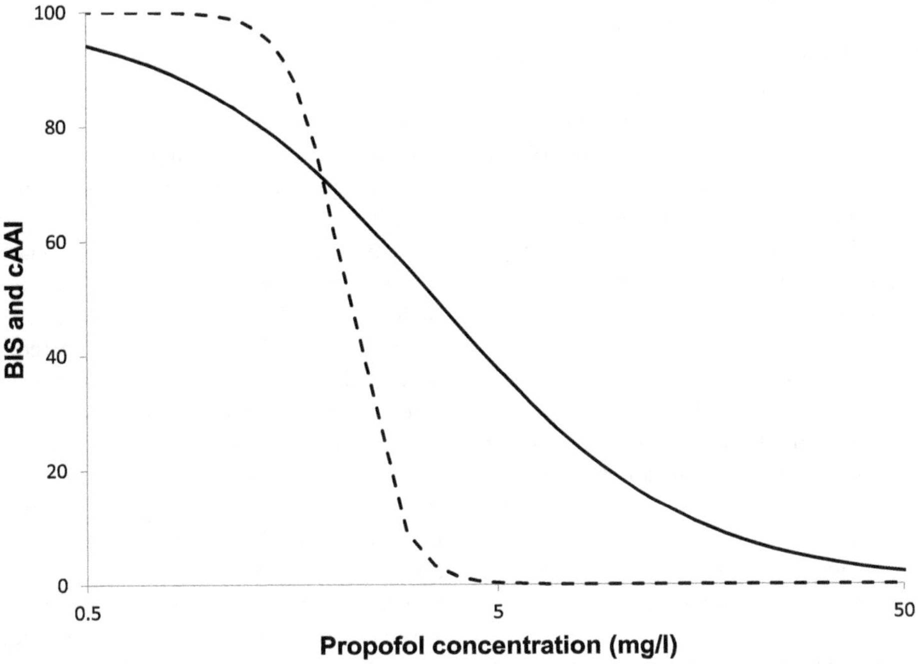

Fig. 4 Propofol concentration – effect relation for Bispectral index (BIS, solid line) and composite A-Line ARX Index (cAAI, dotted line) for the final model

in order to control the concentration at the effect-site. Understanding the pharmacodynamics helps in titrating anesthesia according to individual needs. Simulations based on a PKPD- model will therefore lead to a propofol dosing algorithm that will result in the maintenance of adequate anesthetic depth during propofol anesthesia in each individual patient. The PKPD model that was derived in this study can be used to guide dosing for anesthesia in adolescents, which is a population that is relatively understudied. As such, the results of the current study provide an important step towards addressing propofol dosing challenges in this special population.

Our pharmacodynamic model accurately described BIS and cAAI observations during induction of anesthesia, the intraoperative wakeup test, reinduction and emergence from anesthesia (Fig. 3). Although both monitors have been proposed as pharmacodynamic endpoints, they measure the hypnotic state during anesthesia in a different way. The BIS is an empirically derived multifactorial electroencephalographic parameter that relies on the correlation of the phases between frequency components of the electroencephalogram whereas midlatency auditory evoked potentials (MLAEPS), extracted from the electroencephalogram 10–100 ms after an auditory signal, represent the earliest cortical response to an acoustic stimulus. Amplitudes and latencies of the MLAEPs are influenced by anesthetics and surgical stimuli and are therefore believed to be useful in measuring the level of hypnosis during anesthesia [31]. A monitoring variable indicating the patient's hypnotic state, the composite A-Line ARX Index (cAAI), is then calculated from the MLAEP and the electroencephalogram. Specifically, the cAAI is preferably derived from the MLAEP, but in case of low MLAEP signal quality, it is entirely based on the spontaneous electroencephalogram. Because of these differences in measuring depth of anesthesia it is therefore not surprising that large differences were demonstrated in EC50 and Hill coefficient between both monitors implicating that both monitors measure fundamentally different endpoints in the brain.

For the BIS, depth of anesthesia was best described with a two-compartment biophase distribution model. Theoretically, this two-compartment biophase distribution model for the BIS may represent a redistribution of propofol within the central nervous system. Bjornson et al. showed that a two compartment biophase distribution best described propofol effect measured by BIS in healthy adult volunteers [26]. Earlier Upton and Ludbrook, when defining a physiological PK (PBPK) model of propofol in adult man, found a two-compartment brain model to best describe BIS observations [28].

For the cAAI, depth of sedation was best described by a classic one-compartment effect site model with a sigmodial Emax pharmacodynamic model and no propofol biophase distribution could be characterized for this measure. This finding may be explained by the very steep Hill coefficient (on-off phenomenon) together with low resolution sampling of the pharmacodynamic measurements during the rapid changes in cAAI. Interestingly, the steeper Hill coefficient for cAAI supports our clinical observation that the awaking from propofol remifentanil anesthesia was associated with an 'on/off' cAAI response rather than a gradual progression to awake levels. Further differences between the BIS and cAAI models suggest that they measure significantly different endpoints in the brain, which is reflected by large differences in EC50 (3.51 mg/l for the BIS versus 2.14 mg/l for the cAAI). Research into these differences is needed to elucidate the physiologic- and monitor-based rational of these results.

Although large differences between Emax models of cAAI and BIS measures are found, based on this study there is no evidence that might support the use of one or the other monitor of depth of anesthesia, BIS or cAAI. On the other hand, an instrument of which the value gradually changes with propofol concentration may be of advantage when aiming for an optimal level of anesthesia through titration, which favors the BIS compared to cAAI.

Patients included in this study were instructed to remember a color during the wake/up test, and were postoperatively interviewed for explicit recall. Results from this separate part of our study have been previously published [32]. Although all patients responded adequately to the wake/up test (e.g. by wiggling their toes or feet) and both EEG indices demonstrated patients being awake, no explicit recall or postoperative pain was demonstrated [32]. Furthermore, in this study we reported on the performance of both indices in distinguishing different hypnotic states, as evaluated by the University of Michigan Sedation Scale, during scoliosis surgery with an intraoperative wake-up test [32]. BIS and cAAI were compared at the start of the wake-up test, at purposeful movement to command, and after the patient was reanesthetized. During induction of anesthesia, BIS performed better than cAAI, as indicated by prediction probabilities. Although cAAI was statistically a better discriminator for the level of consciousness during the wake-up test and emergence, these differences do not appear to be clinically meaningful. Both indices increased during the wake-up test, indicating a higher level of consciousness. However, both monitors were not found to be ideal, as considerable overlap in both BIS and cAAI values was present when compared with each level of the UMSS [32].

No covariates could be identified for the pharmacokinetic and for the pharmacodynamic model of propofol, although there was a trend towards an influence of bodyweight on clearance as well as age on the EC50. Another study investigating propofol effects in adolescents studied propofol BIS effect in children (6–13) and adults (13–35 years) [11]. They found, that when pooling adult and children data, the fit with the Schnider model significantly improved when puberty status (child or adult) was added to the model as a covariate, showing that age probably has an influence on the effect of propofol. These results and those of the present study seem to be in line and future studies in a large age range will have to show whether age indeed is of influence for propofol pharmacodynamics. As remifentanil was co-administered with propofol in this study, its potential influence on the pharmacokinetics or pharmacodynamics of propofol was investigated, however no influence could be identified. This seems to be in contrast with literature in adults, in which synergy is reported between remifentanil and propofol, with modest remifentanil concentrations already dramatically reducing the concentrations of propofol required to ablate a response [31]. More specifically, also in children, remifentanil was found to reduce the concentration of propofol required for anesthesia but increasing the remifentanil infusion yielded minimal additional effect [33]. As all children in our study received remifentanil infusions during this prolonged surgical procedure in moderate to high dosages (2–10 mcg.kg-1.h-1), we believe that we have reached maximum synergy at the dose levels used. This may explain why we could not identify an influence of moderate versus high remifentanil infusion rates on the pharmacokinetics and pharmacodynamics of propofol in our patients.

A limitation of our study was that due to ethical considerations, propofol sampling during induction of anesthesia was limited. However, the intraoperative wake-up test during scoliosis surgery allowed for extra propofol sampling after reinduction of anesthesia. Furthermore, because of the relatively small amount of available awake data points in the present study, it was not possible to estimate baseline and Emax for BIS. Therefore, in the final pharmacodynamic model both parameters for BIS were fixed to 100. For cAAI, baseline was estimated at 63.4, and Emax at 49.8. Interestingly, fixing the Emax for cAAI to 100 gave a similar EC50 value, indicating a minimal influence on EC50. Another limitation of the final pharmacodynamic models is that intraoperative stimuli during the wake up test were not accounted for. Model based predictions following the recommended propofol dosing regimen will therefore predict cAAI and BIS values without a stimulus to move legs or arms and may therefore underestimate peak cAAI values (Fig. 3c) and perhaps also BIS values (Fig. 3b), if the wake-up test is accompanied by verbal and surgical stimulation. Finally, although age tended to influence EC50 ($p > 0.05$), no covariates of propofol could be identified in the present study. This is probably due to insufficient statistical power to estimate a continuous influence of age on EC50. Yet, when a separate EC50 for the youngest subject was estimated, a significant decrease in the NONMEM objective function was observed. Future studies in younger individuals will have to explore whether age is of influence to EC50.

Conclusion

In conclusion, a population PKPD model for propofol in adolescents was developed that successfully described the time course and variability of propofol concentration, BIS and cAAI in individuals upon undergoing scoliosis surgery with intraoperative wake-up test and reinduction of anesthesia. Large differences were demonstrated between both monitors. This may imply that BIS and cAAI measure fundamentally different endpoints in the brain.

Comprehensive knowledge of propofol PKPD in this specific age group is of importance, as this will lead to an increased understanding of propofol effects and will eventually lead to evidence-based dosing strategies in this population.

Abbreviations

BIS: Bispectral index; cAAI: composite A-line ARX index; NONMEM: Non-Linear Mixed effect Modeling; NPDE: normalized prediction distribution errors; PD: pharmacodynamics; PK: pharmacokinetics

Acknowledgements

The authors thank Ron Mathôt and Bart Claassen (Department of Clinical Pharmacy, Erasmus MC, Rotterdam, The Netherlands), Gijs Santen (Division of Pharmacology, LACDR, Leiden University, Leiden, The Netherlands), Luuk de Klerk (Department of Orthopedic Surgery, Erasmus MC, Rotterdam, The Netherlands), Tom de Leeuw, Kris Vermeylen, Nadia Kriek, and Bram Valkenburg (Department of Anesthesiology, Erasmus MC – Sophia Children's Hospital, Rotterdam, The Netherlands) for their help and cooperation during the study.

Author details

[1]Department of Anesthesiology, Erasmus Medical Center, Rotterdam, The Netherlands. [2]Department of Anesthesiology, St. Antonius Hospital, Nieuwegein, The Netherlands. [3]Division of Pharmacology, Leiden Academic Center for Drug Research, Leiden University, Leiden, The Netherlands. [4]Department of Clinical Pharmacy, St. Antonius Hospital, P.O. Box 2500, 3430 EM Nieuwegein, The Netherlands. [5]Department of Pediatric Intensive Care, Erasmus Medical Center - Sophia Children's Hospital, Rotterdam, The Netherlands.

References

1. Marsh B, White M, Morton N, Kenny GN. Pharmacokinetic model driven infusion of propofol in children. Br J Anaesth. 1991;67(1):41–8.
2. Rigby-Jones AE, Nolan JA, Priston MJ, Wright PM, Sneyd JR, Wolf AR. Pharmacokinetics of propofol infusions in critically ill neonates, infants, and children in an intensive care unit. Anesthesiology. 2002;97(6):1393–400.
3. Schuttler J, Ihmsen H. Population pharmacokinetics of propofol: a multicenter study. Anesthesiology. 2000;92(3):727–38.
4. Shangguan WN, Lian Q, Aarons L, Matthews I, Wang Z, Chen X, Freemantle N, Smith FG. Pharmacokinetics of a single bolus of propofol in chinese children of different ages. Anesthesiology. 2006;104(1):27–32.
5. Kataria BK, Ved SA, Nicodemus HF, Hoy GR, Lea D, Dubois MY, Mandema JW, Shafer SL. The pharmacokinetics of propofol in children using three different data analysis approaches. Anesthesiology. 1994;80(1):104–22.
6. Wiczling P, Bienert A, Sobczynski P, Hartmann-Sobczynska R, Bieda K, Marcinkowska A, Malatynska M, Kaliszan R, Grzeskowiak E. Pharmacokinetics and pharmacodynamics of propofol in patients undergoing abdominal aortic surgery. Pharmacol Rep. 2012;64(1):113–22.
7. Knibbe CA, Aarts LP, Kuks PF, Voortman HJ, Lie-A-Huen L, Bras LJ, Danhof M. Pharmacokinetics and pharmacodynamics of propofol 6% SAZN versus propofol 1% SAZN and Diprivan-10 for short-term sedation following coronary artery bypass surgery. Eur J Clin Pharmacol. 2000;56(1):89–95.
8. Peeters MY, Bras LJ, DeJongh J, Wesselink RM, Aarts LP, Danhof M, Knibbe CA. Disease severity is a major determinant for the pharmacodynamics of propofol in critically ill patients. Clin Pharmacol Ther. 2008;83(3):443–51.
9. van Kralingen S, Diepstraten J, Peeters MY, Deneer VH, van Ramshorst B, Wiezer RJ, van Dongen EP, Danhof M, Knibbe CA. Population pharmacokinetics and pharmacodynamics of propofol in morbidly obese patients. Clin Pharmacokinet. 2011;50(11):739–50.
10. Przybylowski K, Tyczka J, Szczesny D, Bienert A, Wiczling P, Kut K, Plenzler E, Kaliszan R, Grzeskowiak E. Pharmacokinetics and pharmacodynamics of propofol in cancer patients undergoing major lung surgery. J Pharmacokinet Pharmacodyn. 2015;42(2):111–22.
11. Rigouzzo A, Servin F, Constant I. Pharmacokinetic-pharmacodynamic modeling of propofol in children. Anesthesiology. 2010;113(2):343–52.
12. Jeleazcov C, Schmidt J, Schmitz B, Becke K, Albrecht S. EEG variables as measures of arousal during propofol anaesthesia for general surgery in children: rational selection and age dependence. Br J Anaesth. 2007; 99(6):845–54.
13. Peeters MY, Prins SA, Knibbe CA, DeJongh J, van Schaik RH, van Dijk M, van der Heiden IP, Tibboel D, Danhof M. Propofol pharmacokinetics and pharmacodynamics for depth of sedation in nonventilated infants after major craniofacial surgery. Anesthesiology. 2006;104(3):466–74.
14. Coppens MJ, Eleveld DJ, Proost JH, Marks LA, Van Bocxlaer JF, Vereecke H, Absalom AR, Struys MM. An evaluation of using population pharmacokinetic models to estimate pharmacodynamic parameters for propofol and bispectral index in children. Anesthesiology. 2011;115(1):83–93.
15. Choi BM, Lee HG, Byon HJ, Lee SH, Lee EK, Kim HS, Noh GJ. Population pharmacokinetic and pharmacodynamic model of propofol externally validated in children. J Pharmacokinet Pharmacodyn. 2015;42(2):163–77.
16. Bartkowska-Sniatkowska A, Bienert A, Wiczling P, Owczarek M, Rosada-Kurasinska J, Grzeskowiak M, Matysiak J, Kokot ZJ, Kaliszan R, Grzeskowiak E. Pharmacokinetics and pharmacodynamics of propofol in children undergoing different types of surgeries. Pharmacol Rep. 2014;66(5):821–9.
17. Chidambaran V, Venkatasubramanian R, Sadhasivam S, Esslinger H, Cox S, Diepstraten J, Fukuda T, Inge T, Knibbe CAJ, Vinks AA. Population pharmacokinetic-pharmacodynamic modeling and dosing simulation of propofol maintenance anesthesia in severely obese adolescents. Paediatr Anaesth. 2015;25(9):911–23.
18. Knibbe CA, Koster VS, Deneer VH, Stuurman RM, Kuks PF, Lange R. Determination of propofol in low-volume samples by high-performance liquid chromatography with fluorescence detection. J Chromatogr B Biomed Sci Appl. 1998;706(2):305–10.
19. Zhang L, Beal SL, Sheiner LB. Simultaneous vs. sequential analysis for population PK/PD data I: best-case performance. J Pharmacokinet Pharmacodyn. 2003;30(6):387–404.
20. Beal SL, Boeckmann A, Sheiner LB. NONMEM's User's Guide; 1999.
21. Brendel K, Comets E, Laffont C, Laveille C, Mentre F. Metrics for external model evaluation with an application to the population pharmacokinetics of gliclazide. Pharm Res. 2006;23(9):2036–49.
22. Comets E, Brendel K, Mentre F. Computing normalised prediction distribution errors to evaluate nonlinear mixed-effect models: the npde add-on package for R. Comput Methods Prog Biomed. 2008;90(2):154–66.
23. Sheiner LB, Stanski DR, Vozeh S, Miller RD, Ham J. Simultaneous modeling of pharmacokinetics and pharmacodynamics: application to d-tubocurarine. Clin Pharmacol Ther. 1979;25(3):358–71.
24. Struys MM, Coppens MJ, De Neve N, Mortier EP, Doufas AG, Van Bocxlaer JF, Shafer SL. Influence of administration rate on propofol plasma-effect site equilibration. Anesthesiology. 2007;107(3):386–96.
25. Doufas AG, Bakhshandeh M, Bjorksten AR, Shafer SL, Sessler DI. Induction speed is not a determinant of propofol pharmacodynamics. Anesthesiology. 2004;101(5):1112–21.
26. Bjornsson MA, Norberg A, Kalman S, Karlsson MO, Simonsson US. A two-compartment effect site model describes the bispectral index after different rates of propofol infusion. J Pharmacokinet Pharmacodyn. 2010;37(3):243–55.
27. Diepstraten J, Chidambaran V, Sadhasivam S, Esslinger HR, Cox SL, Inge TH, Knibbe CA, Vinks AA. Propofol clearance in morbidly obese children and adolescents: influence of age and body size. Clin Pharmacokinet. 2012;51(8):543–51.
28. Upton RN, Ludbrook G. A physiologically based, recirculatory model of the kinetics and dynamics of propofol in man. Anesthesiology. 2005;103(2):344–52.
29. Wietasch JKG, Scholz M, Zinserling J, Kiefer N, Frenkel C, Knufermann P,

Brauer U, Hoeft A. The performance of a target-controlled infusion of propofol in combination with remifentanil: a clinical investigation with two propofol formulations. Anesth Analg. 2006;102(2):430–7.

30. Schnider TW, Minto CF, Gambus PL, Andresen C, Goodale DB, Shafer SL, Youngs EJ. The influence of method of administration and covariates on the pharmacokinetics of propofol in adult volunteers. Anesthesiology. 1998; 88(5):1170–82.
31. Mertens MJ, Olofsen E, Engbers FH, Burm AG, Bovill JG, Vuyk J. Propofol reduces perioperative remifentanil requirements in a synergistic manner: response surface modeling of perioperative remifentanil-propofol interactions. Anesthesiology. 2003;99(2):347–59.
32. Blusse van Oud-Alblas HJ, Peters JW, de Leeuw TG, Vermeylen KT, de Klerk LW, Tibboel D, Klein J, Weber F. A comparison in adolescents of composite auditory evoked potential index and bispectral index during propofol-remifentanil anesthesia for scoliosis surgery with intraoperative wake-up test. Anesth Analg. 2008;107(5):1683–8.
33. Drover DR, Litalien C, Wellis V, Shafer SL, Hammer GB. Determination of the pharmacodynamic interaction of propofol and remifentanil during esophagogastroduodenoscopy in children. Anesthesiology. 2004;100(6):1382–6.

6

Validation of noninvasive continuous arterial pressure measurement by clearsight system™ during induction of anesthesia for cardiovascular surgery

Tadashi Tanioku*, Akari Yoshida, Yuichi Aratani, Keisuke Fujii and Tomoyuki Kawamata

Abstract

Background: Since blood pressure tends to be unstable during induction of anesthesia in patients undergoing cardiovascular surgery, an artery catheter is often inserted before induction to continuously monitor arterial pressure during induction of anesthesia. ClearSight System™ enables noninvasive continuous measurement of beat-to-beat arterial pressure via a single finger cuff without pain using photoplethysmographic technology. If ClearSight System™ can replace intra-arterial pressure measurement, blood pressure could be easily and noninvasively assessed. However, the validity of ClearSight System™ during induction of anesthesia in patients undergoing cardiovascular surgery has not been evaluated. The aim of this study was to compare blood pressure measured by ClearSight System™ with intra-arterial pressure during induction of anesthesia for cardiovascular surgery.

Methods: This study was registered retrospectively. Data during induction of anesthesia for elective cardiovascular surgery were obtained for patients in whom noninvasive arterial pressure was measured by ClearSight System™ (APcs) and invasive radial arterial pressure (APrad) was measured simultaneously. According to the widely used criteria formulated by international standards from the Association for the Advancement of Medical Instrumentation, the acceptable bias and precision for arterial pressure measurements were fixed at < 5 mmHg and 8 mmHg, respectively.

Results: Data for 18 patients were analyzed. For 3068 analyzed paired measurements, values of APcs vs APrad bias (precision) were 13.2 (17.5), – 9.1 (7.3) and – 3.9 (7.8) mmHg for systolic, diastolic, and mean arterial pressures, respectively.

Conclusions: Mean arterial pressure measured by ClearSight System™ could be considered as an alternative for mean radial arterial pressure during induction of anesthesia for elective cardiovascular surgery.

Keywords: Cardiovascular surgery, Non-invasive arterial pressure, Monitoring

* Correspondence: ttanioku@wakayama-med.ac.jp
Department of Anesthesiology, Wakayama Medical University School of Medicine, Kimiidera 811-1, Wakayama 641-8509, Japan

Background

Since blood pressure tends to be unstable during induction of anesthesia in patients undergoing cardiovascular surgery, an artery catheter is often inserted before induction to continuously monitor arterial pressure during induction of anesthesia. The success rate of the first attempt at arterial cannulation using palpation has been reported to be less than 50% and sometimes cannulation still fails despite the use of ultrasound [1]. Therefore, arterial cannulation in an awake condition may cause suffering for patients.

ClearSight System™ (previously named ccNexfin system™, Edwards Lifesciences Corp, Irvine CA, USA) enables noninvasive continuous measurement of beat-to-beat arterial pressure via a single finger cuff without pain using photoplethysmographic technology. If ClearSight System™ can replace intra-arterial pressure measurement, blood pressure could be continuously, easily, and noninvasively assessed. Previous studies have shown that this device is reliable in pregnant women [2], children [3], and patients undergoing upper abdominal surgery [4]. On the other hand, it has been reported that it is not reliable in critically ill patients [5] and patients undergoing neurosurgery in a sitting position [6]. Accordingly, the validity of ClearSight System™ may depend on the clinical situation including the type of surgery or the patient's condition. However, the validity of ClearSight System™ during induction of anesthesia in patients undergoing cardiovascular surgery has not been evaluated. The aim of this study was to compare blood pressure measured by ClearSight System™ with intra-arterial pressure during induction of anesthesia for cardiovascular surgery.

Methods

Study design and setting

This retrospective observational study was approved by the medical ethics committee of Wakayama Medical University prior to its initiation (reference number 1919). The study was conducted at Wakayama Medical University Hospital.

Data collection

In this retrospective analysis, data were collected from all patients in whom noninvasive arterial pressure was measured by ClearSight System™ (APcs) and invasive radial arterial pressure (APrad) was measured simultaneously during induction of anesthesia for elective cardiovascular surgery between November 2016 and November 2017 at Wakayama Medical University Hospital. The use of ClearSight System™ depended on the anesthesiologists in charge. Paired values of systolic, diastolic, and mean arterial pressures obtained by both methods were recorded at the rate of 1 sample every 3 s in the institution's Anesthesia Information Management System (PrimeGAIA™, Nihon Kohden Co, Tokyo, Japan). Data from 5 min before tracheal intubation to 5 min after tracheal intubation based on anesthetic records were analyzed.

In our hospital, the induction of cardiovascular anesthesia has been standardized. Two anesthesiologists are generally involved in one case: one anesthesiologist for managing the anesthesia, and other for recording. Before induction of anesthesia, an catheter is inserted into right radial artery in the most of patients to continuously measure blood pressure. Then anesthesia is induced by target-controlled infusion of propofol (1.5–3.0 μg/ml), remifentanil (0.1–0.3 μg/kg/min), and rocuronium (0.6–1.0 mg/kg). The doses of anesthetics depend on the decision of the anesthesiologist in charge. When blood pressure decreases during the induction, ephedrine (4 mg or 8 mg) or phenylephrine (0.1 mg or 0.2 mg) is intravenously administered according to the decision of the anesthesiologist in charge.

Statistical analysis

There is no established knowledge of how many patients should be included and how many measurements should be analyzed for each when performing a repeated measurement. In most of the studies using Bland-Altman analysis, the sample size was not examined. In this study, we collected over 3000 pairs of data based on similar previous studies in which radial arterial pressure was compared with blood pressure measured by ClearSight System™ [7, 8].

Data considered to be artifacts were excluded based on ClearSight auto-calibration, radial artery artifacts, and ClearSight artifacts. Auto-calibration is performed at least once every 70 heartbeats to keep the finger arteries open and of constant diameter. In addition, auto-calibration is performed when the measurement of blood pressure is temporarily interrupted for two or more beats. When auto-calibration is performed, systolic, diastolic and mean blood pressures become the same values, and the values increase step by step. Therefore, it is possible to discriminate such data as artifacts. Radial artery artifacts, which result from blood sampling and flushing, could be discriminated since systolic and diastolic pressures become the same values. ClearSight artifacts, which occur due to external pressure to the ClearSight cuff, can be recognized as extreme outliers.

Data are expressed as means (SD) or medians (interquartile range) as appropriate. For whole repeated paired measurements from all patients, correlations between

APrad and APcs were determined by a linear regression. In addition, Bland-Altman analysis was used to study agreement between APrad and APcs. In this analysis, bias and precision were defined as the mean difference between APrad and APcs and as the SD of bias, respectively. In addition, limits of agreement (LOA) were calculated as bias ±2SD of bias. According to the widely used criteria formulated by international standards from the Association for the Advancement of Medical Instrumentation (AAMI), the acceptable bias and precision for arterial pressure measurements were fixed at < 5 mmHg and 8 mmHg, respectively [9].

For each patient, the SDs of averages of APrad and APcs ("within-subject variability") were calculated to quantify the ranges of different pressures. The SDs of differences between APrad and APcs ("within-subject precision") were also calculated to quantify tracking for systolic arterial pressure (SAP), diastolic arterial pressure (DAP), and mean arterial pressure (MAP). In addition, correlations between APrad and APcs were determined by linear regression.

A two-sided *P*-value of 0.05 was considered statistically significant. All analyses were performed using JMP® statistical software (version 12.2; SAS Institute, Cary NC, USA).

Results

Data for 18 patients were obtained in this study. The characteristics of the patients are shown in Table 1. Given the retrospective nature of this study, all perioperative management was at the direction of the attending clinicians. In all patients, a 22-guage catheter was used for monitoring radial arterial pressure. Both APrad and APcs were measured on the right side in all patients, and noninvasive blood pressure measurement by a cuff was performed on the left arm. Although we obtained 3600 pairs of APcs and APrad, 532 pairs among them were excluded. Of the 532 measurements excluded, 297 measurements were excluded due to ClearSight auto-calibration. In addition, 115 measurements were excluded due to radial artery artifacts, and 120 measurements were excluded due to ClearSight artifacts. The percentage of exclusion data in our data (14.7%) was similar to the percentages in previous prospective studies [7, 8]. Thus, a total of 3068 valid pairs of simultaneous APcs and APrad measurements were analyzed. The median number of paired measurements per patient was 170 (170–200). The ranges of APrad measured during the observational period were 53–225 mmHg for SAP, 27–114 mmHg for DAP, and 41–144 mmHg for MAP. Continuous administration of phenylephrine was started from the beginning of anesthetic induction in 9 of the 18 patients.

Table 1 Baseline characteristics of the subjects

Age (yr)	70 (64–79)
Sex (M/F)	11/7
BMI (kg m^{-2})	24 (21.9–24.9)
Type of surgery (%)	
Coronary artery bypass grafting	11
Aortic valve replacement for aortic valve stenosis	7
Aortic valve replacement for aortic regurgitation	2
Thoracic ascending aortic graft replacement	1
Comorbidities (%)	
Hypertension	18
Diabetes mellitus	9
Renal insufficiency	10
Dialysis	2

N = 18. Values are medians (interquartile range) or numbers
BMI Body mass index

Figure 1 shows individual scatter plots for SAP, DAP, and MAP. Correlation coefficients, within-subject variability, and within-subject precision are summarized in Table 2. Mean differences of pressure in paired data were 13.1 ± 15.5, − 8.5 ± 6.1, and − 3.4 ± 6.2 mmHg for SAP, DAP, and MAP, respectively. Figure 2 shows the correlations between APcs and APrad. APcs for SAP, DAP and MAP were significantly correlated with APrad. The correlation coefficients between APcs and APrad for SAP, DAP, and MAP were 0.85, 0.85 and 0.92, respectively. The results of Bland-Altman analysis between APcs and APrad are shown in Fig. 3. Bias and precision were 13.2 and 17.5 mmHg in SAP, − 9.1 and 7.3 mmHg in DAP, and − 3.9 mmHg 7.8 mmHg in MAP. Upper and lower LOAs were 47.4 and − 21.1 mmHg in SAP, 5.2 and − 23.4 mmHg in DAP, and 11.4 and − 19.2 mmHg in MAP. Accordingly, only MAP fulfilled the criteria of AAMI.

Discussion

In this study, Pearson's correlation coefficients showed that SAP, DAP and MAP measured by ClearSight System™ were significantly correlated with radial arterial pressure. Bland-Altman analysis showed that ClearSight System™ had acceptable bias and precision in MAP but not in SAP and DAP for radial arterial pressure measurements. Our results suggest that changes in SAP, DAP and MAP measured by ClearSight System™ reflect those in radial arterial pressure and that MAP measured by ClearSight System™ is interchangeable with radial arterial pressure during induction of anesthesia for elective cardiovascular surgery.

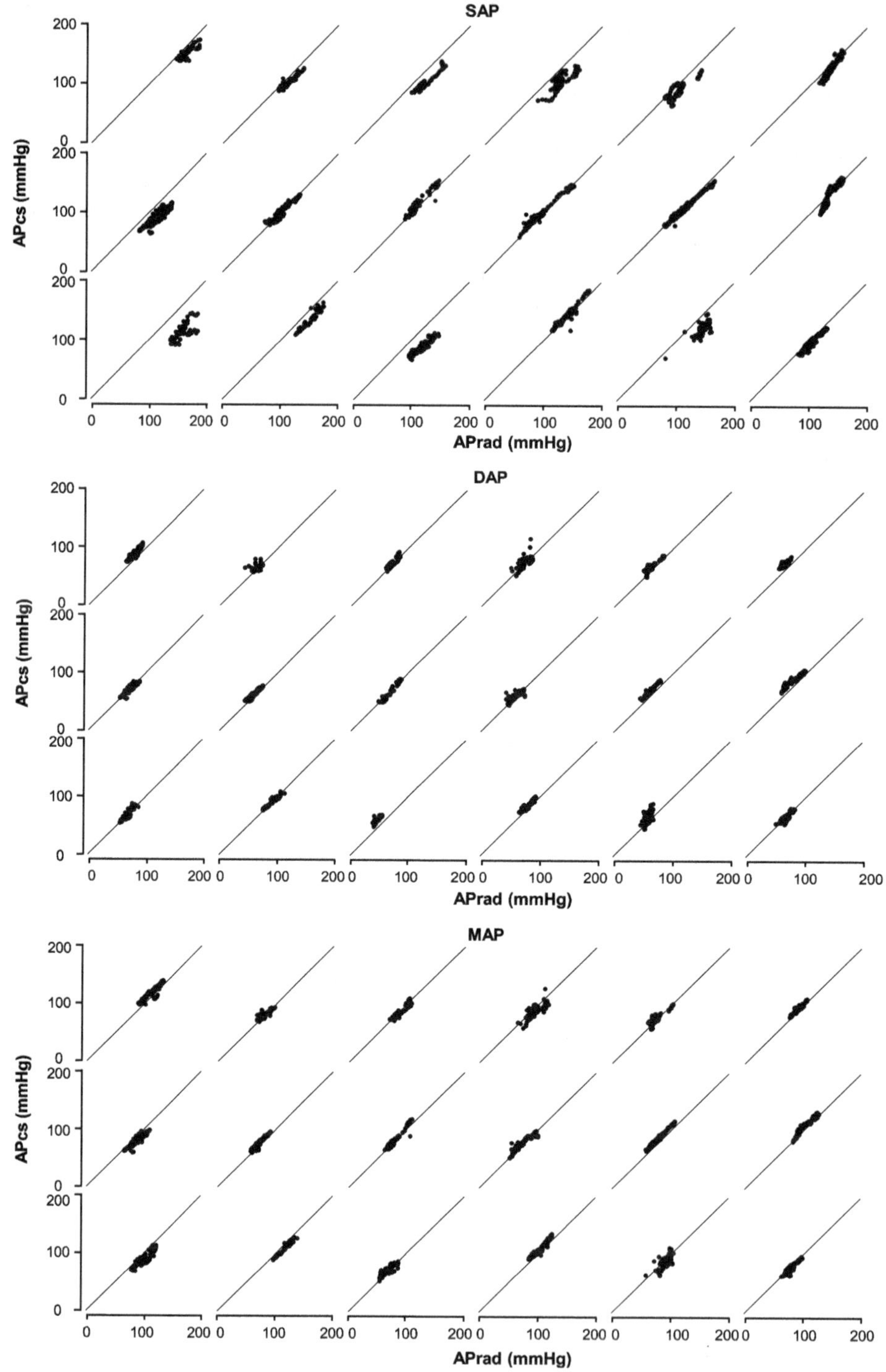

Fig. 1 Individual scatterplots of (**a**) invasive and noninvasive systolic arterial pressure, (**b**) invasive and noninvasive diastolic arterial pressure, and (**c**) invasive and noninvasive mean arterial pressure. SAP, systolic arterial pressure; DAP, diastolic arterial pressure; MAP, mean arterial pressure; APrad, invasive radial arterial pressure; APcs, noninvasive arterial pressure measured by ClearSight System™

Our study showed that MAP measured by ClearSight System™ statistically matched the AAMI criteria. On the other hand, neither SAP nor DAP matched the criteria. A previous study also showed that MAP, but not SAP and DAP, could be considered as an alternative for radial artery blood pressure during carotid endarterectomy, based on AAMI criteria [8]. In general, the arterial pressure waveform

Table 2 Within-subject data averaged over the group

	r, Median (25-75%)	Within-subject Variability	Within-subject Precision
SAP (mmHg)	0.95 (0.89–0.96)	17.3 (4.7)	7.0 (2.6)
DAP (mmHg)	0.91 (0.86–0.95)	8.6 (2.3)	4.1 (1.4)
MAP (mmHg)	0.95 (0.91–0.96)	12.1 (2.7)	4.6 (1.4)

Data are presented as medians (25th-75th percentiles) for correlations and as means (SD) for within-subject variability and within-subject precision in 18 subjects.
r, coefficient of correlation
SAP Systolic arterial pressure, *DAP* Diastolic arterial pressure, *MAP* Mean arterial pressure

changes gradually from the brachial artery to the finger arteries [10]. Accordingly, SAP at a distal site to the heart is higher than that at a proximal site, while DAP at a distal site is lower than that at a proximal site. ClearSight System™ reconstructs brachial artery pressure from finger artery pressure for calculating blood pressure [10]. Therefore, there might be a significant difference between SAP/DAP measured by ClearSight System™ and radial artery pressure. On the other hand, as blood flows from the aorta to the radial artery, mean pressure decreases only slightly because there is little resistance to flow in the major conducting arteries [11]. In our study, the mean difference in MAP between APcs and APrad was − 3.4 ± 6.2 mmHg, which was small compared to the differences in SAP and DAP (13.1 ± 15.5 and − 8.5 ± 6.1 mmHg, respectively).

The aim of managing hemodynamics is to maintain adequate organ perfusion. MAP is widely used as an index for optimal blood pressure, and it reflects driving pressure at the organ level [12]. MAP is the value that has most often been used for assessing autoregulation of renal blood flow [13] and cerebral blood flow [14]. Measurement of MAP by ClearSight System™ would be useful for maintaining organ perfusion during induction of anesthesia for cardiovascular surgery. During induction of anesthesia for patients with coronary artery disease, maintain of DAP is also important. Our results showed that diastolic pressure measured by ClearSight System™ is not interchangeable with radial diastolic pressure but correlates well with it. Therefore, we can pay attention to coronary perfusion by assessing the change in diastolic pressure but not absolute values measured by ClearSight System™.

The limitation of this study would result from a retrospective nature. The quality of data in a prospective study are generally higher than that in a retrospective study. When APcs is compared to APrad, the advantage of a prospective study is that study conditions including patient's bias, data collection period, and exclusion of data influenced by artifacts can be controlled. In this study, we decided to analyzed preserved data for the following reasons. First, when we reviewed our preserved data from 18 patients before data analysis, the characteristics of patients were similar to those in previous prospective studies. The exclusion criteria in previous studies

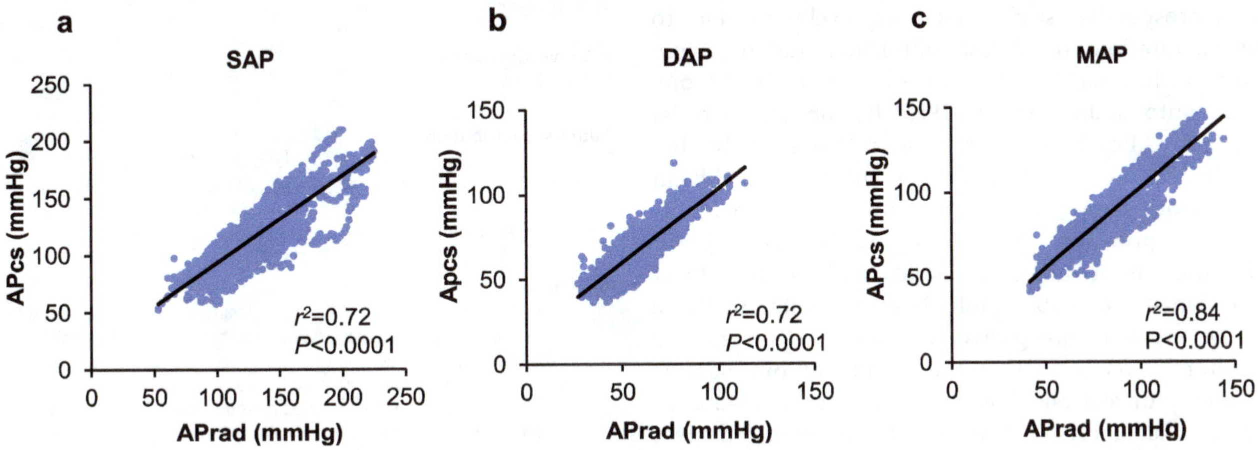

Fig. 2 Relationships between absolute values of (**a**) invasive and noninvasive systolic arterial pressure (3084 paired data points), (**b**) invasive and noninvasive diastolic arterial pressure (3084 paired data points), and (**c**) invasive and noninvasive mean arterial pressure (3084 paired data points). r2, coefficient of determination; SAP, systolic arterial pressure; DAP, diastolic arterial pressure; MAP, mean arterial pressure; APrad, invasive radial arterial pressure; APcs, noninvasive arterial pressure measured by ClearSight System™

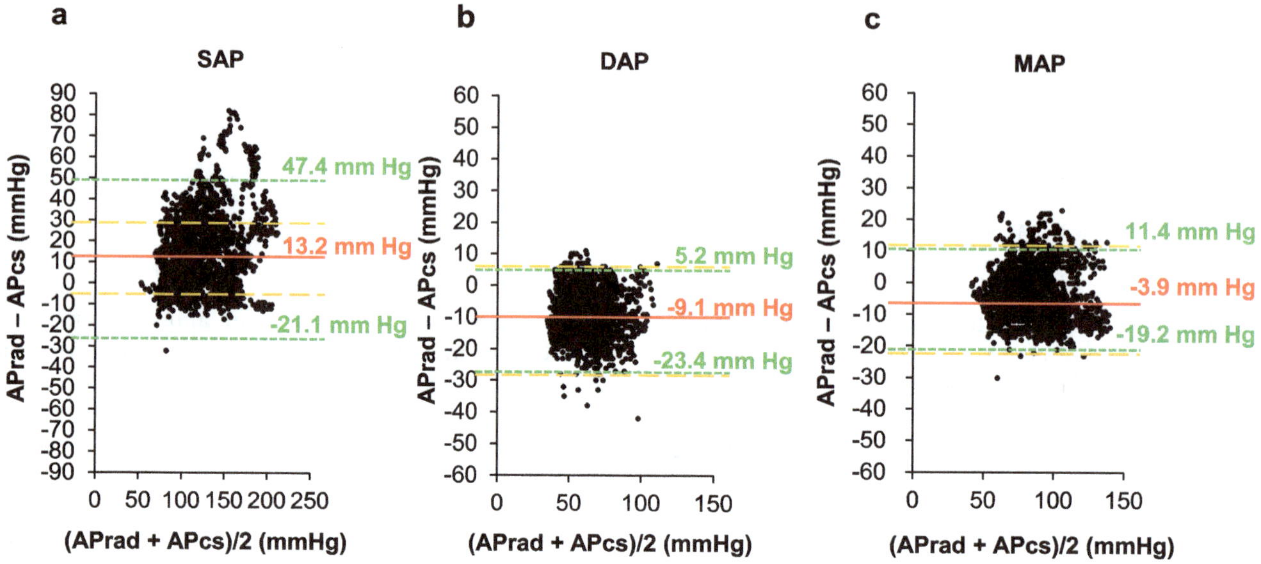

Fig. 3 Bland-Altman graphical representation of agreement for individual values of (**a**) systolic arterial pressure between invasive and noninvasive measurements, (**b**) diastolic arterial pressure between invasive and noninvasive measurements, and (**c**) mean arterial pressure between invasive and noninvasive measurements. The red continuous line represents the bias and dotted green lines represent the upper and lower LOA, respectively. Dashed orange lines represent LOA recommended by AAMI for validation of NIAP devices. SAP, systolic arterial pressure; DAP, diastolic arterial pressure; MAP, mean arterial pressure; APrad, invasive radial arterial pressure; APcs, noninvasive arterial pressure measured by ClearSight System™

included peripheral arterial disease, preoperative atrial fibrillation, and obesity (> BMI 30) [4, 7, 15, 16], and such patients were also not included in our study. Second, when data are collected from the anesthetic record, the time to intubate may not be accurate. In our hospital, two anesthesiologists are generally involved in one case: one anesthesiologist for managing the anesthesia, and other for recording. Therefore, we considered the time of events and data collection period (from 5 min before intubation to 5 min after intubation) would be accurate. Third, in a prospective study, data are excluded due to auto-calibration of APcs, unreliable radial artery wave, flushing arterial line, or APcs artifacts. Among them, auto-calibration of APcs, flushing an arterial line and APcs artifacts can be retrospectively discriminated. Accordingly, the percentage of exclusion data in our data (14.7%) was similar to the percentages in previous prospective studies [7, 8]. In addition, within-subject variability and within-subject precision in our data (Table 2) were similar to those in the previous prospective studies [8, 17], and we therefore considered that the quality of our data is adequate for analysis. For the above reasons, we considered that analysis of preserved data would be less inferior to analysis of prospective data when APcs is compared to APrad. However, a prospective study will be needed to obtain a more precise evaluation of ClearSight System™.

Conclusions

MAP measured by ClearSight System™ could be considered as an alternative for mean radial arterial pressure during induction of anesthesia for elective cardiovascular surgery. SAP and DAP may be useful for inferring changes in systolic and diastolic radial arterial pressures.

Abbreviations

APcs: Noninvasive arterial pressure measured by ClearSight System™; APrad: Invasive radial arterial pressure; LOA: Limits of agreement; SAP: Systolic arterial pressure; DAP: Diastolic arterial pressure; MAP: Mean arterial pressure; AAMI: Association for the Advancement of Medical Instrumentation

Acknowledgements

Not applicable.

Authors' contributions

TT: data collection, data analysis, study design; YA: data collection, drafting of the manuscript; AY: data collection, drafting of the manuscript; FK: data collection, drafting of the manuscript; KT: study design, drafting of the manuscript. All authors have read and approval the manuscript.

References

1. Shiloh AL, Savel RH, Paulin LM, Eisen LA. Ultrasound-guided catheterization of the radial artery: a systematic review and meta-analysis of randomized controlled trials. Chest. 2011;139:524–9.
2. Akkermans J, Diepeveen M, Ganzevoort W, van Montfans GA, Westerhof BE, Wolf H. Continuous non-invasive blood pressure monitoring, a validation study of Nexfin in a pregnant population. Hypertens Pregnancy. 2009;28:230–42.
3. Garnier RP, van der Spoel AG, Sibarani-Ponsen R, Markhorst DG, Boer C. Level of agreement between Nexfin non-invasive arterial pressure with invasive arterial pressure measurements in children. Br J Anaesth. 2012;109: 609–15.
4. de Wilde RB, de Wit F, Geerts BF, van Vliet AL, Aarts LP, Vuyk J, Jansen JR. Non-invasive continuous arterial pressure and pulse pressure variation

measured with Nexfin® in patients following major upper abdominal surgery: a comparative study. Anaethesia. 2016;71:788–97.

5. Ameloot K, Van De Vijver K, Van Regenmortel N, De Laet I, Schoonheydt K, Dits H, Broch O, Bein B, Malbrain ML. Validation study of Nexfin® continuous non-invasive blood pressure monitoring in critically ill adult patients. Minerva Anestesiol. 2014;80:1294–301.
6. Schramm P, Tzanova I, Gööck T, Hagen F, Schmidtmann I, Engelhard K, Pestel G. Noninvasive hemodynamic measurements during neurosurgical procedures in sitting position. J Neurosurg Anesthesiol. 2017;29:251–7.
7. Weiss E, Gayat E, Dumans-Nizard V, Le Guen M, Fischler M. Use of the Nexfin™ device to detect acute arterial pressure variations during anaesthesia induction. Brit J Anaesth. 2014;113:52–60.
8. Heusdens JF, Lof S, Pennekamp CW, Specken-Welleweerd JC, de Borst GJ, van Klei WA, van Wolfswinkel L, Immink RV. Validation of non-invasive arterial pressure monitoring during carotid endarterectomy. Br J Anaesth. 2016;117:316–23.
9. Vos JJ, Poterman M, Mooyaart EAQ, Weening M, Struys MMRF, Scheeren TWL, Kalmar AF. Comparison of continuous non-invasive finger arterial pressure monitoring with conventional intermittent automated arm arterial pressure measurement in patients under general anaesthesia. Br J Anaesth. 2014;113:67–74.
10. Gizdulich P, Prentza A, Wesseling KH. Models of brachial to finger pulse wave distortion and pressure decrement. Cardiovasc Res. 1997;33:698–705.
11. Schroeder B, Barbeito A, Bar-Yosef S, Mark JB. Cardiovascular monitoring. In: Miller RD, editor. Miller's anesthesia eighth edition. Philadelphia: WB Saunders; 2015. p. 1356.
12. Leone M, Asfar P, Radermacher P, Vincent JL, Martin C. Optimizing mean arterial pressure in septic shock: a critical reappraisal of the literature. Crit Care. 2015;101:1–7.
13. Bersten AD, Holt AW. Vasoactive drugs and the importance of renal perfusion pressure. New Horiz. 1995;3:650–61.
14. Strandgaard S. Autoregulation of cerebral blood flow in hypertensive patients. The modifying influence of prolonged antihypertensive treatment on the tolerance to acute, drug-induced hypotension. Circulation. 1976;53:720–7.
15. Rogge DE, Nicklas JY, Schon G, Grothe O, Haas SA, Reuter DA, Saugel B. Continuous noninvasive arterial pressure monitoring in obese patients during bariatric surgery: an evaluation of the vascular unloading technique. Anesth Analg. 2019;128:477–83.
16. Blazer F, Habicher M, Sander M, Sterr J, Scholz S, Feldheiser A, Muller M, Perka C, Treskatsch S. Comparison of the non-invasive Nexfin® monitor with conventional methods for the measurement of arterial blood pressure in moderate risk orthopaedic surgery patients. J Int Med Res. 2016;44:832–43.
17. Martina JR, Westerhof BE, van Goudoever J, de Beaumont EMFH, Truijen J, Kim YS, Immink RV, Jobsis DA, Hollmann MW, Lahpor JR, de Mol BAJM, van Lieshout JJ. Noninvasive continuous arterial blood pressure monitoring with Nexfin®. Anesthesiology. 2012;116:1092–103.

7

Induction techniques that reduce redistribution hypothermia: a prospective, randomized, controlled, single blind effectiveness study

Jonathan V. Roth[1,2,3*], Leonard E. Braitman[4] and Lacy H. Hunt[4]

Abstract

Background: While much effort has been devoted to correcting intraoperative hypothermia, less attention has been directed to preventing redistribution hypothermia. In this study, we compared three different anesthetic induction techniques to standard IV propofol inductions (control) in their effect on reducing redistribution hypothermia.

Methods: Elective, afebrile patients, age 18 to 55 years, were randomly assigned to one of four groups ($n = 50$ each). Group "INH/100" was induced with 8% sevoflurane in 100% oxygen, Group "INH/50" with 8% sevoflurane in 50% oxygen and 50% nitrous oxide, Group "PROP" with 2.2 mg/kg propofol, and Group "Phnl/PROP" with 2.2 mg/kg propofol immediately preceded by 160 mcg phenylephrine. Patients were maintained with sevoflurane in 50% nitrous oxide and 50% oxygen in addition to opioid narcotic. Forced air warming was used. Core temperatures were recorded every 15 min after induction for 1 h.

Results: Compared to control group PROP, the mean temperatures in groups INH/100, INH/50, and Phnl/PROP were higher 15, 30, 45 and 60 min after induction ($p < 0.001$ for all comparisons), averaging between 0.39 °C and 0.54 °C higher. In group PROP, 60% of patients had at least one temperature below 36.0 °C in the first hour whereas only 16% did in each of groups INH/100, INH/50, and Phnl/PROP ($p < 0.0001$ in each group compared to PROP).

Conclusions: In this effectiveness trial, inhalation inductions with sevoflurane or with prophylactic phenylephrine bolus prior to propofol induction reduced the magnitude of redistribution hypothermia by an average of 0.4 to 0.5 °C in patients aged 18 to 55 years.

Keywords: Hypothermia, Redistribution hypothermia, Intraoperative hypothermia, Perioperative hypothermia, Postoperative hypothermia, Anesthesia induction, Inhalation induction, Intravenous induction, Inhalation anesthesia induction, Intravenous anesthesia induction

* Correspondence: jvroth1@aol.com
[1]Department of Anesthesiology, Albert Einstein Medical Center, 5501 Old York Road, Philadelphia, PA, USA
[2]Albert Einstein Healthcare Network, Philadelphia, PA, USA

Prior presentations

1) Roth JV, Braitman LE: Induction techniques that can reduce redistribution hypothermia. Abstract presented at the American Society of Anesthesiologists Annual Meeting, October 23, 2016.
2) Roth JV, Braitman LE, Hunt LH: Induction techniques that can reduce redistribution hypothermia. Abstract presented at the International Anesthesia Research Society Annual Meeting, #1135, May 2017.

The Pennsylvania Society of Anesthesiologists has published a non-peer reviewed summary letter of this work in their newsletter based upon data from the abstract submissions. There is a very small amount of text recycling.

What we already know about this topic

Propofol causes significant redistribution hypothermia, and intraoperative hypothermia is common in the first hour of anesthesia.

What this article tells us that is new

Either inhalation inductions with sevoflurane or the administration of phenylephrine immediately prior to intravenous induction with propofol can reduce the degree of redistribution hypothermia by an average of 0.4 to 0.5 °C during the first hour of anesthesia. The degree and duration of intraoperative hypothermia can be reduced by using these alternative induction techniques.

Background

Hypothermia has multiple adverse consequences and should be avoided [1, 2]. Anesthesia induction with propofol is known to cause a rapid and clinically important temperature decrease due to redistribution hypothermia, typically by about 1.5 °C [3]. Ikeda et al. showed there is on average 0.7 °C less redistribution hypothermia when patients are induced with an inhalation induction rather than with intravenous propofol [3]. However, the use of inhalation inductions has not been widely adapted. Sun et al. documented that hypothermia is routine during the first hour of anesthesia [4]. While there is great effort expended to warm patients intraoperatively, relatively little attention has been directed to preventing redistribution hypothermia.

In studies assessing whether patients were hypothermic, two methods have been used. First, the "end of case" temperature has been used to assess hypothermia and its association with complications [5]. In the United States, the SCIP (Surgical Care Improvement Project) guideline for body temperature management uses end of case temperature as its measure of compliance [5]. However, this method has limitations in assessing intraoperative hypothermia. Some hypothermia complications occur intra-operatively (e.g., coagulopathy, increased transfusion requirements), some post-operatively (e.g., shivering, delayed emergence) and some likely both (e.g., infection risk) [4, 6, 7]. End of case hypothermia indicates intraoperative hypothermia. End of case normothermia does not imply intraoperative normothermia. A patient may have been hypothermic intraoperatively, having suffered the consequences of intraoperative hypothermia, achieving normothermia only at the end of the case. Thus, the contribution of intraoperative hypothermia to postoperative complications may be unrecognized.

Because of the limitations of using end of case temperature as an indication of intraoperative hypothermia, more current literature focuses on the area under the core temperature vs time curve. The magnitude of the area under the time vs core temperature curve below a threshold, typically 36.0 °C, is used as an indicator of the degree of hypothermia. The greater the area under 36.0 °C, the greater the amount of intraoperative hypothermia. It is plausible that if redistribution hypothermia can be reduced, there will be less intraoperative hypothermia (assessed by less area under the curve) and thus fewer intraoperative and postoperative complications associated with hypothermia.

Vasodilation causes redistribution hypothermia by increasing blood flow to the cooler peripheral and dermal thermal compartments. This results in heat transfer away from the warmer core. We hypothesized that anesthetic inductions causing less vasodilation (than propofol alone inductions) will result in less redistribution hypothermia. The purpose of this effectiveness study is to compare the effect of three such alternative induction techniques to standard propofol inductions on core temperature during the first hour of anesthesia.

Methods

This study and consent forms were approved by our IRB (Albert Einstein Healthcare Network IRB #1) and submitted to clinical-trials.gov as NCT02331108 by Jonathan V. Roth on November 20, 2014. Written informed consent was obtained by the first author from all participating patients. (The consents were all dated and timed and signed by the patient and the first author. A copy of the consent was provided to the patient. The original signed consent was maintained in the research file.) The manuscript complies with the CONSORT requirements. This study was performed at the Albert Einstein Healthcare Network in Philadelphia, Pennsylvania during 2014 and 2015.

Four groups (described below and summarized in Table 3 in Appendix 1) of 50 patients each were studied. The major inclusion criteria were: age 18 to 55 years inclusive; supine or lithotomy positioning; scheduled for general anesthesia where 50% nitrous oxide would be used; endotracheal intubation or laryngeal mask airway insertion would be used; afebrile (preoperative oral or temporal scan temperature between 36.2 and 37.4 °C inclusive); forced air warming would be used; and expected duration of anesthetic to be at least 60 min. A complete list of inclusion and exclusion criteria are presented in Table 4 in Appendix 2. After enrollment, random assignments were contained in opaque envelopes that were opened immediately before induction of anesthesia. Each of the envelopes contained one of the four group designations, 50 envelopes for each group. Randomization was achieved by putting the envelopes in a basket and mechanically mixing the envelopes within the basket. When a patient was entered into the study, an opaque envelope was selected arbitrarily from any location in the stack.

For all patients, operating rooms were kept between 21 °C and 24 °C with a target of 22 °C. No patients were prewarmed. Upon entering the operating room, cotton blankets were placed on all patients covering their lower extremities, abdomen, and thorax. These blankets were removed after induction to allow for forced air warming (FAW) blanket placement and surgical positioning, preparation, and draping. All operating rooms had the same air flow design. Patients were administered 2 mg IV midazolam prior to entering the operating room. No opioid narcotics were administered until after the airway was secured with either a laryngeal mask airway (LMA) or endotracheal tube. Heat and moisture exchangers were used on all patients. Patients could receive up to 300 mL room temperature intravenous crystalloid before fluid was warmed (Ranger, Arizant Healthcare, Eden Prairie, MN) to 41 °C. All inductions, nasal temperature probe placement, and application of a FAW blanket were performed in the same manner by the first author. (Nasal temperature was used as a surrogate for core temperature for all patients since it could be used for patients having either an LMA or endotracheal intubation [8].) Either an upper or lower body FAW blanket (SW-2010 Snuggle Warm Small Upper Body Convective Warming Blanket, or SW-2001 Snuggle Warm Adult Full Body Convective Warming Blanket, Level 1, Smiths Medical ASD, Rockland, MA) was used. The face was not directly covered by the FAW blanket in order to avoid the possibility that a collection of warm air could affect the nasal temperature measurements. Cotton blankets were placed on top of the warming blankets. The FAW (Equator Convective Warmer, Level 1, Smiths Medical ASD, Rockland, MA) was turned on to 44 °C as soon as the patient was prepped and draped; the time duration from the start of induction (T_0) until the time the FAW was turned on was recorded. Neurophysiologic monitors to measure "depth of anesthesia" were not used. Preinduction core temperatures were not measured. All doses of propofol were based on actual (not ideal) body weight.

Group INH/100 – inhalation induction with sevoflurane in 100% oxygen (O_2)

A baseline blood pressure was taken prior to induction. No formal preoxygenation regimen was performed. The patients were asked to breath for a few breaths via the face mask with 100% O_2 just to confirm reservoir bag movement and capnograph detection of carbon dioxide. At time T_0, with an unprimed circuit, the O_2 flow meter was set at 6 LPM and the sevoflurane vaporizer was turned on at 8%. Blood pressures were recorded every minute starting 1 min after T_0 (T_1) until airway intervention commenced. At the discretion of the first author, an LMA was inserted when the patient was assessed to be adequately deep, determined by masseter muscle relaxation, typically just 2 min after T_0 (T_2). Alternatively, if the patient was to be endotracheally intubated, muscle relaxant (vecuronium, rocuronium, or succinylcholine) was administered when the patient was assessed as being unconscious, typically at T_1. Positive pressure ventilation was performed as required until endotracheal intubation. If necessary, to avoid hypotension, the Sevoflurane concentration was decreased while waiting for adequate muscle relaxation. If the systolic blood pressure dropped below 85 mmHg prior to airway intervention, the patient would be treated immediately either with phenylephrine or airway intervention if ready. After securing either the LMA or endotracheal tube, anesthesia was maintained with sevoflurane in 50% nitrous oxide (1 LPM) and 50% O_2 (1 LPM). Opioid narcotics (fentanyl, hydromorphone, methadone), neuromuscular reversal agents (glycopyrrolate, neostigmine), dexamethasone, and ketamine were administered as per the discretion of the attending anesthesiologist.

A skin temperature probe (Skin Temperature Sensor, 400 Series, DeRoyal Industries, Inc., Lane Powell, TN) was modified by removing the skin adhesive portion, bending the probe 90° 8 cm from the tip (to assure insertion depth would be 8 cm), and straightening the probe from the bend to the tip. Previous work has shown a close agreement between the nasal technique used in this study and distal esophageal temperature measurements [8]. Within 10 min of T_0, the blunt tipped nasal temperature probe was inserted 8 cm into one naris [8–10]. This provided a minimum of 5 min for thermal equilibration of the temperature probe before the first measurement (T_{15}), 15 min after T_0. Either naris was used arbitrarily. Starting at T_{15}, nasal temperatures were recorded every 15 min (T_{15}, T_{30}, T_{45}, T_{60}). If the core temperature reached 37.5 °C, the FAW was turned off. The patient's data were included in the analysis if there were at least two temperature measurements (T_{15} and T_{30}). If the anesthetic ended before 30 min or if there was a protocol violation, that patient's data were not analyzed; a replacement envelope assigning another future patient to that group was generated and inserted randomly back into the envelope stack. All patients received 4 mg ondansetron within 15 min of emergence. Temperature data collection ceased at the initiation of IV acetaminophen administration or if there was any event that could have a substantial impact on patient temperature. All cystoscopy procedures were conducted with warmed bladder irrigation.

Group INH/50 - inhalation induction with sevoflurane in 50% nitrous oxide (N_2O) / 50% O_2

The protocol was identical to group INH/100 except that induction was performed with 3 LPM N_2O and 3 LPM O_2 (instead of 6 LPM O_2) with 8% sevoflurane.

Group PROP – intravenous induction with 2.2 mg/kg intravenous propofol

The induction differed from group INH/100 in the following manner. Two mL of 2% lidocaine (40 mg) were added to 20 mL of 1% propofol. After preoxygenation with 100% O_2 for a minimum of 2 min, 3 mL of 2% lidocaine (60 mg) was administered followed immediately by 2.2 mg/kg propofol (rounded to the nearest 5 mg) at T_0. If the patient was to receive an LMA, one blood pressure was taken at T_1 and then the LMA was inserted. If the patient was to be endotracheally intubated, muscle relaxant was administered immediately after propofol administration, blood pressures were measured every minute, and positive pressure ventilation with 100% O_2 was performed as required. After securing the airway, the protocol continued in the same manner as in Group INH/100.

Group Phnl/PROP – intravenous induction with 2.2 mg/kg intravenous propofol preceded by 160 mcg phenylephrine

The protocol differed from group PROP only in that 2 mL of 80 mcg/mL phenylephrine (160 mcg) was administered immediately after the administration of 3 mL 2% lidocaine but before the 2.2 mg/kg propofol.

Statistical methods

To address the lack of pre-test core temperature measurements, we used the post-test only, single blind randomized trial. This is a "true experimental design" [11]. The primary

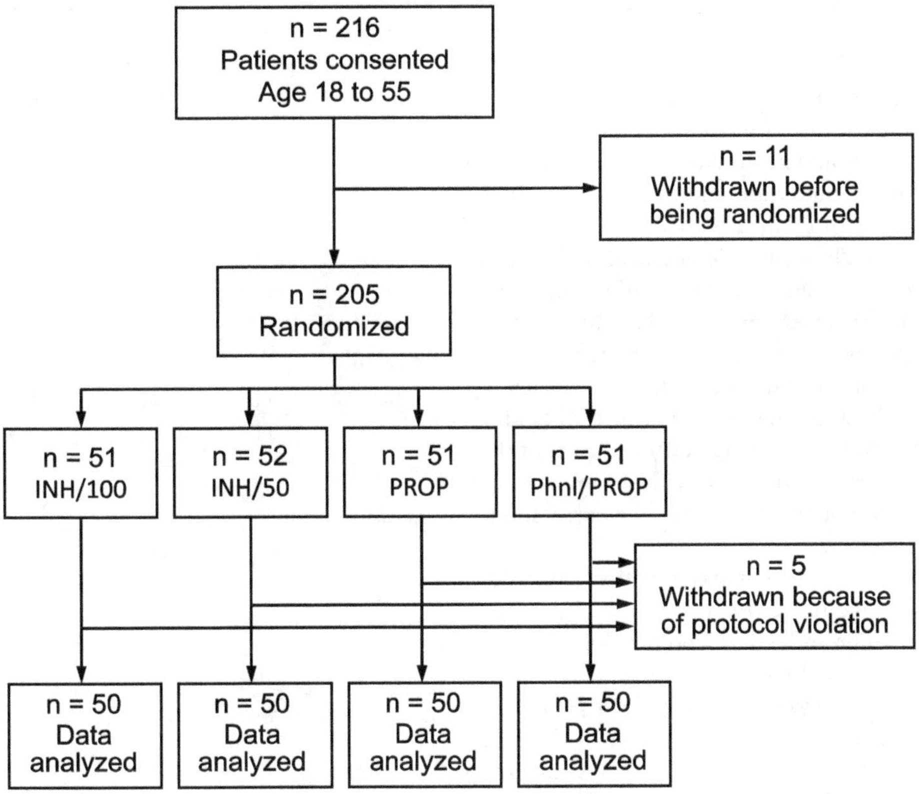

Fig. 1 Consort Diagram. Eleven patients consented but were never randomized and not studied: 9: The first author was not available to perform the induction. 1: The case changed from a general anesthetic to a sedation case. 1: The surgeon did not want that patient to be in a clinical study. Five patients were induced and then withdrawn from analysis* because of protocol violations: 1: Airway difficulty during induction. 1: Additional propofol required; 2: Patients received more than 300 mL unwarmed IV fluid. 1: Forced air warming malfunction. *Four patients were withdrawn before T_{15} so that they had no post-induction temperature measurements. In one patient, there was only one temperature measurement at T_{15}. This patient received more than 300 mL unwarmed IV fluid

outcomes were the nasal (core) temperatures at 4 time points after induction (not changes from pre-induction baseline). In bivariate analyses, we compared differences in mean core temperature between the propofol only induction control group (PROP) and each of 3 groups administered alternative induction techniques (INH/100, INH/50, and Phnl/PROP). Specifically, analyses of the mean temperature differences (and 95%CIs) for 1) INH/100 vs. PROP, 2) INH/50 vs. PROP, and 3) Phnl/PROP vs. PROP were performed at each of 15, 30, 45, and 60 min (T_{15}, T_{30}, T_{45}, and T_{60}) after induction. These differences in mean core temperatures at T_{15}, T_{30}, T_{45}, and T_{60} among groups were assessed using unpaired t-tests and corresponding 95% confidence intervals (95% CIs). Bonferroni's correction was used to adjust for these 12 multiple comparisons. Core temperature data were tested for normality by the Shapiro-Wilk test.

The random assignment of 50 patients per group made it likely that the treatment groups would be balanced in both measured and unmeasured characteristics (including pre-induction core temperatures). However, imbalances did occur in BMI and sex. Those imbalances and the lack of pre-induction core temperature measurements necessitated a multivariable analysis comparing the average core temperatures at T_{15}, T_{30}, T_{45}, and T_{60}; the covariates were BMI, sex, age, ASA classification, and time to initiating FAW. (Upper vs lower FAW were not covariates because the rates of heat transfers are similar [12].) This multivariable analysis was a linear mixed model with random intercepts and random slopes and unstructured covariance. This model fit better than a model with random intercepts alone nested within it ($p < 0.0001$ by the likelihood ratio test) [13]. There was no statistically significant interaction between group and time ($p = 0.15$). Since the results of the bivariate and multivariable analyses were similar and led to the same conclusions, we present the simpler bivariate results. The differences in the secondary outcomes, the percentages of patients who had at least one temperature < 36.0 °C (and ≤ 35.5 °C) between the control group (PROP) and each of the other three groups were evaluated by Fisher's exact tests. Although the resulting p values were exact; the corresponding 95% CIs were approximate.

Interval estimates of the percentages of patients that developed hypotension requiring treatment and of patients undergoing an inhalation induction who developed apnea were computed using exact binomial 95% CIs.

In a statistical power analysis, assuming alpha = 0.05 and beta = 0.2, 17 patients per group were needed to detect a 0.5 °C difference between means of any two compared groups as statistically significant in a two tailed test. We enrolled patients who were expected to have a surgical procedure lasting at least 60 min after the induction of anesthesia. However, we had no way to estimate the percentage of cases that would end early and therefore not provide data at T45 and T60. We increased the size of the study groups to 50 in order to be reasonably sure there were at least 17 patients in all groups at T60.

All statistical analyses compared patients as treated using two-sided tests with alpha = 0.05 and were performed using Stata, version 14 (Stata Press, College Station, Texas).

Results

After randomization and withdrawals, 50 patients in each group were analyzed (Fig. 1). Demographic and forced air warming data are presented in Table 1. The surgical procedures are presented in Table 5 Appendix 3.

Compared to group PROP, the three alternative induction groups each had higher mean core temperatures and fewer patients having at least one core temperature measurement < 36.0 °C in the first hour. At all four time points (T_{15}, T_{30}, T_{45}, T_{60}), the mean temperatures in group PROP were between 0.39 and 0.54 °C lower than in groups INH/100, INH/50 and Phnl/PROP (all $p \leq 0.0042$ adjusted for multiple comparisons, Fig. 2,

Table 1 Demographics and forced air warming data of the 200 patients analyzed

Group	INH/100	INH/50	PROP	Phnl/PROP
Age (years)				
Mean (SD)	42.8 (10.1)	43.0 (8.6)	39.0 (11.2)	40.6 (9.1)
Range	22 to 55	26 to 55	18 to 55	20 to 55
Sex				
Male n(%)	20 (40)	31 (62)	20 (40)	21 (42)
ASA classification				
1 n (%)	1 (2)	3 (6)	10 (20)	2 (4)
2 n (%)	23 (46)	23 (46)	29 (58)	33 (66)
3 n (%)	16 (52)	24 (48)	11 (22)	15 (30)
BMI (kg/m^2)				
Mean (SD)	31.9 (7.5)	31.2 (6.7)	26.8 (5.6)	29.9 (6.4)
Range	21.7 to 48.9	18.9 to 44.2	17.2 to 43.0	15.1 to 44.4
Preoperative screening temperature (°C)				
Mean (SD)	36.8 (0.3)	36.8 (0.3)	36.8 (0.3)	36.7 (0.3)
Use of upper body forced air warming (FAW) blanket (remaining patients used lower body FAW)				
n	32	39	29	30
(%)	(64)	(78)	(58)	(60)
Time from T_0 until FAW turned on, (minutes)				
Mean (SD)	16.4 (7.0)	14.7 (7.0)	15.9 (7.9)	17.1 (7.7)
Range	5 to 45	4 to 45	4 to 44	6 to 40

Mean Temperature ± SD and Number (n) in Each Group at Each Time Point (°C)

	T15	T30	T45	T60
INH/100	36.42 ± 0.49 (50)	36.41 ± 0.49 (50)	36.47 ± 0.53 (37)	36.52 ± 0.56 (27)
INH/50	36.44 ± 0.44 (50)	36.48 ± 0.44 (50)	36.50 ± 0.45 (41)	36.57 ± 0.42 (28)
PROP	35.96 ± 0.40 (50)	35.95 ± 0.41 (50)	36.00 ± 0.45 (43)	36.03 ± 0.53 (32)
Phnl/PROP	36.35 ± 0.38 (50)	36.36 ± 0.40 (50)	36.45 ± 0.40 (45)	36.51 ± 0.40 (40)

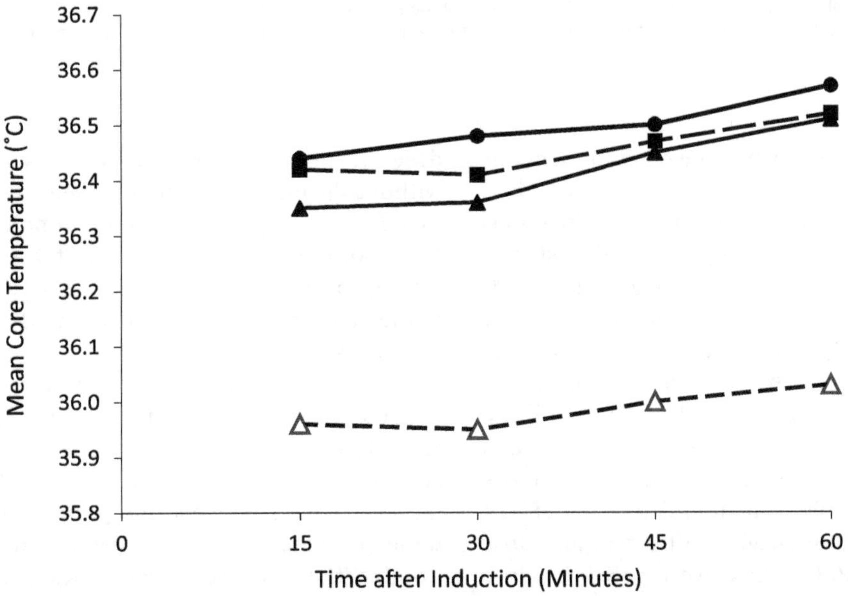

Fig. 2 Mean Temperature ± SD and Number (n) in Each Group at Each Time Point (°C). In the three successive time intervals (T_{15} to T_{30}, T_{30} to T_{45}, and T_{45} to T_{60}), the percentage of patients (all groups combined) whose temperature decreased were (37.5, 14.4, and 14.2% respectively). The percentage of patients whose temperature increased were (39.0, 55.4, and 59.1% respectively). The remaining patients had no temperature changes within these time intervals

Table 2). There were no statistically significant differences in the mean temperatures between groups INH/100 and INH/50, INH/100 and Phyl/PROP, and INH/50 and Phyl/PROP at any time point (all $p > 0.18$). In group PROP, 60% of patients had at least one temperature < 36.0 °C in the first hour compared to 16% in each of groups INH/100, INH/50, and Phnl/PROP (all with an identical 44 percentage point difference, 95% CI 27% to 61%, $p < 0.0001$). In group PROP, 22% of patients had at least one temperature ≤ 35.5 °C, compared to 8% in group INH/100 ($p = 0.09$), 4% in INH/50 ($p = 0.015$), and 2% in Phnl/PROP ($p = 0.004$).

No patient in any of these 4 groups had a core temperature > 37.5 °C at any time point. Apnea did not occur in either group INH/100 or INH/50 (0%, 95% CI 0% to 7.1% for each group).

Only blood pressures at T_1 (and T_2 if prior to airway intervention) were considered. In the first 2 min, treatment of hypotension (systolic BP < 85 mmHg) was required in 2 patients in Group PROP (4%, 95% CI 0.5% to 13.7%) and 1 patient in group Phnl/PROP (2%, 95% CI 0.05% to 10.6%). In group Phnl/PROP, only 1 patient's blood pressure increased to a value > 180 mmHg and no patient suffered a reflex bradycardia ≤40 beats per minute. No patients in groups INH/100 or INH/50 (0%, 95% CI 0% to 7.1% for each group) required treatment for hypotension.

Discussion

This effectiveness study found that in patients aged 18 to 55 years, inhalation inductions with sevoflurane or the administration of 160 mcg phenylephrine immediately prior to 2.2 mg/kg propofol each caused less

Table 2 Differences between the mean core temperature (°C) of each of three alternative induction groups and the standard propofol alone group at each time point*

Comparison groups	T_{15}	T_{30}	T_{45}	T_{60}
INH/100 minus PROP				
Difference (°C)	0.46	0.46	0.47	0.49
95% CI of difference	0.28 to 0.64	0.28 to 0.64	0.25 to 0.69	0.20 to 0.77
INH/50 minus PROP				
Difference (°C)	0.47**	0.52**	0.50	0.54
95% CI of difference	0.31 to 0.64	0.36 to 0.69	0.31 to 0.69	0.28 to 0.79
Phnl/PROP minus PROP				
Difference (°C)	0.39	0.41	0.45	0.47**
95% CI of difference	0.24 to 0.54	0.25 to 0.57	0.27 to 0.63	0.25 to 0.70

*Applying Bonferroni's correction for the 12 multiple comparisons (3 groups compared to propofol only group at 4 time points) results in $\alpha = 0.05/12 = 0.0042$. All 12 comparisons achieved statistical significance as $p \leq 0.001 < \alpha = 0.0042$ for each of the above comparisons

**These differences are correct to 2 decimal places. Because of rounding to two decimal places in Fig. 2, they differ by 0.01 from those that would be calculated using Fig. 2

redistribution hypothermia than intravenous inductions with propofol alone.

This study's results are consistent with previous work [3, 4] and thus provide support for this study's conclusion. Ikeda found a 0.7 °C average thermal advantage of sevoflurane inhalation inductions over intravenous propofol [3]. We found a slightly smaller (0.4 °C to 0.5°) advantage. That may reflect the use of forced air warming whereas Ikeda did not use FAW [3]. Also, Ikeda used a larger dose of propofol, which might have caused more vasodilation and thus more redistribution hypothermia. Sun found 64% of 58,814 patients had a temperature < 36 °C after 45 min, close to the 60% in group PROP; 29% were < 35.5 °C, close to the 22% in group PROP [4]. The small differences in results in these studies may in part reflect Sun's patients having a higher mean age than study group PROP and/or random variation. Older patients have an increased risk for hypothermia [9, 14, 15].

Without patient warming, temperature decreases can continue for 3 h [16]. With the prompt initiation of forced air warming, we found most of the redistribution hypothermia occurred in the first 15 min. Within each group, the differences in mean core temperature between T_{15} and T_{30}, T_{30} and T_{45}, and T_{45} and T_{60} were small and clinically insignificant (Fig. 2).

We found a bolus dose of phenylephrine reduced redistribution hypothermia. Ikeda et al. found intraoperative phenylephrine infusion decreased the magnitude of redistribution hypothermia [17]. Ikeda concluded that even a short period of vasodilation can result in redistribution hypothermia [3]. The phenylephrine bolus opposed enough of the propofol induced vasodilation to reduce the amount of redistribution hypothermia. We administered a prior bolus dose of phenylephrine (about 10 s before propofol) without an infusion. Whether phenylephrine would be as effective if given after the propofol is not known. First, some vasodilation and heat transfer might have already occurred, and second, it is unknown if there is the same resultant vasodilation when phenylephrine is given after propofol.

Techniques that can reduce redistribution hypothermia now include prewarming [18–22], ketamine [23], etomidate [24], phenylephrine infusions [17], amino acid infusions [25], fructose [26], inhalation inductions [3], and bolus phenylephrine prior to propofol. None of these techniques solve the hypothermia problem fully. Combinations of these techniques may result in additional thermal benefit but have not been studied.

Inhalation inductions were performed gradually (i.e., without a primed circuit) for two reasons. First, apnea is unlikely to occur. Apnea never occurred in the 100 inhalation patients. Second, gradually increasing anesthetic depth likely contributes to hemodynamic stability, a potential benefit of inhalation inductions. Thwaites concluded that inhalation inductions were more hemodynamically stable than IV propofol inductions [27]. Retrospective studies found that adverse outcomes were associated with even short periods of hypotension, but not hypertension [28, 29]. Maheshwari et al. recently found that a substantial fraction of all hypotension occurred before surgical incision as a result of anesthetic management; this hypotension was associated with postoperative kidney injury [30]. We observed no hypotension (systolic BP < 85 mmHg) in any inhalation induction patient. Hypotension can occur rapidly with intravenous propofol inductions. Decreases in blood pressure with inhalation inductions are usually more gradual. Such gradual decreases could be addressed earlier, or prophylactically, before there is clinically important hypotension.

We found 160 mcg phenylephrine to be an effective dose in most Phnl/PROP patients. Small percentages of Phnl/PROP patients had a post-induction systolic blood pressure either < 85 mmHg or > 180 mmHg. An optimal phenylephrine dose (e.g., weight based) would minimize hypotensive and hypertensive events and still maintain the thermal benefit. We studied only one dose of phenylephrine.

In the multivariable analysis, neither BMI nor sex was associated with the degree of redistribution hypothermia. This indicates that differences in BMI and sex between treatment groups were not responsible for the differences in mean core temperatures (redistribution hypothermia) between groups. We found patients were susceptible to redistribution hypothermia regardless of BMI. Because it takes more heat transfer to change the temperature of a heavier patient, it is commonly believed that obese patients are more resistant to temperature change. However, a different process is dominant during the initial redistribution hypothermia phase. Many obese patients have substantial muscle mass in their periphery to move their heavy body parts. The relatively little blood flow in adipose tissue may prevent meaningful temperature buffering during the redistribution hypothermia phase.

Limitations

We studied hypothermia during surgery, not surgical outcome. Since hypothermia causes adverse outcomes [1, 2], it is plausible that the studied alternative induction techniques will result in superior clinical outcomes than propofol by keeping patients warmer. It remains to conduct randomized controlled trials addressing all major aspects of anesthesia care (e.g., hemodynamics, post-operative nausea and vomiting) and whether clinical outcomes improve using any of the alternative induction techniques.

Although our results suggest a possible hemodynamic benefit of these alternative induction techniques, many more patients need to be studied to demonstrate that benefit.

In randomization, allocation of treatment to individuals is left purely to chance and not systematically biased by deliberate selection of patients. Despite randomization, there were imbalances in sex and BMI. These imbalances may have been due either to chance or to insufficient group size. Increasing the size of the study reduces the probability of baseline differences in both measured and unmeasured variables, but cannot assure balanced groups. Baseline differences are only important if they affect the study conclusions. In this study, these imbalances did not provide an alternative explanation to the three treatments' thermal advantage over propofol. In bivariate analyses, neither sex nor BMI were associated with the observed temperature differences. Their inclusion in the multivariable analysis did not affect the temperature differences between propofol and the other treatment groups, Thus, despite baseline differences, neither sex nor BMI provides an alternative explanation. Although there may be unmeasured confounding, the large and consistent differences between propofol and the alternative treatment groups makes it unlikely that the study conclusions will change.

Although the study design reduced the risk of selection bias, the possibility of measurement bias still exists. Having one caregiver (the first author) performing the randomization, providing anesthetic care, and recording outcomes is a potential source of bias. However, since the next study patient was already in the operating room at the time of random assignment, the caregiver could not affect the random allocation. By having a single caregiver, the manner of induction and all the tasks performed at the beginning of the case were more uniform than if the tasks were performed by multiple caregivers. The temperatures recorded were objective and not affected by who recorded the data.

We did not control for "depth of anesthesia". A greater depth of anesthesia likely results in more vasodilation and thus more redistribution hypothermia (and hypotension). If inductions achieve only the minimum necessary depth, it is plausible there may be less redistribution hypothermia (and hypotension). In this effectiveness study, we titrated the maintenance dose of anesthetic by vital signs, as is common in clinical practice. Titrating anesthetic doses to anesthetic depth may yield different results. A given depth of anesthesia can be achieved by varying the type and dose of anesthesia. We studied only one dose of propofol. It is plausible that using a lower dose of propofol and/or sevoflurane for induction will result in less redistribution hypothermia. Kazama et al. demonstrated that anesthetic inductions can be accomplished with a smaller dose of propofol than used in this study [31].

There were a variety of different surgeries, but no major intraabdominal or intrathoracic surgeries (with their greater potential for intraoperative heat loss). Since patients with different surgeries were treated similarly and had comparable thermal exposure in the first 15 min post induction, the impact of the specific surgery should be minor.

We did not study intrathoracic or major intraabdominal surgeries where there is greater thermal stress. We can make no statement as to whether the initial thermal benefit is well maintained in such cases.

We did not measure pre-induction (baseline) core temperatures. Although studies similar to this one often compare the changes from baseline temperature, we did not. We measured the core temperatures at 4 times after induction. To address the lack of pre-test core temperature measurements, we used a post-test only randomized trial. Since the randomization makes it likely that the baseline temperatures are similar in the four groups, the observed post-induction differences are probably due to the different induction techniques. Our experimental design, while less common, is a standard design that "contains no threats to internal validity" [11].

We performed "as treated" analyses on 200 of the 205 (97.6%) randomized patients. Those 5 excluded patients provided no valid temperature data. Four patients had no post-induction temperature measurements because they were withdrawn before T_{15}. In one patient, there was only one temperature measurement at T_{15}. This patient received more than 300 mL unwarmed IV fluid. This makes it very unlikely that the results differ substantially from an intention-to-treat analysis. With the exclusion of these five patients, the 200 patients presented in Table 1 are exactly those we analyzed. Thus, the randomization combined with the bivariate and multivariable statistical results support the study conclusion that the three alternative inductions produced higher intraoperative temperatures than propofol alone.

Conclusions

This study makes evident the thermal benefits of inhalation inductions and prophylactic bolus phenylephrine administration over standard intravenous propofol alone inductions in adults age 18 to 55 inclusive. This offers quick, simple, and easy to use partial solutions to the on-going problem of intraoperative hypothermia.

Appendix 1

Table 3 Study groups

Group	Induction technique
INH/100	Inhalation: 8% sevoflurane in 100% oxygen
INH/50	Inhalation: 8% sevoflurane in 50% oxygen and 50% nitrous oxide
PROP	Intravenous: 2.2 mg propofol
Phyl/PROP	Intravenous: 2.2 mg propofol preceded by 160 mcg phenylephrine

Appendix 2

Table 4 Inclusion and exclusion criteria

Inclusion criteria
Age 18 to 55 years inclusive
Scheduled for general anesthesia where 50% nitrous oxide in oxygen would be used
Endotracheal intubation or laryngeal mask airway insertion would be used
Afebrile (preoperative oral or temporal scan temperature between 36.2 and 37.4 °C inclusive)
Positioned supine or lithotomy
Forced air warming would be used
Expected duration of anesthetic to be at least 60 min
Exclusion criteria
Emergency surgery or any other aspiration risk
Age < 18 years or > 55 years
Pregnant
Incarceration
Febrile illness
Anticipated difficult airway
Contraindication to nitrous oxide use
Contraindication to nasal instrumentation
Nasal surgery
Current or recent epistaxis
Requirement for foreign language interpreter
Allergy to propofol
Malignant hyperthermia risk
Inability to oxygenate on less than 50% oxygen
Cardiac surgery
Neuro-surgery
Receiving vasoactive infusions
Significant valvular heart disease
Unstable cardiac disease
Requiring prone or lateral positioning
Inability to provide informed consent
Inability to use forced air warming
Untreated hypo- or hyper-thyroidism
ASA class 4, 5 or 6[a]
Anticipated inability to tolerate any of the 4 different anesthetic induction options in this study

[a]Patients with end stage renal disease on dialysis were classified as ASA 3

Appendix 3

Table 5 List of surgeries

Procedure	Groups having at least one patient having the listed procedure are denoted by an x			
	INH/100	INH/50	PROP	Phnl/PROP
UROLOGIC				
Cystoscopic surgery	x	x	x	x
Penile procedures	x	x	x	
Suprapubic tube placement	x			
Scrotal procedures	x			
Urethroplasty		x	x	x
ORTHOPEDIC				
Lower extremity orthopedics	x	x	x	x
Upper extremity orthopedics	x	x	x	x
Anterior cervical discectomy and fusion				x
GYNECOLOGIC				
Vulvoplasty or excision of lesion	x	x		
Dilation and curettage, hysteroscopy	x	x	x	x
Loop endocervical excision procedure	x	x		
Endocervical curettage	x	x		
Hysterectomy	x	x		x
Myomectomy		x	x	x
VASCULAR				
Dialysis access related procedures	x	x	x	x
Lower extremity vascular – open procedures		x		
Radiofrequency ablation and/or Lower extremity phlebectomies	x	x	x	
Lower extremity amputations	x	x		
DENTAL/ENT	x	x	x	
THORACIC				
Endobronchial ultrasound	x	x	x	
GENERAL SURGERY				
Vacuum assisted closure change	x			
Non-cavitary procedures	x	x		x
Inguinal hernia	x			x
Breast	x	x	x	x

Abbreviations

BMI: Body mass index; BP: Blood pressure; C: Centigrade; CI: Confidence interval; FAW: Forced air warming; Hg: Mercury; INH/100: Study group induced with 100% oxygen; INH/50: Study group induced with 50% oxygen and 50% nitrous oxide; IV: Intravenous; kg: Kilogram; LMA: Laryngeal mask airway; LPM: Liters per minute; m: Meter; mcg: Microgram; mg: Milligram; mL: Milliliter; mm: Millimeter; N_2O: Nitrous oxide; O_2: Oxygen; Phnl/PROP: Study group induced with 160 mcg phenylephrine followed by 2.2 mg/kg IV propofol; PROP: Study group induced with 2.2 mg/kg IV propofol; SCIP: Surgical Care Improvement Project; SD: Standard deviation; T_x: Time x minutes after the start of anesthetic induction

Acknowledgements

We thank Dr. Daniel I Sessler for his helpful comments.

Authors' contributions

LEB: Power study back in 2014. Statistical calculations. Wrote the statistical methods section and much of the results section. Overall review and edits for clarity. Made suggestions for tables and figures. Response to reviewers. LHH: Statistical calculations. Suggestions for methods and results sections, tables, and figures. Overall review and edits for clarity. JVR: (Everything else.) Background research. Generation of idea. Generated protocol. IRB approval. Periodic reporting to IRB. Registered on clinical-trials.gov. Creation of randomized envelopes. Obtained consent for every patient. Performed induction and other required tasks for every patient. Data collection and entered into EXCEL worksheets. Basic analysis and data preparation/organization for statisticians. Writing of manuscript. Submission to journal. *Response* to reviewers. All authors have read and approved this manuscript.

Author's information
None

Author details
[1]Department of Anesthesiology, Albert Einstein Medical Center, 5501 Old York Road, Philadelphia, PA, USA. [2]Albert Einstein Healthcare Network, Philadelphia, PA, USA. [3]Sidney Kimmel Medical School of Thomas Jefferson University, Philadelphia, PA, USA. [4]Office for Research and Technology Development, Albert Einstein Medical Center, 5501 Old York Road, Philadelphia, PA, USA.

References

1. Sessler DI. Complications and treatment of mild hypothermia. Anesthesiology. 2001;95:531–43.
2. Stewart PA, Liang SS, Li QS, Huang ML, Bilgin AB, Kim D, Phillips S. The impact of residual neuromuscular blockade, oversedation, and hypothermia on adverse respiratory events in a postanesthetic care unit: a prospective study of prevalence, predictors, and outcomes. Anesth Analg. 2016;123(4): 859–68.
3. Ikeda T, Sessler DI, Kikura M, Kazama T, Ikeda K, Sato S. Less core hypothermia when anesthesia is induced with inhaled sevoflurane than with intravenous propofol. Anesth Analg. 1999;88:921–4.
4. Sun Z, Honar H, Sessler DI, Dalton JE, Yang D, Panjasawatwong K, Deroee AF, Salmasi V, Saager L, Kurz A. Intraoperative core temperature patterns, transfusion requirement, and hospital duration in patients warmed with forced air. Anesthesiology. 2015;122:276–85.
5. Scott AV, Stonemetz JL, Wasey JO, Johnson DJ, Rivers RJ, Koch CG, Frank SM. Compliance with surgical care improvement project for body temperature management (SCIP Inf-10) is associated with improved clinical outcomes. Anesthesiology. 2015;123(1):116–25.
6. Winkler M, Akca O, Birkenberg B, Hetz H, Scheck T, Arkilic CF, Kabon B, Marker E, Gru A, Czepan R, Greher M, Goll V, Gottsauner-Wolf F, Kurz A, Sessler DI. Aggressive warming reduces blood loss during hip arthroplasty. Anesth Analg. 2000;91:978–84.
7. Rajagopalan S, Mascha E, Na J, Sessler DI. The effects of mild perioperative hypothermia on blood loss and transfusion requirement. Anesthesiology. 2008;108:71–7.
8. Roth JV, Braitman LE. Nasal temperature can be used as a reliable surrogate measure of core temperature. J Clin Monit Comput. 2008;22:309–14.
9. Sessler DI. Temperature monitoring and perioperative thermoregulation. Anesthesiology. 2008;109(2):318–38.
10. Wang M, Singh A, Qureshi H, Leone A, Mascha EI, Sessler DI. Optimal depth for nasopharyngeal temperature probe positioning. Anesth Analg. 2016;122: 1434–8.
11. Campbell DT, Stanley JC. Experimental and Quasi-experimental designs for research. Boston: Houghton Mifflin Company; 1963. p. 8.
12. Giesbrecht GG, Ducharme MB, McGuire JP. Comparison of forced-air warming systems for perioperative use. Anesthesiology. 1994;80:671–9.
13. Hoffman L. Longitudinal Analysis- Modelling Within-Person Fluctuation and Change. New York: Routledge; 2015. p. 101–3. 152–3
14. Vaughan MS, Vaughan RW, Cook RC. Postoperative hypothermia in adults: relationship of age, anesthesia, and shivering to rewarming. Anesth Analg. 1981;60:746–51.
15. Ozaki M, Sessler DI, Suzuki H, Ozaki K, Tsunoda C, Atarashi K. Nitrous oxide decreases the threshold for vasoconstriction less than sevoflurane or isoflurance. Anesth Analg. 1995;80:1212–6.
16. Matsukawa T, Sessler DI, Sessler AM, Schroeder M, Ozaki M, Kurz A, Cheng C. Heat flow and distribution during induction of general anesthesia. Anesthesiology. 1995;82:662–73.
17. Ikeda T, Ozaki M, Sessler DI, Kazama T, Ikeda K, Sato S. Intraoperative phenylephrine infusion decreases the magnitude of redistribution hypothermia. Anesth Analg. 1999;89(2):462–5.
18. Just B, Trevien V, Lelva E, Lienhart A. Prevention of intraoperative hypothermia by preoperative skin-surface warming. Anesthesiology. 1993; 79:214–8.
19. Andrzejowski J, Hoyle J, Eapen G, Turnbull D. Effect of prewarming on post-induction core temperature and the incidence of inadvertent perioperative hypothermia in patients undergoing general anaesthesia. Br J Anaesth. 2008;101:627–31.
20. Bock M, Muller J, Bach A, Bohrer H, Martin E, Motsch J. Effects of preinduction and intraoperative warming during major laparotomy. Br J Anaesth. 1998;80:159–63.
21. Camus Y, Delva E, Sessler DI, Lienhart A. Pre-induction skin-surface warming minimizes intraoperative core hypothermia. J Clin Anesth. 1995;7:384–8.
22. Hynson JM, Sessler DI, Moayeri A, McGuire J, Schroeder BS. The effects of pre-induction warming on temperature and blood pressure during propofol-nitrous oxide anesthesia. Anesthesiology. 1993;79:219–28.
23. Ikeda T, Kazama T, Sessler DI, Toriyama S, Niwa K, Shimada C, Sato S. Induction of anesthesia with ketamine reduces the magnitude of redistribution hypothermia. Anesth Analg. 2001;93:934–8.
24. Park HP, Kang JM, Jeon YT, Choi IY, Oh YS, Hwang JW. Comparison of the effects of etomidate and propofol on redistribution hypothermia during general anesthesia. Korean J Anesthesiol. 2006;50:S19–24.
25. Aoki Y, Aoshima Y, Atsumi K, Kaminaka R, Nakau R, Yanagida K, Kora M, Fujii S, Yokoyama J. Perioperative amino acid infusion for preventing hypothermia and improving clinical outcomes during surgery Unger general anesthesia: a systematic review and meta-analysis. Anesth Analg. 2017;125:793–802.
26. Mizobe T, Nakajima Y, Ueno H, Sessler DI. Fructose administration increases intraoperative core temperature by augmenting both metabolic rate and the vasoconstriction threshold. Anesthesiology. 2006;104:1124–30.
27. Thwaites A, Edmends S, Smith I. Inhalation induction with sevoflurane: a double –blind comparison with propofol. Br J Anaesth. 1997;78:356–61.
28. Monk TG, Bronsert MR, Henderson WG, Mangione MP, Sum-Ping ST, Bentt DR, Nguyen JD, Richman JS, Mequid RA, Hammermeister KE. Association between intraoperative hypotension and hypertension and 30-day postoperative mortality in noncardiac surgery. Anesthesiology. 2015;123:307–19.
29. Walsh M, Devereaux PJ, Garg AX, Kurz A, Turan A, Rodseth RN, Cywinski J, Thabane L, Sessler DI. Relationship between intraoperative mean arterial blood pressure and clinical outcomes after noncardiac surgery: toward an empirical definition of hypotension. Anesthesiology. 2013;119:507–15.
30. Maheshwari K, Turan A, Mao G, Yang D, Niazi AK, Agarwal D, Sessler DI, Kurz A. The association of hypotension during non-cardiac surgery, before and after skin incision, with postoperative acute injury: a retrospective cohort analysis. Anaesthesia. 2018;73:1223–8.
31. Kazama T, Ikeda K, Morita K, Kikura M, Ikeda T, Kurita T, Sato S. Investigation of effective anesthesia induction doses using a wide range of infusion rates with undiluted and diluted propofol. Anesthesiology. 2000;92:1017–28.

8

Optimal crystalloid volume ratio for blood replacement for maintaining hemodynamic stability and lung function

Gergely H. Fodor[1], Walid Habre[2], Adam L. Balogh[3], Roberta Südy[3], Barna Babik[3] and Ferenc Peták[1*]

Abstract

Background: Crystalloids are first line in fluid resuscitation therapy, however there is a lack of evidence-based recommendations on the volume to be administered. Therefore, we aimed at comparing the systemic hemodynamic and respiratory effects of volume replacement therapy with a 1:1 ratio to the historical 1:3 ratio.

Methods: Anesthetized, ventilated rats randomly included in 3 groups: blood withdrawal and replacement with crystalloid in 1:1 ratio (Group 1, $n = 11$), traditional 1:3 ratio (Group 3, $n = 12$) and a control group with no interventions (Group C, $n = 9$). Arterial blood of 5% of the total blood volume was withdrawn 7 times, and replaced stepwise with different volume rations of Ringer's acetate, according to group assignments. Airway resistance (Raw), respiratory tissue damping (G) and tissue elastance (H), mean arterial pressure (MAP) and heart rate (HR) were assessed following each step of fluid replacement with a crystalloid (CR1-CR6). Lung edema index was measured from histological samples.

Results: Raw decreased in Groups 1 and 3 following CR3 ($p < 0.02$) without differences between the groups. H elevated in all groups ($p < 0.02$), with significantly higher changes in Group 3 compared to Groups C and 1 (both $p = 0.03$). No differences in MAP or HR were present between Groups 1 and 3. Lung edema was noted in Group 3 ($p < 0.05$).

Conclusions: Fluid resuscitation therapy by administering a 1:1 blood replacement ratio revealed adequate compensation capacity and physiological homeostasis similar with no lung stiffening and pulmonary edema. Therefore, considering this ratio promotes the restrictive fluid administration in the presence of continuous and occult bleeding.

Keywords: Fluid resuscitation, Respiratory mechanics, Pulmonary edema, Lung function, Fluid replacement

Background

With the increased awareness of the potential harmful effect of colloids on the organs, crystalloids are considered as first line fluid resuscitation therapy. Moreover, goal-directed fluid therapy is now a well-established strategy in routine clinical practice in the perioperative period. The main feature of this strategy is to reduce the amount of fluid administered to the patients while maintaining optimal cardiac output and adequate organ perfusion [1, 2]. However, crystalloids have short hemodynamic beneficial effect due to the extravasation into the interstitial space [3] with a very low (less than 20%) intravascular volume effect [4].

There are various clinical situations where continuous and occult bleeding (such as liver surgery and trauma, transplants, scoliosis surgery, etc.) may occur and the clinicians may have to face higher ratio of fluid replacement to maintain hemodynamic stability. Despite the routine use of crystalloids in these clinical situations, the optimal volume to be administered to re-establish blood

* Correspondence: petak.ferenc@med.u-szeged.hu
[1]Department of Medical Physics and Informatics, University of Szeged, 9 Koranyi fasor, Szeged H-6720, Hungary

volume and maintain optimal cardiac output and end-organ perfusion is arbitrary. This ambiguity arises from the lack of evidence-based recommendations with regard to the volume of crystalloid solution to be administered in order to compensate for the same blood lost volume. Historically, 3- to 4-fold ratio is recommended in various textbooks as a traditional approach to counterweigh blood loss [5]. Despite the recent European guidelines to use a restricted volume replacement [6], closer to a 1:1 ratio, there have been no studies providing evidence for the choice of the optimal crystalloid volume to be administered to maintain hemodynamic stability with minimal adverse effect due to interstitial water extravasation.

We recently demonstrated that measurements of respiratory mechanics provide sensitive indices of lung water extravasation as a consequence of fluid replacement therapy in an experimental model of acute hemorrhage [7, 8]. Therefore, we aimed at using a similar approach to clarify the debate on the optimal crystalloid volume ratio following occult and continuous bleeding. We hypothesized that when compared to the historical ratio of 1:3, crystalloid fluid replacement in a 1:1 ratio is sufficient to ensure hemodynamic stability with little effect on lung function as a surrogate for interstitial edema development.

Methods

Ethics

The experimental procedures were approved by the institutional ethics committee for experimental research of the University of Szeged (no. I-74-50/2012) and by the National Food Chain Safety and Animal Health Directorate of Csongrád County, Hungary (no. XIV/152/2013). The procedures were performed according to the guidelines of the Scientific Committee of Animal Experimentation of the Hungarian Academy of Sciences (updated Law and Regulations on Animal Protection: 40/2013. (II. 14.) Government of Hungary), following the EU Directive 2010/63/EU on the protection of animals used for scientific purposes, and reported in compliance with the ARRIVE guidelines.

Animal preparations

Anesthesia of 32 male adult Wistar rats (330 [285–388] g from the animal facility of Faculty of Pharmacy, University of Szeged, Hungary) was induced with an intraperitoneal injection of sodium pentobarbital (45 mg/kg). Tracheostomy was performed after subcutaneous administration of lidocaine (2–4 mg/kg) and a polyethylene cannula was introduced into the trachea (16 G, B. Braun Melsungen AG, Melsungen, Germany). A small animal ventilator (Model 683, Harvard Apparatus, South Natick, MA, USA) was used to ventilate the animals in a supine position with room air (70 breaths/min, tidal volume 7 ml/kg) through the tracheal tube. The left femoral vein was cannulated (Abbocath 22 G) for drug delivery and fluid replacement. This line was used to maintain anesthesia by repeated injections of sodium pentobarbital (12 mg/kg, every 30 min) and muscle relaxation was achieved by regular administration of pipecuronium (0.1 mg/kg, every 30 min, Arduan, Richter-Gedeon, Budapest, Hungary). The left femoral artery was catheterized (Abbocath 22 G) and connected to a pressure transducer (Model TSD104A, Biopac, Santa Barbara, CA, USA) for continuous systemic blood pressure monitoring to assess mean arterial pressure (MAP), and to allow blood withdrawal, as part of the experimental protocol. A data collection and acquisition system (Biopac, Santa Barbara, CA, USA) was used to monitor the MAP, ECG and heart rate (HR) continuously. Body temperature was kept in the 37 ± 0.5 °C range by utilizing a heating pad.

Measurement of respiratory mechanical parameters

The forced oscillation technique was applied in short (6-s-long) end-expiratory pauses, as detailed previously [9, 10] to obtain the input impedance of the respiratory system (Zrs). Briefly, ventilation was ceased at end-expiration and the tracheal cannula was switched to a loudspeaker-in-box system by means of a three-way tap. A computer-generated small amplitude (< ±1 cmH_2O) pseudorandom signal composed of 23 non-integer multiples ranging 0.5–20.75 Hz was delivered by the loudspeaker through a 100-cm-long, 2-mm-internal diameter polyethylene wave-tube. The lateral pressures were measured at the loudspeaker end (P_1) and at the tracheal end (P_2) of the wave-tube by using two identical pressure transducers (model 33NA002D, ICSensors, Milpitas, CA, USA). The signals P_1 and P_2 were low-pass filtered at 25 Hz, and digitized by a data acquisition board (NI USB-6211, National Instruments, Austin, TX) at a rate of 256 Hz. Pressure transfer functions (P_1/P_2) were calculated with fast Fourier transformation (4-s time windows and 95% overlapping) from each 6-s recordings. Zrs was calculated as the load impedance of the wave-tube [11]. The input impedance of the ET tube and the connections was also determined, and was subtracted from each Zrs spectrum.

A model containing a frequency-independent resistance (Raw) and inertance (Iaw) and a constant-phase tissue compartment consisting of tissue damping (G) and elastance (H) was fitted to the Zrs spectra by minimizing the weighted difference between the measured and the modelled impedance data [12]. G describes the dissipative (damping or resistive) properties, while H reflects stiffness (elastance) of the respiratory tissues. Raw and Iaw characterize mainly the resistance and inertance of the airways, since the contribution of the chest wall to these parameters in rats is minor [13].

Pulmonary edema assessments

At the end of the experimental protocol the animals were euthanized with an intravenous overdose of pentobarbital sodium (300 mg/kg), then a midline thoracotomy was performed. The right lungs were fixed by instilling 4% formaldehyde at a hydrostatic pressure of 20 cmH_2O via the tracheal cannula. The lungs were excised in one piece and placed into 4% buffered formalin until further processing. After complete fixation, transhilar horizontal sections (perpendicular to the longitudinal axes of the lung from the hilum) were embedded in paraffin. Two 5-μm sections were prepared in each lung specimen and were stained with hematoxylin-eosin. Digitized images of 10 non-overlapping fields of view were used to obtain the edema index around randomly selected pulmonary vessels by dividing the lumen area by the total area of the pulmonary vessel (edema cuff area + vessel lumen area). Histological images were analyzed by the same investigator in a blind fashion and in a random sequence by using JMicroVision image analysis software (version 1.2.7).

Three-to-four tissue samples were dissected from the different lobes of the non-fixated left lungs; these samples were weighed to establish the wet-to-dry weight ratio (W/D) as an index of the lung water content.

Study protocol

The rats were assigned to the protocol groups randomly and the same experimental protocol was applied to both treatment groups apart from the volume of replaced fluid (as depicted in Fig. 1). Following animal preparations and reaching a steady-state condition, a lung hyperinflation was applied by occluding the expiratory port of the ventilator for 1 respiratory cycle to standardize the lung volume history. Baseline respiratory mechanical parameters were determined by measuring 4 reproducible Zrs data sets. Blood loss was achieved by withdrawing 5% (approximately 1 ml) of total estimated blood volume (TBV) [14] via the femoral artery, then after 7 min, withdrawal of blood was repeated once again identically. Following these two withdrawals of arterial blood, fluid replacement was carried out by a rapid injection of Ringer's acetate solution (Ringerfundin B. Braun, B. Braun Melsungen AG, Melsungen, Germany) into the femoral vein in accordance with the group allocation: Group 1 ($n = 11$) received 5% of TBV (1:1 ratio) and Group 3 ($n = 12$) received 15% of TBV (1:3 ratio) at each replacement. A set of Zrs data was recorded three minutes later. The blood withdrawal-replacement was repeated five more times (until a total of 7 withdrawal and 6 replacement steps) with additional Zrs recordings after each replacement maneuvers. Blood gas analyses were performed from the first, fourth and sixth withdrawn arterial blood samples (epoc Reader and Host, Epocal Inc., Ottawa, ON, Canada) to determine hematocrit (Hct), pH and partial pressures of oxygen (PaO_2) and carbon dioxide ($PaCO_2$). Arterial oxygen content (CaO_2) of the blood was calculated based on the following equation: $CaO_2 = SaO_2 \times Hb \times 1.39 + (PaO_2 \times 0.03)$ with hemoglobin estimated from the hematocrit level based on the formula Hb (g/dl) = Hct (%)/3 [15]. At the end of the experimental protocol the lungs were processed for assessment of pulmonary edema as detailed above. Each withdrawal-replacement step lasted about 12–15 min, resulting in a total duration of the fluid resuscitation period of around 90 min.

A control group (Group C, $n = 9$) was also used with identical timing of the measurements, but no withdrawal and replacement, apart from approximately 0.3 ml for each arterial blood gas sample at the same time as in the protocol groups.

Statistical analyses

Group mean averages with SE values are reported. Normality was checked with the Shapiro-Wilk test. Considering the mean values of the primary outcome, H (4800 cmH_2O/l) and its variability (650 cmH_2O/l) established in earlier studies in rats [7], sample size estimation revealed that 10 rats are necessary in each group to detect 20% difference in the three groups with 80%

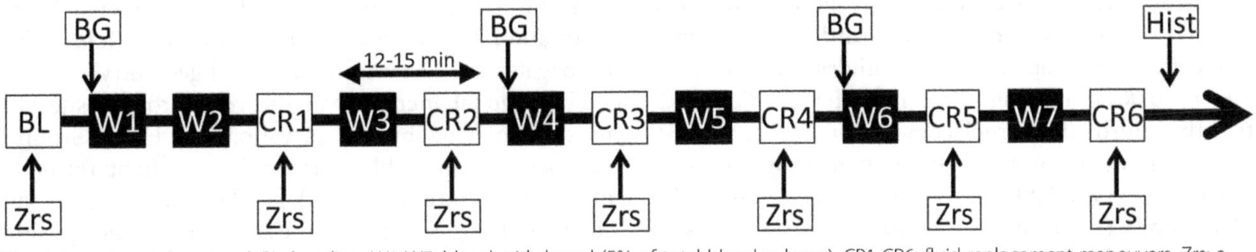

Fig. 1 Experimental protocol. BL: baseline, W1-W7: blood withdrawal (5% of total blood volume), CR1-CR6: fluid replacement maneuvers, Zrs: a set of respiratory impedance measurements, BG: arterial blood gas measurements. Each withdrawal-replacement step lasted about 12–15 min, resulting in a total duration of the fluid resuscitation period of around 90 min

power at significance level of 0.05. Two-way repeated measures analysis of variance (ANOVA) was used with the variables group assessment and time to establish the effects of these factors on respiratory mechanical, blood gas and hemodynamic parameters. The Holm-Sidak multiple comparison procedure was employed to compare the mechanical, blood gas and hemodynamic parameters under different conditions versus controls of both group assessment (Group C) and time (BL or first blood gas measurement). One-way ANOVA with the factor group assessment was used to assess effects of fluid volume on edema indices and to assess differences of final responses (those obtained at CR6). The Holm-Sidak multiple comparison procedure was applied for post hoc tests. The statistical tests were performed with SigmaPlot statistical software package (Version 13, Systat Software, Inc. Chicago, IL, USA). In each test, a significance level of $p < 0.05$ was applied.

Results

Body weights of the rats did not differ significantly between the groups (335 [285–386] g for Group C, 333 [285–388] g for Group 1 and 324 [285–380] g for Group 3).

Changes in respiratory mechanical parameters following each fluid replacement maneuver are demonstrated in Fig. 2. No significant changes in Raw were observed in Group C. While significant decreases in Raw were observed in Groups 1 (CR2–CR6, each $p < 0.02$) and 3 (CR3–CR6, each $p < 0.02$), there was no evidence for a difference in the relative changes in Raw between the groups. No significant changes were observed in G in any of the groups apart from slight increases from CR4 in Group 1 (CR4–CR6, each $p < 0.03$). Respiratory elastance worsened in all groups with mild changes in groups C and 1 (CR2–CR6, each $p < 0.01$ and CR1–CR6, each $p < 0.01$ for group C and group 1, respectively), whereas a significantly more severe deterioration was observed with time in group 3 (CR1–CR6, each $p < 0.03$).

Parameters assessed from arterial blood gas analyses are demonstrated in Table 1. The study protocol led to a significant decrease in Hct in both Groups 1 ($p < 0.001$ at W4 and W6) and 3 ($p < 0.001$ at W4 and W6). However, in comparison to Group C and 1, fluid replacement with a 1:3 ratio resulted in significantly lower values of Hct from the fourth blood withdrawal maneuver (W4, $p < 0.001$), implying lowered Hct in Group 3 after the third fluid replacement maneuver (CR3). Slight decrements of pH were obtained in Group 1 ($p = 0.019$ and $p < 0.001$ at W4 and W6, respectively) and Group 3 ($p = 0.049$ and $p < 0.001$ at W4 and W6, respectively) during the fluid replacement protocol, however no significant differences were detected between the groups. No significant changes were detected in PaO_2 and $PaCO_2$ in any of the protocol groups. Significant decreases were observed in CaO_2 both in Group 1 and Group 3 at fourth (W4) and sixth (W6) blood withdrawal maneuvers ($p < 0.001$ for all) with significantly lower values in Group 3 compared to Group C at W6 ($p = 0.004$).

Figure 3 exhibits the changes of systemic hemodynamic parameters. No significant changes in MAP or HR were detected in Group C, however, significantly lower values of MAP were observed in Group 1 and Group 3 from the fifth blood withdrawal (W5–CR6, each $p < 0.05$). The relative decreases in MAP at the end of the protocol were significantly greater in both Group 1 and Group 3 than those observed in Group C ($p = 0.03$ for both). No significant changes of HR were detected during the protocol.

The results of lung edema assessments obtained from the protocol groups are summarized in Fig. 4. Wet-to-dry lung weight ratio was significantly greater in Group 3 than those obtained in Groups C ($p = 0.05$) and 1 ($p = 0.048$). Histological lung edema index was significantly elevated in Group 1 compared to Group C ($p < 0.001$), with even more severe elevations observed in Group 3 compared to Group 1 ($p = 0.05$).

Discussion

We demonstrated in the present experimental study that compensating blood loss with crystalloids in a ratio of 1:1 led to lack of adverse alterations in the lung with maintenance of physiological homeostasis. Conversely, the use of a historical ratio of 1:3 resulted in a deterioration in respiratory tissue stiffness as a consequence of perivascular edema development. Moreover, fluid replacement in a ratio of 1:3 induced greater hemodilution as expressed in the significant decrease in the oxygen content of the blood.

In agreements with our previous study when the blood loss was replaced with normal saline [7], a slight decrease was observed in Raw in Group 1 and Group 3 following fluid resuscitations. While this bronchodilation is presumably caused by a catecholamine-release induced by a loss of blood volume [8], the lack of differences at the final replacement maneuver suggests that this catecholamine-release is counteracted by the restoration of vascular filling with crystalloid, which propagates the recovery of bronchial geometry.

The gradual increases in the respiratory tissue stiffness manifested by the elevations of H in Group C can be most probably attributed to a slight formation of atelectatic areas in the dependent lung regions subsequent to general anesthesia and supine position leading to lung volume loss [16]. Interestingly, fluid replacement with crystalloid at 1:1 ratio resulted in a similar trend in H, indicating that such intervention

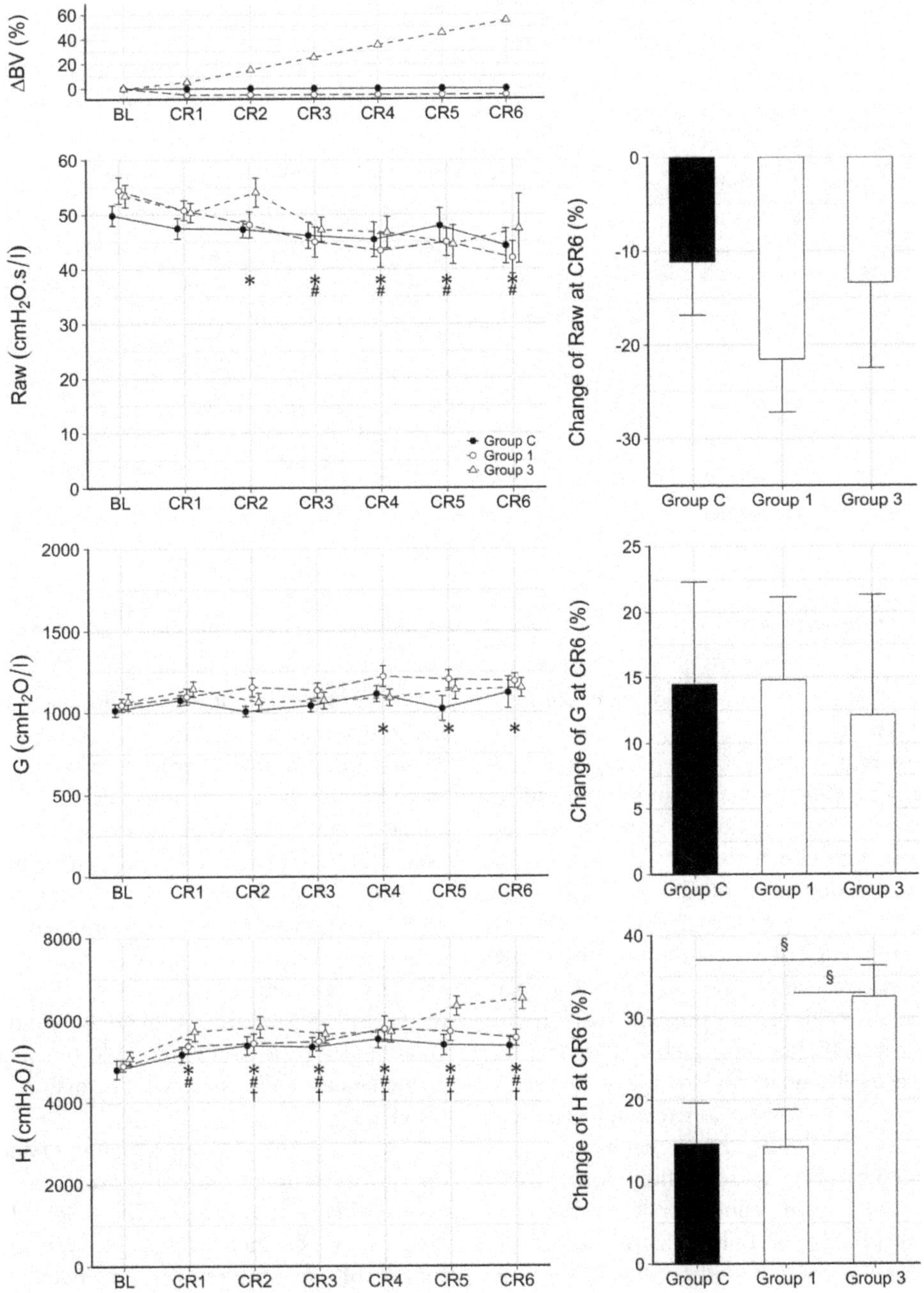

Fig. 2 Mean (±SE) values of respiratory mechanical parameters during the experimental protocol. ΔBV: changes of total blood volume. The absolute values of airway resistance (Raw), tissue damping (G) and tissue elastance (H) over the experimental protocol (left) and their changes following the last fluid replacement maneuver relative to their corresponding baseline (right). BL: baseline. CR1-CR6: replacement maneuvers. *: $p < 0.05$ in Group 1 vs BL, #: $p < 0.05$ in Group 3 vs BL, †: $p < 0.05$ in Group C vs BL. §: $p < 0.05$ in the relative changes

has no deleterious consequences in the lung tissue mechanics. In contrast with these mild changes, fluid replacement therapy with the larger crystalloid volume (1:3) led to severe respiratory tissue stiffening when the circulatory blood volume was increased above 140% of baseline. These adverse respiratory mechanical changes can be attributed to a significant increase in the pulmonary edema extent subsequent to severe hemodilution manifested in the significant drop in Hct level. The excessive edema development in the animals of Group 3 may lead ultimately to deterioration in gas exchange [17–19], and may be a risk factor for the development of acute respiratory distress syndrome [20]. Hypoxemia was not observed in the present study due to the relatively limited drop in CaO_2 and Hct that allowed the maintenance of

Table 1 Mean ± SE values of parameters obtained from arterial blood gas measurements

		W1	W4	W6
Hematocrit (%)	Group C	35.60 ± 0.77	34.24 ± 1.29	33.04 ± 1.88
	Group 1	36.64 ± 0.72	32.26 ± 0.81*	29.63 ± 1.23*$
	Group 3	36.39 ± 0.77	30.30 ± 1.09*$	27.09 ± 0.60*$§
pH	Group C	7.50 ± 0.01	7.45 ± 0.01	7.45 ± 0.03
	Group 1	7.52 ± 0.02	7.45 ± 0.03*	7.41 ± 0.02*
	Group 3	7.54 ± 0.02	7.47 ± 0.02*	7.41 ± 0.03*
PaO_2 (mmHg)	Group C	70.75 ± 2.10	63.21 ± 2.86	67.35 ± 1.73
	Group 1	74.24 ± 2.84	69.06 ± 3.55	75.43 ± 3.22
	Group 3	75.28 ± 2.55	67.00 ± 4.10	71.06 ± 1.15
$PaCO_2$ (mmHg)	Group C	30.51 ± 1.74	30.63 ± 1.57	27.57 ± 3.08
	Group 1	30.08 ± 1.55	31.07 ± 1.34	31.21 ± 1.49
	Group 3	27.94 ± 0.97	29.71 ± 0.97	23.52 ± 2.34
CaO_2 (ml O_2/100 ml)	Group C	15.67 ± 0.38	14.36 ± 0.56	14.37 ± 0.94
	Group 1	16.29 ± 0.35	14.00 ± 0.36*	12.97 ± 0.48*
	Group 3	16.21 ± 0.43	12.91 ± 0.48*	11.78 ± 0.22*$

PaO_2 and *$PaCO_2$*: arterial partial pressures of O_2 and CO_2, respectively. *CaO_2*: arterial oxygen content. *W* blood withdrawal.*: $p<0.05$ vs. W1, $: $p<0.05$ vs. Group C, §: $p<0.05$ vs. Group 1.

physiological homeostasis and the short duration of the experiment (90 min).

The mechanisms responsible for the changes in the respiratory mechanics following hemodilution are still to be fully characterized. In an earlier in vitro model, we demonstrated that decreased hematocrit values resulted in no change of Raw and decreases of G and H [21]. The contradiction between the previous in vitro and the current in vivo results suggest that although hematocrit content and blood viscosity affect the mechanical properties of the respiratory system, our present findings are governed mainly by systemic factors, such as the systemic catecholamine-release subsequent to blood loss [8].

There is still no clear consensus on the optimal fluid replacement therapy. Colloids have been used as volume-sparing agents for large-scale fluid losses [22], however due to the recent controversies related to hydroxyethyl-starch [23, 24] and albumin [24, 25], crystalloids are still highly recommended for fluid resuscitation [6, 26]. In clinical practice, not only the type of the applied solution, but the applied volume is also under debate. It is commonly accepted that although crystalloids are recommended in a goal-directed manner [27], these solutions are still applied in higher volumes compared to colloids [28]. There is increasing evidence for the benefit of intravenous fluid restriction during the perioperative period on patient recovery and outcome [29, 30]. Our findings support the clinical concept of reducing the administered crystalloids volume to a ratio of 1:1 to avoid any additional detrimental effects on the lungs, which may further contribute to the major postoperative complications [3, 31, 32].

While no significant differences in the systemic hemodynamic parameters were observed between Group 1 and Group 3, the magnitude of the significant decrease in MAP was similar in both Groups 1 and 3. This result suggests an equality of 1:1 and 1:3 ratios in terms of systemic hemodynamic effects. In addition, our findings are in line with the goal-oriented therapy concept, which promotes fluid restriction associated with early onset of vasopressors to maintain perfusion pressure [32, 33]. Therefore, comparing the traditional 1:3–1:4 ratios for crystalloids implied by textbooks [5] with a smaller, 1:1 ratio is already able to ensure physiological homeostasis without compromising the respiratory function.

The choice of the replacement crystalloid was based on the current recommendations of favoring balanced crystalloids over normal saline (0.9% NaCl) [26, 27, 34]. The use of balanced solutions results in lower occurrences of hypochloremia and metabolic acidosis [35]. This may be reflected in the maintenance of normal physiological pH in the animals of Group 1 in the present study, as opposed to development of acidosis in a similar earlier protocol by using normal saline [7].

As concerns the changes of Raw and H following fluid resuscitation, the present findings demonstrate similar trends to those observed previously [7]. However, the results of the present study differs from the previous findings for H, with an increase of approximately 15% detected in our present study opposed to as high as ~ 40% when fluid replacement was performed with 1:1 crystalloid [7]. These differences were also consistent with the development of more severe of lung edema.

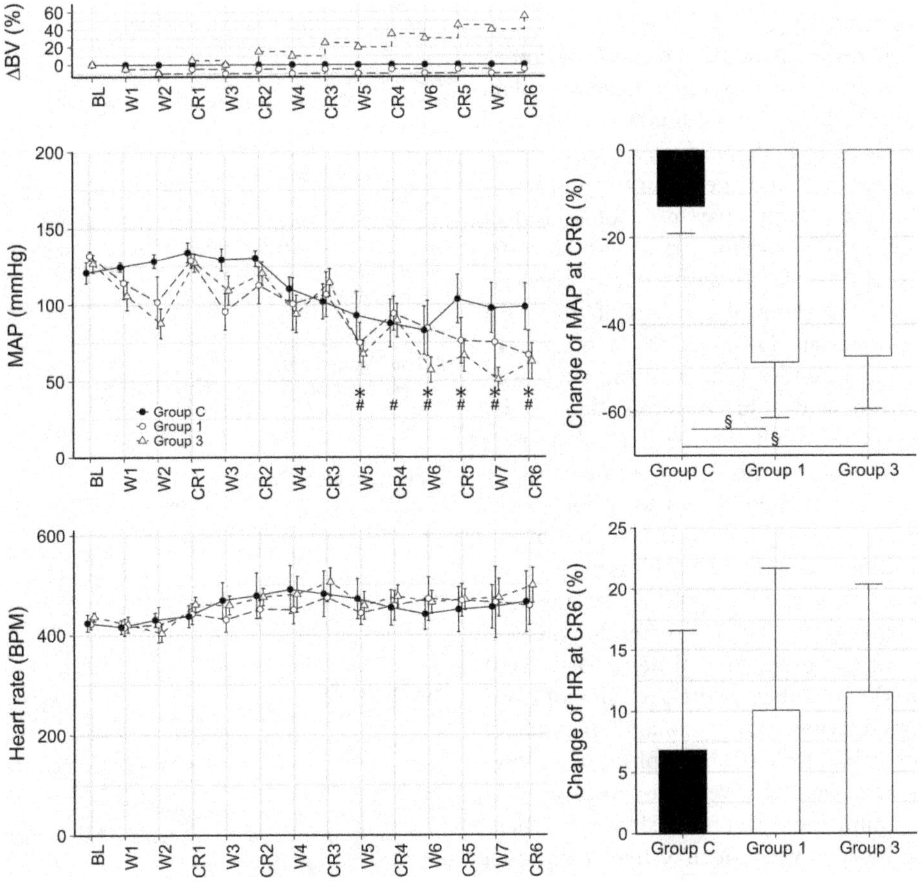

Fig. 3 Mean (±SE) values of hemodynamic parameters during the experimental protocol (both at replacement and withdrawal steps). ΔBV: changes of total blood volume. Absolute values of mean arterial pressure (MAP) and heart rate (HR) over the experimental protocol (left) and their changes following the last replacement compared to baseline (right). BL: baseline. CR1-CR6: replacement maneuvers, W1-W7: blood withdrawal steps. *: $p < 0.05$ in Group 1 vs BL, #: $p < 0.05$ in Group 3 vs BL. §: $p < 0.05$ in the relative changes

The primary reason for these differences can also be attributed to the use of different crystalloid solutions in the two studies: normal saline in the previous one and a balanced solution (Ringer's acetate) in the current study. It has been previously reported that higher levels of body surface indexed extravascular lung water (EVLWI) can be detected in a swine model of fluid resuscitation of hemorrhagic shock when normal saline is used as opposed to a balanced crystalloid solution (Ringer's lactate) [36]. Our results also support that balanced crystalloids

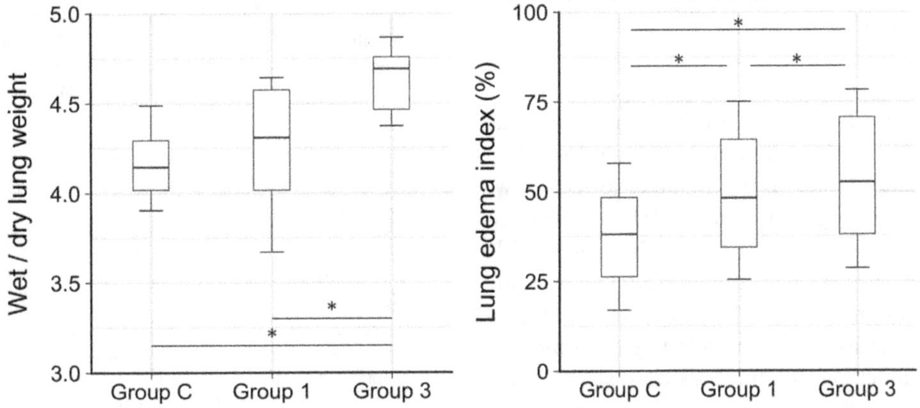

Fig. 4 Edema index obtained by ratio of perivascular edema cuff and vascular area from the histological samples. *: $p < 0.05$

are more favorable opposed to normal saline in terms of pulmonary edema formation [27, 34].

A limitation of our results is related to the experimental setting. The total respiratory system impedance data comprises contributions from the pulmonary system and the surrounding tissues (e.g. diaphragm and the chest wall) [13]. This means that the mechanical parameters obtained in the present study may not solely reflect changes in the pulmonary system, particularly for the tissue parameters [13]. We are not aware of any previous studies addressing the mechanical changes of the chest wall following hemodilution, however, no changes were reported in the resistance and elastance of the chest wall following severe oleic acid-induced interstitial edema [37]. Therefore, we believe that the mechanical properties of the chest wall would not change substantially following hemodilution and the changes we detected are mainly of pulmonary origin. However, due to the masking effects of the fairly constant extrapulmonary tissue mechanical compartments, the real pulmonary mechanical changes are expected to be of greater magnitude. Another limitation of our experimental design is related to the lack of injured tissues like in the presence of traumatism, where hemodilution with crystalloids may affect coagulation factors with subsequent rebleeding. However, our primary aim was to investigate intravascular volume expansion mimicking a clinical situation where the coagulation pathway is functional. While our model did not aim at maintaining the colloid-osmotic pressures or the level of coagulation factors, it still represents clinical approaches resulting from continuous occult bleeding and/or application of stable coagulation factors with crystalloids avoiding fresh frozen plasma. Accordingly, our findings do not allow any conclusions regarding volume replacement under trauma conditions. A further limiting factor is related to the lack of direct monitoring of cardiac output as an indicator of optimal organ perfusion. However, the homeostasis remained physiological (Table 1) despite the drop in MAP, which indicated that anaerobic metabolism did not occur.

Conclusions

In summary, the results of the present study provide evidence for the optimal fluid replacement ratio when considering crystalloids for fluid replacement following blood loss. Accordingly, a ratio of 1:1 is more appropriate than the historical approach since it is able to meet the needs for maintaining homeostasis while avoiding the adverse effects related to fluid extravasation. With the limitations of extrapolating experimental results to clinical practice, our findings may suggest that considering crystalloid fluid replacement in a ratio of 1:1 to compensate continuous occult bleeding maintains appropriate organ perfusion without the adverse consequences of fluid extravasation.

Abbreviations

ANOVA: Analysis of variances; BL: Baseline; CaO_2: Arterial oxygen content; CR1–6: Crystalloid replacement steps; EVLWI: Extravascular lung water; G: Tissue damping; H: Tissue elastance; Hb: Hemoglobin; Hct: Hematocrit; HR: Heart rate; Iaw: Airway inertance; MAP: Mean arterial pressure; P_1: Pressure at the loudspeaker end; P_2: Pressure at the tracheal end; $PaCO_2$: Arterial partial pressures of carbon dioxide; PaO_2: Arterial partial pressures of oxygen; pH: Arterial pH; Raw: Airway resistance; TBV: Total blood volume; W/D: Wet-to-dry weight ratio; W1–7: Blood withdrawal steps; Zrs: Impedance of the respiratory system

Acknowledgements

The authors wish to thank Orsolya Ivánkovitsné Kiss for her technical assistance during the experiments.

Authors' contributions

GHF: study design, data collection, data analyses and article drafting. WH: study design, interpretation of the results and article drafting. ALB: data collection and data analyses. RS: data collection and data analyses. BB: study design, interpretation of the results and article drafting. FP: study design, data analyses, interpretation of the results and article drafting. All authors have read, critically revised and accepted the final manuscript.

Author details

[1]Department of Medical Physics and Informatics, University of Szeged, 9 Koranyi fasor, Szeged H-6720, Hungary. [2]Unit for Anesthesiological Investigations, Department of Anesthesiology, Pharmacology and Intensive Care, University Hospitals of Geneva, University of Geneva, 1 Rue Michel Servet, CH-1205 Geneva, Switzerland. [3]Department of Anesthesiology and Intensive Therapy, University of Szeged, 8 Semmelweis str, Szeged H-6725, Hungary.

References

1. Rivers E, Nguyen B, Havstad S, Ressler J, Muzzin A, Knoblich B, Peterson E, Tomlanovich M. Early goal-directed therapy collaborative G: early goal-directed therapy in the treatment of severe sepsis and septic shock. N Engl J Med. 2001;345(19):1368–77.
2. Goepfert MS, Richter HP, Zu Eulenburg C, Gruetzmacher J, Rafflenbeul E, Roeher K, von Sandersleben A, Diedrichs S, Reichenspurner H, Goetz AE, et al. Individually optimized hemodynamic therapy reduces complications and length of stay in the intensive care unit: a prospective, randomized controlled trial. Anesthesiology. 2013;119(4):824–36.
3. Hahn RG, Lyons G. The half-life of infusion fluids: an educational review. Eur J Anaesthesiol. 2016;33(7):475–82.
4. Jacob M, Chappell D, Hofmann-Kiefer K, Helfen T, Schuelke A, Jacob B, Burges A, Conzen P, Rehm M. The intravascular volume effect of Ringer's lactate is below 20%: a prospective study in humans. Crit Care. 2012;16(3):R86.
5. Puyana JC. Resuscitation of hypovolemic shock. In: Fink MP, editor. Textbook of critical care. 5th ed. Philadelphia: Elsevier Saunders; 2005. p. 1939–40.
6. Rossaint R, Bouillon B, Cerny V, Coats TJ, Duranteau J, Fernandez-Mondejar E, Filipescu D, Hunt BJ, Komadina R, Nardi G, et al. The European guideline on management of major bleeding and coagulopathy following trauma: fourth edition. Crit Care. 2016;20:100.
7. Fodor GH, Babik B, Czovek D, Doras C, Balogh AL, Bayat S, Habre W, Petak F. Fluid replacement and respiratory function: comparison of whole blood with colloid and crystalloid: a randomised animal study. Eur J Anaesthesiol. 2016;33(1):34–41.
8. Bayat S, Albu G, Layachi S, Portier F, Fathi M, Petak F, Habre W. Acute hemorrhagic shock decreases airway resistance in anesthetized rat. J Appl Physiol. 2011;111(2):458–64.
9. Petak F, Hantos Z, Adamicza A, Asztalos T, Sly PD. Methacholine-induced bronchoconstriction in rats: effects of intravenous vs. aerosol delivery. J Appl Physiol. 1997;82(5):1479–87.

10. Petak F, Banfi A, Toth-Szuki V, Barati L, Bari F, Szekely E, Novak Z. Airway responsiveness and bronchoalveolar lavage fluid profiling in individual rats: effects of different ovalbumin exposures. Respir Physiol Neurobiol. 2010;170(1):76–82.
11. Franken H, Clement J, Cauberghs M, Van de Woestijne KP. Oscillating flow of a viscous compressible fluid through a rigid tube: a theoretical model. IEEE Trans Biomed Eng. 1981;28(5):416–20.
12. Hantos Z, Daroczy B, Suki B, Nagy S, Fredberg JJ. Input impedance and peripheral inhomogeneity of dog lungs. J Appl Physiol. 1992;72(1):168–78.
13. Petak F, Hall GL, Sly PD. Repeated measurements of airway and parenchymal mechanics in rats by using low-frequency oscillations. J Appl Physiol. 1998;84(5):1680–6.
14. Lee HB, Blaufox MD. Blood volume in the rat. J Nucl Med. 1985;26(1):72–6.
15. Bain BJ, Bates I. Basic haematological techniques. In: Bain BJ, Lewis SM, Bates I, editors. Practical Haematology. Edinburgh: Churchill Livingstone; 2001. p. 19–46.
16. Camilo LM, Avila MB, Cruz LF, Ribeiro GC, Spieth PM, Reske AA, Amato M, Giannella-Neto A, Zin WA, Carvalho AR. Positive end-expiratory pressure and variable ventilation in lung-healthy rats under general anesthesia. PLoS One. 2014;9(11):e110817.
17. Kudoh I, Segawa Y, Numata K, Kitamura H. PaO2 change during progressive pulmonary edema in dogs. Crit Care Med. 1985;13(12):1020–4.
18. Perlman CE, Lederer DJ, Bhattacharya J. Micromechanics of alveolar edema. Am J Respir Cell Mol Biol. 2011;44(1):34–9.
19. Robinson BRH, Cohen MJ, Holcomb JB, Pritts TA, Gomaa D, Fox EE, Branson RD, Callcut RA, Cotton BA, Schreiber MA *et al*: Risk factors for the development of acute respiratory distress syndrome following hemorrhage. Shock. 2017. https://www.ncbi.nlm.nih.gov/pubmed/29194339.
20. Robinson BR, Cotton BA, Pritts TA, Branson R, Holcomb JB, Muskat P, Fox EE, Wade CE, del Junco DJ, Bulger EM, et al. Application of the Berlin definition in PROMMTT patients: the impact of resuscitation on the incidence of hypoxemia. J Trauma Acute Care Surg. 2013;75(1 Suppl 1):S61–7.
21. Petak F, Fodor GH, Babik B, Habre W. Airway mechanics and lung tissue viscoelasticity: effects of altered blood hematocrit in the pulmonary circulation. J Appl Physiol. 2016;121(1):261–7.
22. Allen SJ. Fluid therapy and outcome: balance is best. J Extra Corpor Technol. 2014;46(1):28–32.
23. Mutter TC, Ruth CA, Dart AB. Hydroxyethyl starch (HES) versus other fluid therapies: effects on kidney function. Cochrane Database Syst Rev. 2013;7:CD007594.
24. Skhirtladze K, Base EM, Lassnigg A, Kaider A, Linke S, Dworschak M, Hiesmayr MJ. Comparison of the effects of albumin 5%, hydroxyethyl starch 130/0.4 6%, and Ringer's lactate on blood loss and coagulation after cardiac surgery. Br J Anaesth. 2014;112(2):255–64.
25. Finfer S, Bellomo R, Boyce N, French J, Myburgh J, Norton R, Investigators SS. A comparison of albumin and saline for fluid resuscitation in the intensive care unit. N Engl J Med. 2004;350(22):2247–56.
26. Lira A, Pinsky MR. Choices in fluid type and volume during resuscitation: impact on patient outcomes. Ann Intensive Care. 2014;4:38.
27. Myburgh JA, Mythen MG. Resuscitation fluids. N Engl J Med. 2013;369(13): 1243–51.
28. Orbegozo Cortes D, Gamarano Barros T, Njimi H, Vincent JL. Crystalloids versus colloids: exploring differences in fluid requirements by systematic review and meta-regression. Anesth Analg. 2015;120(2):389–402.
29. Boland MR, Noorani A, Varty K, Coffey JC, Agha R, Walsh SR. Perioperative fluid restriction in major abdominal surgery: systematic review and meta-analysis of randomized, clinical trials. World J Surg. 2013;37(6):1193–202.
30. Aga Z, Machina M, McCluskey SA. Greater intravenous fluid volumes are associated with prolonged recovery after colorectal surgery: a retrospective cohort study. Br J Anaesth. 2016;116(6):804–10.
31. Brandstrup B, Tonnesen H, Beier-Holgersen R, Hjortso E, Ording H, Lindorff-Larsen K, Rasmussen MS, Lanng C, Wallin L, Iversen LH, et al. Effects of intravenous fluid restriction on postoperative complications: comparison of two perioperative fluid regimens: a randomized assessor-blinded multicenter trial. Ann Surg. 2003;238(5):641–8.
32. Navarro LH, Bloomstone JA, Auler JO Jr, Cannesson M, Rocca GD, Gan TJ, Kinsky M, Magder S, Miller TE, Mythen M, et al. Perioperative fluid therapy: a statement from the international fluid optimization group. Perioper Med (Lond). 2015;4:3.
33. Della Rocca G, Vetrugno L, Tripi G, Deana C, Barbariol F, Pompei L. Liberal or restricted fluid administration: are we ready for a proposal of a restricted intraoperative approach? BMC Anesthesiol. 2014;14:62.
34. Smorenberg A, Ince C, Groeneveld AJ. Dose and type of crystalloid fluid therapy in adult hospitalized patients. Perioper Med (Lond). 2013;2(1):17.
35. Burdett E, Dushianthan A, Bennett-Guerrero E, Cro S, Gan TJ, Grocott MP, James MF, Mythen MG, O'Malley CM, Roche AM, et al. Perioperative buffered versus non-buffered fluid administration for surgery in adults. Cochrane Database Syst Rev. 2012;12:CD004089.
36. Phillips CR, Vinecore K, Hagg DS, Sawai RS, Differding JA, Watters JM, Schreiber MA. Resuscitation of haemorrhagic shock with normal saline vs. lactated Ringer's: effects on oxygenation, extravascular lung water and haemodynamics. Crit Care. 2009;13(2):R30.
37. Barnas GM, Stamenovic D, Lutchen KR. Lung and chest wall impedances in the dog in normal range of breathing: effects of pulmonary edema. J Appl Physiol. 1992;73(3):1040–6.

9

Systematic review and bibliometric analysis of african anesthesia and critical care medicine research: hierarchy of evidence and scholarly productivity

Ulrick Sidney Kanmounye[1,2*], Joel Noutakdie Tochie[3,4], Aimé Mbonda[5,6,7], Cynthia Kévine Wafo[3], Leonid Daya[3,7], Thompson Hope Atem[8], Arsène Daniel Nyalundja[1,9] and Daniel Cheryl Eyaman[3]

Abstract

Background: Research is an essential component of Anesthesia, and the contributions of researchers and institutions can be appreciated from the analysis of scholarly outputs. Such analyses help identify major contributors and trends in publication. Little is known about the state of Anesthesia and Critical Care Medicine (A.C.C.M.) research in Africa. We aimed to describe African A.C.C.M. research's current landscape by determining its productivity per country and point towards possible ideas for improvement.

Methods: The authors searched PubMed, Embase, Web of Science, and Cumulative Index to Nursing and Allied Health Literature (CINAHL) from inception to May 4, 2020, for articles on or about A.C.C.M. in Africa. Studies were selected based on their titles and abstracts. Rayyan software was later on used for data management in the review selection process. Then, the full-text of eligible articles were screened. Data were extracted, and the number of articles per physician anesthesia providers and provider density were calculated. Kruskal Wallis test and Spearman's correlation were used, and a P-value < 0.05 was considered statistically significant.

Results: Of the 4690 articles, only 886 (18.9%) were included in the analysis. The articles were published between 1946 and 2020 in 278 target journals. 55 (6.2%) articles were published in the South African Journal of Surgery, 51 (5.8%) in Anesthesia and Analgesia, and 46 (5.2%) in Anaesthesia. 291 (32.8%) studies were cross-sectional. 195 (22.0%) first authors were from Nigeria, 118 (13.3%) from South Africa, and 88 (9.9%) from the U.S.A. Malawi (1.67), Togo (1.06), and Sierra Leone (1.00) had the highest number of articles per provider. Whereas Ethiopia (580.00), Nigeria (336.21), and Malawi (333.33) had the highest number of articles per provider density.

Conclusion: We identified the most and least productive African countries in A.C.C.M. research and a low-quality hierarchy of evidence in these publications. Hence, the study's findings may aid in driving the A.C.C.M. research agenda and capacity building in Africa.

Keywords: Africa, Anesthesia, Bibliometrics, Global anesthesia, Research

* Correspondence: ulricksidney@gmail.com
[1]Department of Research, Association of Future African Neurosurgeons, Kinshasa, Democratic Republic of Congo
[2]Department of Neurosurgery, Faculty of Medicine, Bel Campus University of Technology, Kinshasa, Democratic Republic of Congo

Background

African anesthesia and critical care medicine (A.C.C.M.) face numerous challenges: delayed patient presentations, lack of equipment, lack of an adequate specialist workforce, poor information management infrastructure, and lack of funding [1–3]. These barriers hamper the development of A.C.C.M. practice, education, and research. Out of the three components of A.C.C.M., research has the greatest potential to change the status quo. First, research can help identify the barriers of universal A.C.C.M. access in Africa [4]. Research has been used, for example, to map the workforce deficit and to identify obstacles to the development of A.C.C.M. services in Africa [5, 6]. Also, research can help design, monitor, and evaluate context-specific solutions to previously identified problems [4]. This has been the case with the World Health Organization surgical safety checklist, the LifeBox pulse oximeter, and oxygen provision in low-resource settings [3, 7, 8].

Research can equally improve the career trajectory of individuals and the academic standing of institutions. Their colleagues respect high academic performers, get promoted, and be recruited to more prestigious institutions [9–11]. Similarly, prolific academic institutions attract talented researchers, secure more funding, and gain recognition from the research community and the public [12].

We aimed to describe the landscape of AACM research in Africa, and we hypothesized that the most significant contributions to African A.C.C.M. were from South Africa and Western countries.

Methods

Search strategy

A protocol was developed and can be accessed online (https://doi.org/10.13140/RG.2.2.28999.32167). PubMed, Embase, Web of Science, and Cumulative Index to Nursing and Allied Health Literature (CINAHL) were searched from inception to May 4, 2020, using a systematic Boolean search strategy (Additional File 1) developed by an author (U.S.K.). The search was developed without language limits, and it covered articles on or about anesthesia and critical care practice in Africa. Articles in languages none of the authors understood were sent to a professional medical translator on ProZ (http://www.proz.com, ProZ, Syracuse, New York, U.S.A.). After the database search, Google Scholar, ResearchGate, and ORCiD were searched. This hand search was informed using forward and backward citation analyses, i.e., the articles cited by the studies found during the database search and the articles that cited the studies found during the database search.

Screening

The citations were exported then uploaded on the free online review platform - Rayyan (https://rayyan.qcri.org/, Doha, Qatar). First, duplicates were excluded, then each article was (title and abstract) screened by at least two reviewers (J.T.N., AM, C.W.S., L.D., TA, A.D.N., and D.C.E.). Next, conflicts were resolved by the authors concerned, and if the two authors could not agree, a third author (U.S.K.) was sought for arbitration.

Data extraction and analysis

Metadata of all the articles included were extracted - article title, year of publication, author affiliations, study design. The data were stored on Google Forms (Google, Menlo Park, CA, U.S.A.) then imported into SPSS v26 (I.B.M., Armonk, NY, U.S.A.). The publication trends, author contributions, and hierarchy of evidence frequencies were calculated and visualized using Tableau Public (Salesforce, Mountain View, CA, U.S.A.).

The absolute number of published articles is a good measure of academic proficiency and research aptitude; however, it does not factor individual contributions at the level of a nation. Countries with more physician anesthesia providers (P.A.P.s) are expected to have higher research outputs. To account for this, the authors chose to calculate the number of articles per African P.A.P.s. This metric was calculated by dividing the number of first author articles by the number of P.A.P.s from each African country. A major barrier to A.C.C.M. research is the lack of protected research time [13]. The P.A.P. density (P.A.P.s per 100,000 population) was used to account for the clinical workload's effect on research output.

The data on the P.A.P.s (total P.A.P.s and P.A.P.s per 100,000 population) was obtained from a 2015/2016 survey of the World Federation of Societies Anaesthesiologists [14]. Also, correlations were computed between the number of articles and the P.A.P. data. The P.A.P. data of six countries (Botswana, Djibouti, Gambia, Lesotho, Seychelles, and Sudan) was not available, so they were excluded from the analysis. The bivariate analyses (Kruskal Wallis test and Spearman's correlation) were run and considered statistically significant when the P-value < 0.05.

Results

The search strategy returned 4690 articles: 4688 from databases and 22 from the supplementary hand search. We excluded 705 duplicates and reviewed 3985 non-duplicate articles. After the title and abstract screening, we excluded 2922 more articles because they were irrelevant. Most irrelevant articles returned articles from Papua New Guinea and animal research on guinea pigs in non-African countries (Fig. 1).

Publication trends and target journals

The final 886 citations were published between 1946 and 2020. The publication trend had three primary

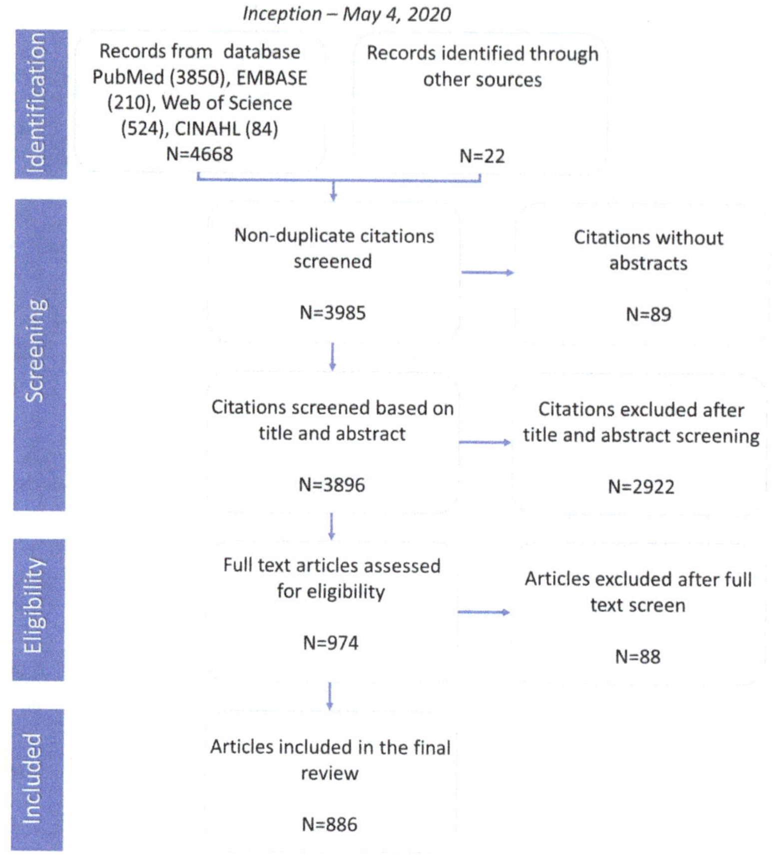

Fig. 1 Flow diagram illustrating the search strategy

cycles with peaks in 1981 (11 articles), 1993 (14 articles), and 2018 (71 articles) ($P = 0.48$) (Fig. 2).

The articles were published in 278 journals. South African Journal of Surgery (55 articles, 6.2%), Anesthesia and Analgesia (51, 5.8%), and Anaesthesia (46, 5.2%) were the top contributors. The top 50 journals are displayed in Table 1.

Hierarchy of evidence

Most (291, 32.8%) studies had a cross-sectional design. The next most common study designs were cohort studies (172, 19.4%) and randomized controlled trials (76, 8.6%). There were a few animal studies (2, 0.2%) and published guidelines (1, 0.1%) (Additional File 2 Table).

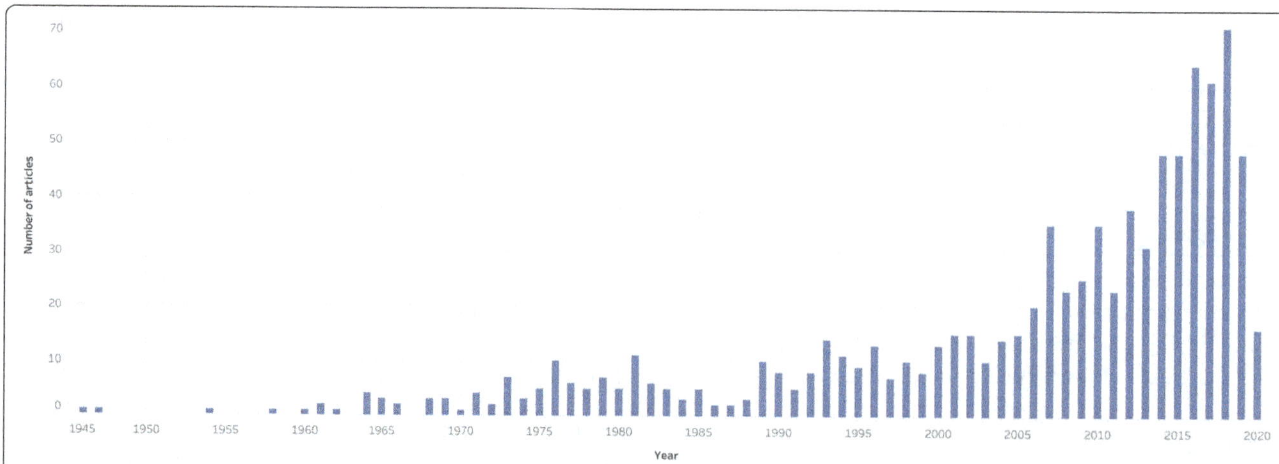

Fig. 2 Publication trends in African anesthesia

Table 1 Top 50 target journals for African anesthesia research

Journal	Frequency (*N* = 886)	Percentage (%)
1. South African Journal of Surgery	55	6.2
2. Anesthesia and Analgesia	51	5.8
3. Anaesthesia	46	5.2
4. East African Medical Journal	33	3.7
5. West African Medical Journal	31	3.5
6. Pan African Medical Journal	26	2.9
7. Tropical Doctor	26	2.9
8. Annales Francaises d'Anesthesie et de Réanimation	23	2.6
9. Canadian Journal of Anaesthesia	21	2.4
10. World Journal of Surgery	21	2.4
11. British Journal of Anaesthesia	16	1.8
12. Médecine Tropicale	16	1.8
13. African Journal of Medicine and Medical Sciences	15	1.7
14. International Journal of Gynaecology and Obstetrics	13	1.5
15. The Nigerian Postgraduate Medical Journal	13	1.5
16. African Health Sciences	12	1.4
17. PLoS One	11	1.2
18. La Tunisie Médicale	10	1.1
19. Nigerian Journal of Medicine	10	1.1
20. International Journal of Obstetric Anesthesia	8	0.9
21. Middle East Journal of Anaesthesiology	8	0.9
22. South African Medical Journal	8	0.9
23. Lancet	7	0.8
24. Nigerian Journal of Clinical Practice	7	0.8
25. Dakar Medical	6	0.7
26. Paediatric Anaesthesia	6	0.7
27. African Journal of Paediatric Surgery	5	0.6
28. Anesthesiology	5	0.6
29. B.M.C. Anesthesiology	5	0.6
30. Journal of Obstetrics and Gynaecology	5	0.6
31. Médecine et Santé Tropicales	5	0.6
32. Nigerian Quarterly Journal of Hospital Medicine	5	0.6
33. Anesthesiology Research and Practice	4	0.5
34. B.M.C. Health Services Research	4	0.5
35. B.M.C. Research Notes	4	0.5
36. British Journal of Nursing	4	0.5
37. Journal Français d'Ophtalmologie	4	0.5
38. Journal of Clinical Anesthesia	4	0.5
39. South African Dental Journal	4	0.5
40. Southern African Journal of Anaesthesia and Analgesia	4	0.5
41. The Central African Journal of Medicine	4	0.5
42. Trials	4	0.5
43. African Journal of Reproductive Health	3	0.3
44. Anaesthesia and Intensive Care	3	0.3

Table 1 Top 50 target journals for African anesthesia research *(Continued)*

Journal	Frequency (*N* = 886)	Percentage (%)
45. Annals of The Royal College of Surgeons of England	3	0.3
46. Cahiers d'Anesthésiologie	3	0.3
47. Central African Journal of Medicine	3	0.3
48. Ethiopian Journal of Health Sciences	3	0.3
49. Ethiopian Medical Journal	3	0.3
50. International Anesthesiology Clinics	3	0.3

First author academic output

The first authors were affiliated with institutions of 62 countries. Most (36, 58.1%) countries were African, and the median number of first author articles by Africans was 8.5 (IQR = 16.25). The most productive first authors were affiliated with institutions from Nigeria (195, 22.0%), South Africa (118, 13.3%), U.S.A. (88, 9.9%), UK (65, 7.3%), and Ethiopia (29, 3.3%) (Fig. 3).

The median number of articles per African P.A.P.s was 0.13 (IQR = 0.38), while the median number of articles per African P.A.P. density was 30.65 (IQR = 88.29) articles. Malawi had the highest number of articles per African P.A.P.s (1.67), followed by Togo (1.06), and Sierra Leone (1.00). When taking into account the P.A.P. density, Ethiopia (580.00), Nigeria (336.21), and Malawi (333.33) were the most significant contributors (Table 2). The number of articles was correlated significantly with the number of African P.A.P.s ($R = 0.40$, $P = 0.03$) but not with the African P.A.P. density ($R = 0.23$, $P = 0.22$).

Second and senior author contributions

There were 245 (27.5%) single-author articles. Similarly to the first authorship, Nigeria was a major contributor among second authors (133, 15.0%). South Africa (77, 8.7%) and the U.S.A. (72, 8.1%) were the second and third major contributors to second author positions.

While Nigeria remained the major contributor among first authors (89, 10.0%), South Africa dropped to the third place (47, 5.3%) behind the U.S.A. 74 (8.4%) (Fig. 4).

Discussion

This study is the first comprehensive analysis of A.C.C.M. research in Africa. African A.C.C.M. publication had cycles of increasing amplitude organized around three peaks. Also, we noted an essential increase in the scholarly output over the last 20 years. The articles were published in a variety of journals, and most studies had an observational study design. Moreover, researchers from Nigeria and South Africa contributed the most to the scholarly output.

Academic output

Malawi, Sierra Leone, and Togo had the highest number of articles per P.A.P. Malawi ranked among the highest contributors in publications, publications per P.A.P.s, and publications per P.A.P. density. This indicates that Malawian P.A.P.s are proficient researchers despite a higher workload. Both Sierra Leone and Togo have median articles per P.A.P. density below the African median. Moreover, Sierra Leone was adversely affected by the Ebola virus disease and benefited from international aid [15]. This aid fostered the creation of

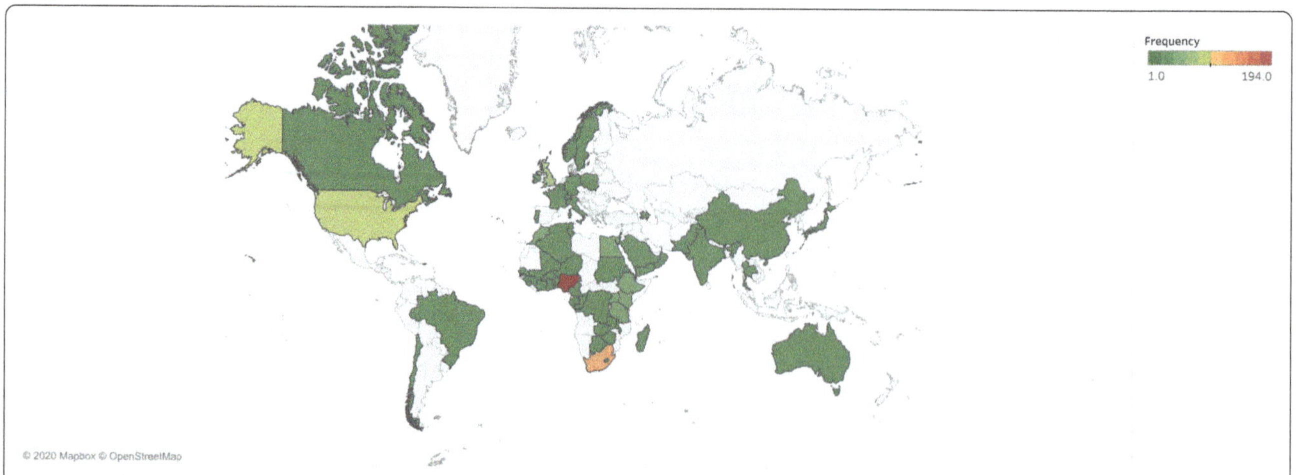

Fig. 3 Heat map showing the affiliations of first authors. This map is not under copyright and is freely available to use

Table 2 Scholarly output per physician anesthesia provider and physician anesthesia provider density

Country	Articles per physician anesthesia provider	Articles per physician anesthesia provider density
Algeria	0.00	0.26
Benin	0.88	93.33
Botswana	NA	NA
Burkina Faso	0.04	7.14
Cameroon	0.42	100.00
Congo, Rep.	0.22	10.53
Côte d'Ivoire	0.04	9.46
Djibouti	NA	NA
D.R.C.	0.05	38.50
Egypt	0.00	3.99
Eritrea	NAN	NAN
Ethiopia	0.57	580.00
Gabon	0.05	0.78
Gambia	NA	NA
Ghana	0.13	35.00
Guinea	0.67	100.00
Kenya	0.12	56.82
Lesotho	NA	NA
Madagascar	0.13	30.43
Malawi	1.67	333.33
Mali	0.02	3.33
Morocco	0.04	14.29
Niger	0.07	14.29
Nigeria	0.19	336.21
Rwanda	0.33	38.24
Senegal	0.20	30.65
Seychelles	NA	NA
Sierra Leone	1.00	66.67
South Africa	0.01	7.29
Sudan	NA	NA
Tanzania	0.42	233.33
Togo	1.06	78.26
Tunisia	0.03	0.04
Uganda	0.31	122.22
Zambia	0.13	20.41
Zimbabwe	0.09	13.25

NA Data not available, *NAN* Not a number value

partnerships between local PAPS and foreign P.A.P.s. On the other hand, Togo has trained local P.A.P.s and P.A.P.s from neighboring French-speaking countries, thereby increasing the quantity of Anesthesia research and researchers [16]. Furthermore, Togo and Sierra Leone have relatively small populations (less than 9 million) than other African countries. Hence, increases in the absolute number of articles and P.A.P.s lead to more remarkable changes in the number of articles per P.A.P.s and P.A.P. density.

One-third (18, 33.3%) of African countries did not have first-author publications. This finding is not surprising because African researchers face numerous barriers to publication.

Barriers faced by African A.C.C.M. researchers include lack of funding, institutional support, inexperience, and

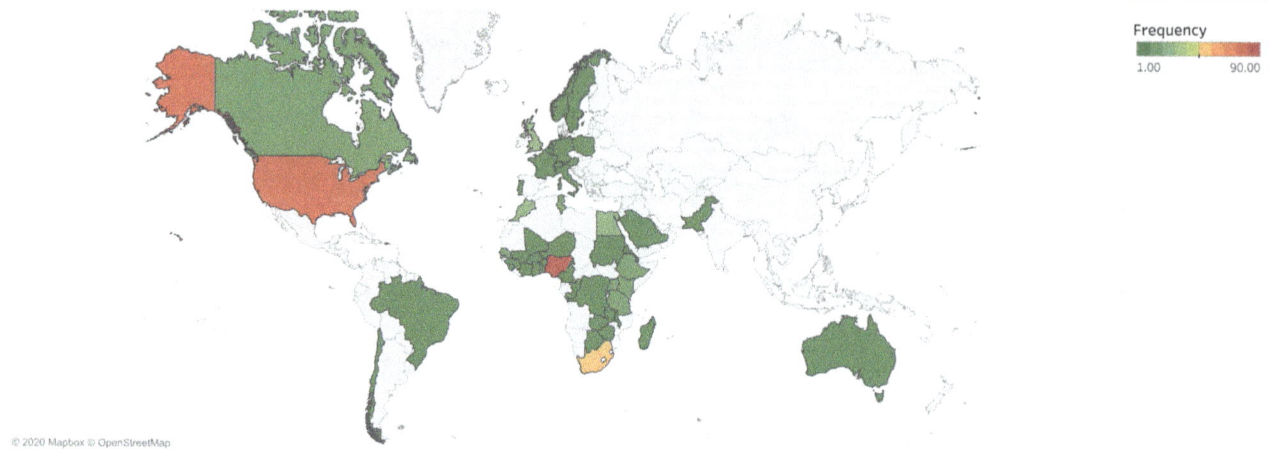

Fig. 4 Heat map showing the affiliations of the last authors. This map is not under copyright and is freely available to use

lack of mentorship [13]. Researchers lack funding to conduct research and to pay for the time spent away from clinical duties. Fortunately, most high impact open access journals offer a sizable discount to researchers from low- and middle-income countries.

African countries, without first author publications, should collaborate with higher-performing countries. The more experienced African researchers can mentor and build capacity among less experienced researchers in neighboring countries. The African Perioperative Research Collaborative is an excellent example of the potential of inter-African A.C.C.M. research collaboratives. The African Perioperative Research Collaborative is a group led by members of the South African Perioperative Research Collaborative that has facilitated A.C.C.M. clinical research among African researchers via technical support, mentorship, and capacity building [4, 17].

A sizable proportion (25, 40.3%) of the first authors were affiliated to non-African institutions, most of them from high-income countries. This might explain why some countries did not have first-author publications. African researchers often assume the role of middle authors when they collaborate with researchers from high-income countries [18]. The lack of first author publications could equally be due to publications in journals that are not indexed in the major databases. Young African researchers often target foreign journals to increase their articles' visibility because most local journals have low impact factors and small readerships [19–22]. However, African researchers face numerous barriers to publish in international journals, especially if they have high impact factors, and some researchers eventually resort to publishing in predatory journals [22]. These predatory journals do not offer transparent and rigorous peer-review and do not meet the indexation criteria in major databases [23]. Further research is needed to understand the causes of the non-representation of the 18 countries.

The most substantial increase in publications occurred during the early 2000s, and they can be explained by increased interest in Global Anesthesia. Global Anesthesia is a field at the crossroads between anesthesia and public health that focuses on access to safe, timely, and affordable anesthesia care in the world. The World Federation of Societies of Anesthesiologists (W.F.S.A.) and prominent specialty journals supported research on access to and safety in anesthesia care. For example, the W.F.S.A. was a founding member and a sponsor of LifeBox and the World Health Organization Safe Surgery checklist, respectively [3, 5, 7]. Moreover, the W.F.S.A., high-income country academic centers, and non-governmental organizations have developed global anesthesia fellowships in South Africa, Ethiopia, Kenya, and Tanzania, contributing significantly to A.C.C.M. research in Africa. This is evidenced by the sizeable contribution of authors affiliated with non-African institutions to African A.C.C.M. research.

Hierarchy of evidence

There were few systematic reviews and guidelines among the African A.C.C.M. articles. These two forms of information synthesis are among the highest forms of scientific evidence and should inform practice [24]. The integration of evidence-based medicine to A.C.C.M. is common practice today [25]. However, the implementation of international guidelines to A.C.C.M. practice in Africa is faced with numerous challenges that require adaptation [26, 27]. The adaptation of international guidelines is necessary because the guidelines are based on evidence generated in resource-rich milieus, and there is a dearth of evidence-based and context-specific

African guidelines [28, 29]. African researchers must develop these context-specific African guidelines from high-quality scientific evidence. To increase the quality of the evidence generated, African researchers must hone existing skills and acquire new ones. In systematic reviews, researchers can train using the Cochrane Interactive Learning online resource that offers free access to most African nationals [30].

Also, there were few animal studies among the African A.C.C.M. publications. Although animal studies generate lower-grade scientific evidence, they are essential to the development of A.C.C.M.. For example, animal research played an essential role in developing the Guedel cannula, curarisation, and motor blocks [31]. Africa's rich biodiversity and ethnopharmacology are likely to house the next essential drug in A.C.C.M [32]. This untapped potential could lead to the discovery and production of more affordable drugs for African patients. Unfortunately, African basic science researchers face more barriers than clinical researchers. Researchers are challenged by lack of funding, difficulties obtaining ethical approvals, and inadequate infrastructure [33, 34]. Balogun et al. have proposed the engagement of local and international funding agencies by researchers, the use of invertebrates, and innovative low-cost research methods [35].

Journals

A significant proportion of the top 50 journals were specialty journals, and only one of the specialty journals was African. Unsustainable financial models can explain the dearth of African specialty journals, lack of editorial expertise, and low submissions quality [36]. All these factors precipitate the failure of young journals. Young specialty journals can curtail the effects of these challenges if they collaborate with more experienced journals. The African Journal Partnership Program provides mentorship and capacity from leading journals of high-income countries to African journals' editorial teams [37].

The African Journal Partnership Program model should be supplemented by inter-African partnerships between more and less experienced journals. The top contributing journal was South African, and the only African specialty journal was equally South African and emphasized the critical role of South African journals in A.C.C.M. research. The prominence of South African journals is an opportunity for other journals to learn from a successful African editorial staff.

A considerable number of articles were published in non-local high impact factor specialty journals. Similar trends have been observed in Europe and South Asia [38, 39]. Publication in a high impact journal does not guarantee visibility or recognition [40]. Citation metrics are better measures of visibility and recognition [41]; however, we did not collect data on citations. Future studies should evaluate the quantitative and qualitative impact of African A.C.C.M. research. Notwithstanding, the publication of African articles in high impact factor journals attests to the quality of research emanating from the continent.

The future of A.C.C.M. research in Africa

Going forward, African A.C.C.M. research must adopt a "no woman/man left behind" approach. Continental-level professional groups like the Africa Regional Section of the World Federation of Societies of Anesthesiologists should oversee a continental research agenda focused on capacity-building, especially in countries without first author publications. The capacity-building could be organized online and in-person (concomitantly with continental meetings). These training sessions should be opened not only to specialist physicians but equally to nurse anesthetists, residents, and medical students. Nurse anesthetists, residents, and medical students can help decrease the research workload by contributing to data curation, project administration, and writing of original manuscript drafts. In the absence of protected research time, this strategy can "buy" some time for specialist physicians and build capacity among non-physicians.

Limitations

We acknowledge the following limitations in our study: our definition of African research excluded Africans' research about A.C.C.M. in other continents. Next, we considered studies to be equal irrespective of their citation metrics or study design. Therefore, we did not factor the impact of the studies into the contributions. Hence, a letter to the editor with lower citation metrics was considered equal to a systematic review with higher citation metrics. Finally, we limited our analysis to prominent author positions. As such, we failed to capture a detailed picture of the contributors to African A.C.C.M. research. In addition, our search strategy could have been more explicit. We initially opted for a more comprehensive search strategy, but the results returned many irrelevant results. Given our limited resources, we opted for a less broad search. Despite these limitations, we believe our study adds value to existing research.

Conclusion

This study analyzed the publication trends, study designs, target journals, and contributions to A.C.C.M. research in Africa. There has been an increase in article publication over the past two decades, and the greatest contributors are Nigeria and Malawi. This analysis helped to identify less productive countries, subspecialties, and study designs. As such, our findings can be used to set the A.C.C.M. research agenda in Africa.

Abbreviations

A.C.C.M: Anesthesia and critical care medicine; P.A.P.s: Physician anesthesia providers

Acknowledgments

We wish to thank Daniel S. Nteranya for his help during the initial stages of the investigation.

Authors' contributions

U.S.K. conceptualized the study, investigated, curated, analyzed, and visualized the data, wrote the original draft of the manuscript, and administered the project. J.N.T., A.M., C.K.W., L.D., T.H.A., A.D.N., and D.C.E. investigated, validated, and wrote the original manuscript draft. All authors have read and approved the manuscript

Author details

[1]Department of Research, Association of Future African Neurosurgeons, Kinshasa, Democratic Republic of Congo. [2]Department of Neurosurgery, Faculty of Medicine, Bel Campus University of Technology, Kinshasa, Democratic Republic of Congo. [3]Department of Anesthesiology and Critical Care Medicine, Faculty of Medicine and Biomedical Sciences, University of Yaounde I, Yaounde, Cameroon. [4]Human Research Education and Networking, Yaounde, Cameroon. [5]Faculty of Medicine and Biomedical Sciences, University of Yaounde I, Yaounde, Cameroon. [6]Surgery Unit, District Hospital of Batouri, Batouri, Cameroon. [7]Department of Research, International Student Surgical Network, Yaounde, Cameroon. [8]Department of Internal Medicine, Faculty of Medicine, Bel Campus University of Technology, Kinshasa, Democratic Republic of Congo. [9]Faculty of Medicine, Catholic University of Bukavu, Bukavu, Democratic Republic of Congo.

References

1. Epiu I, Tindimwebwa JVB, Mijumbi C, Chokwe TM, Lugazia E, Ndarugirire F, et al. Challenges of anesthesia in low- and middle-income countries: A cross-sectional survey of access to safe obstetric anesthesia in East Africa. Anesth Analg. 2017;124:290–9.
2. Epiu I, Wabule A, Kambugu A, Mayanja-Kizza H, Tindimwebwa JVB, Dubowitz G. *Key* bottlenecks to the provision of safe obstetric anaesthesia in low- income countries; a cross-sectional survey of 64 hospitals in Uganda. BMC Pregnancy Childbirth. 2017;17:387.
3. Epiu I, Tindimwebwa JVB, Mijumbi C, Ndarugirire F, Twagirumugabe T, Lugazia ER, et al. Working towards safer surgery in Africa; a survey of utilization of the WHO safe surgical checklist at the main referral hospitals in East Africa. BMC Anesthesiol. 2016;16:60.
4. Biccard BM. Priorities for peri-operative research in Africa. Anaesthesia. 2020; 75:e28–33.
5. Dubowitz G, Detlefs S, McQueen KAK. Global anesthesia workforce crisis: a preliminary survey revealing shortages contributing to undesirable outcomes and unsafe practices. World J Surg. 2010;34:438–44.
6. Ho M, Livingston P, Bould MD, Nyandwi JD, Nizeyimana F, Uwineza JB, et al. Barriers and facilitators to implementing a regional anesthesia service in a low-income country: a qualitative study. Pan Afr Med J. 2019;32. https://doi.org/10.11604/pamj.2019.32.152.17246.
7. Dubowitz G, Breyer K, Lipnick M, Sall JW, Feiner J, Ikeda K, et al. Accuracy of the Lifebox pulse oximeter during hypoxia in healthy volunteers. Anaesthesia. 2013;68:1220–3.
8. Walker IA, Bashford T, Fitzgerald JE, Wilson IH. Improving anesthesia safety in low-income regions of the world. Curr Anesthesiol Rep. 2014;4:90–9.
9. Swaminathan M, Glas KE, Heller L, Augoustides JGT, Culp WC, Sniecinski RM. Mission possible: successful careers in adult cardiothoracic anesthesiology- what I wish I had known in the first 5 years after fellowship. J Cardiothorac Vasc Anesth. 2017;31:321–8.
10. Culley DJ, Fahy BG, Xie Z, Lekowski R, Buetler S, Liu X, et al. Academic productivity of directors of ACGME-accredited residency programs in surgery and anesthesiology. Anesth Analg. 2014;118:200–5.
11. Ahmad S, De Oliveira GS, McCarthy RJ. Status of anesthesiology resident research education in the United States: structured education programs increase resident research productivity. Anesth Analg. 2013;116:205–10.
12. Wood M. Maintaining and fostering the future success of academic anesthesia: recruiting and training the next generation of academic anesthesiologists. Anesth Analg. 2013;116:1–3.
13. Elobu AE, Kintu A, Galukande M, Kaggwa S, Mijjumbi C, Tindimwebwa J, et al. Research in surgery and anesthesia: challenges for post-graduate trainees in Uganda. Educ Health Abingdon Engl. 2015;28:11–5.
14. Kempthorne P, Morriss WW, Mellin-Olsen J, Gore-Booth J. The W.F.S.A. Global anesthesia workforce survey. Anesth Analg. 2017;125:981–90.
15. Bolkan HA, van Duinen A, Samai M, Bash-Taqi DA, Gassama I, Waalewijn B, et al. Admissions and surgery as indicators of hospital functions in Sierra Leone during the west-African Ebola outbreak. B.M.C. Health Serv Res. 2018;18:1–9.
16. Maman A, Zoumenou E, Zéminkandé J, Kaboré F, Bula Bula I, Tagirumugabe T, et al. Anaesthesia training: where and how it is conducted in French-speaking sub-Saharan Africa? Update Ahesthesia. 2008;24:42–4.
17. Biccard BM, Madiba TE, Kluyts H-L, Munlemvo DM, Madzimbamuto FD, Basenero A, et al. Perioperative patient outcomes in the African surgical outcomes study: a 7-day prospective observational cohort study. Lancet. 2018;391:1589–98.
18. Hedt-Gauthier BL, Jeufack HM, Neufeld NH, Alem A, Sauer S, Odhiambo J, et al. Stuck in the middle: a systematic review of authorship in collaborative health research in Africa, 2014–2016. BMJ Glob Health. 2019;4:e001853.
19. Kokwaro G, Kariuki S. Medical research in Africa: problems and some solutions. Malawi Med J J Med Assoc Malawi. 2001;13:40.
20. Rusakaniko S, Makanga M, Ota MO, Bockarie M, Banda G, Okeibunor J, et al. Strengthening national health research systems in the WHO African region - progress towards universal health coverage. Glob Health. 2019;15:50.
21. Dhalla KA, Guirguis M. Barriers and incentives for conducting research amongst the ophthalmologists in sub-Sahara Africa. PLoS One. 2018;13:e0197945.
22. Tarkang EE, Bain LE. The bane of publishing a research article in international journals by African researchers, the peer-review process and the contentious issue of predatory journals: a commentary. Pan Afr Med J. 2019;32. https://doi.org/10.11604/pamj.2019.32.119.18351.
23. Huh S. How to add a journal to the international databases, science citation index expanded and medline. Arch Plast Surg. 2016;43:487–90.
24. Schulman SR, Schardt C, Erb TO. Evidence-based medicine in anesthesiology. Curr Opin Anaesthesiol. 2002;15:661–8.
25. Myles PS, Bain DL, Johnson F, McMahon R. Is anaesthesia evidence-based? A survey of anaesthetic practice. Br J Anaesth. 1999;82:591–5.
26. Chica HO, Okello E. Evidence-based medicine practice in Africa: is it feasible? Trop Dr. 2009;39:61–2.
27. Mellins CA, Nestadt D, Bhana A, Petersen I, Abrams EJ, Alicea S, et al. Adapting evidence-based interventions to meet the needs of adolescents growing up with H.I.V. in South Africa: the VUKA case example. Glob Soc Welf Res Policy Pract. 2014;1:97–110.
28. Motani P, Van de Walle A, Aryeetey R, Verstraeten R. Lessons learned from evidence-informed decision-making in Nutrition & Health (EVIDENT) in Africa: a project evaluation. Health Res Policy Syst. 2019;17:12.
29. Aryeetey R, Holdsworth M, Taljaard C, Hounkpatin WA, Colecraft E, Lachat C, et al. Evidence-informed decision making for nutrition: African experiences and way forward. Proc Nutr Soc. 2017;76:589–96.
30. Cochrane Interactive Learning. Cochrane Training. Cochrane Training. 2020. https://training.cochrane.org/. Accessed July 8 2020.
31. Goyal R. Animal testing in the history of anesthesia: now and then, some stories, some facts. J Anaesthesiol Clin Pharmacol. 2015;31:149–51.
32. Malterud KE. Ethnopharmacology, chemistry and biological properties of four Malian medicinal plants. Plants. 2017;6. https://doi.org/10.3390/plants6010011.
33. Nyika A. Animal research ethics in Africa: an overview. Acta Trop. 2009; 112(Suppl 1):S48–52.
34. Grants awarded to support small animal research in Africa. Vet Rec. 2016; 178:432. https://veterinaryrecord.bmj.com/content/178/18/432.2.
35. Balogun WG, Cobham AE, Amin A, Seeni A. Advancing neuroscience research in Africa: invertebrate species to the rescue. Neuroscience. 2018; 374:323–5.
36. Goehl TJ, Flanagin A. Enhancing the quality and visibility of African medical and health journals. Environ Health Perspect. 2008;116:A514–5.
37. Bickton FM, Manda-Taylor L, Hamoonga R, Mwenda AS. Challenges facing sub-Saharan African health science journals and benefits of international collaborations and partnerships. Sci Ed. 2019;42:116–9.
38. Figueredo E, Muñoz BF. Evaluation and evolution of the scientific production by Spanish anesthesiology departments. Rev Esp Anestesiol Reanim. 2002;49:306–13.
39. Chen S-Y, Wei L-F, Ho C-M. Trend of academic publication activity in anesthesiology: A 2-decade bibliographic perspective. Asian J Anesthesiol. 2017;55:3–8.

40. Brink PA. Article visibility: journal impact factor and availability of full text in PubMed central and open access. Cardiovasc J Afr. 2013;24:295–6.
41. Baltussen A, Kindler CH. Citation classics in anesthetic journals. Anesth Analg. 2004;98:443–51 table of contents.

10

PreAnaesThesia Computerized Health (PATCH) assessment: development and validation

Tarig Osman[1], Eileen Lew[2*], Elaine Pooi-Ming Lum[1,3], Louise van Galen[1,4], Rajive Dabas[2], Ban Leong Sng[2] and Josip Car[1,5]

Abstract

Background: Technological advances in healthcare have enabled patients to participate in digital self-assessment, with reported benefits of enhanced healthcare efficiency and self-efficacy. This report describes the design and validation of a patient-administered preanaesthesia health assessment digital application for gathering medical history relevant to preanaesthesia assessment. Effective preoperative evaluation allows for timely optimization of medical conditions and reduces case cancellations on day of surgery.

Methods: Using an iterative mixed-methods approach of literature review, surveys and panel consensus, the study sought to develop and validate a digitized preanaesthesia health assessment questionnaire in terms of face and criterion validity. A total of 228 patients were enrolled at the preoperative evaluation clinic of a tertiary women's hospital. Inclusion criteria include: age ≥ 21 years, scheduled for same-day-admission surgery, literacy in English and willingness to use a digital device. Patient perception of the digitized application was also evaluated using the QQ10 questionnaire. Reliability of health assessment questionnaire was evaluated by comparing the percentage agreement of patient responses with nurse assessment.

Results: Moderate to good criterion validity was obtained in 81.1 and 83.8% of questions for the paper and digital questionnaires respectively. Of total 3626 response-pairs obtained, there were 3405 (93.4%) concordant and 221 (6.1%) discrepant response-pairs for the digital questionnaire. Discrepant response-pairs, such as ""no/yes" and "unsure/yes", constitute only 3.7% of total response-pairs. Patient acceptability of the digitized assessment was high, with QQ10 value and burden scores of 76 and 30%, respectively.

Conclusions: Self-administration of digitized preanaesthesia health assessment is acceptable to patients and reliable in eliciting medical history. Further iteration should focus on improving reliability of the digital tool, adapting it for use in other languages and incorporating clinical decision tools.

Keywords: Preanaesthesia assessment, Computer-assisted history-taking system, Digital health

Background

Current practice guidelines mandate that patients undergo preanaesthesia assessment prior to surgery and anaesthesia, defined as the process of clinical assessment that precedes the delivery of anaesthesia care for surgery and non-surgical procedures [1]. Its goal is to allow for timely identification and optimization of medical conditions, thereby reducing perioperative morbidity and mortality. Effective preoperative evaluation can also decrease case delays and cancellations on day of surgery [2].

Traditionally, preanaesthesia assessment is conducted by a health care provider via a face-to-face interview with the patient. Studies suggest that self-administration of digital assessment questionnaires is a feasible means of gathering

* Correspondence: eileen.lew@singhealth.com.sg
[2]Department of Women's Anaesthesia, KK Women's and Children's Hospital (Singapore), 100 Bukit Timah Road, Singapore 229899, Singapore

medical information for preanaesthesia assessment [3–12]. Compared with in-person interviews, these digital self-assessment tools are associated with patient acceptance and satisfaction, reliability of information and improved efficiency of assessment [4, 6, 9].

At the preoperative evaluation clinic of our hospital, a 33-item preanaesthesia health assessment paper questionnaire is currently administered to elective surgical patients by nurses to gather medical information pertinent to preanaesthesia assessment [13]. Based on pre-determined criteria, responses help to identify patients with medical issues who require outpatient anaesthetic review 2 to 4 weeks in advance of surgery. Relatively healthy patients are allowed to bypass outpatient referral and undergo standard anaesthetic review on the day of surgery. The questionnaire has served our purpose well, but is not designed for patient self-administration as it contained technical language and medical terms.

In line with global advances in information technology, healthcare institutions are increasingly leveraging on digital health technologies for care delivery. Local hospital statistics indicate that an average 900 patients are scheduled for elective surgeries every month and this number is expected to increase, as disease burden increases with an aging population. To cope with this demand, we postulate that a patient self-administered digital health assessment tool can be developed and implemented for the purpose of gathering medical history relevant for preanaesthesia assessment. The virtual tool allows remote access, so that assessment questionnaires can be completed at a time, place and pace convenient to the patient. The present study describes our experience in the development and validation of a patient-administered digital preanaesthesia health assessment questionnaire on a tablet device at a tertiary hospital.

Methods

The study was conducted at a preoperative evaluation clinic that provides care for women scheduled for elective surgery at a tertiary hospital. A working group comprising three consultant anaesthetists, six clinic nurses and five digital health researchers from a local medical school sought to develop a patient self-administered digital preanaesthesia health assessment application through an iterative process. Ethics approval was granted by the Nanyang Technological University Institutional Review Board (Ref: IRB-2017-12-011) and the SingHealth Institutional Review Board (Ref: 2017/3002).

A mixed-methods approach was adopted. A paper version of the questionnaire was first designed and validated, before conversion to a digital prototype. We hereby refer to the paper versions as Forms 1 and 2 and the digital version as Form 3. All versions of the questionnaire were developed in English and iteratively, each version was an improvement over the previous. Figure 1 describes the phases of development and validation of the questionnaires from paper to digital formats.

Phase 1: development and assessment of form 1

The self-administered paper questionnaire, Form 1, was designed after an extensive review of relevant literature via Pubmed and Google Scholar. Search terms used include (*preanaesthesia* or *preanesthesia* or *pre-anaesthetic* or *pre-anesthetic* or *preoperative* or *pre-operative*) and *(health assessment* or *screening* or *questionnaire)* and/or *(validation)*. Shortlisted questionnaires were further examined for scope and relevance of domains and items, options of response types (i.e. binary/non-binary/free-text response), and design format of questions. Through consensus, the working group also determined the clinically relevant domains and corresponding items to be included in Form 1.

First draft of Form 1 was then presented to twelve attending anaesthetists of the hospital for evaluation of its face validity. While the domains were deemed adequate, the anaesthetists suggested the addition of follow-up questions to qualify some items e.g. number of pack-years as a follow-up to a positive history of cigarette smoking.

The draft of Form 1 was also evaluated at a workshop, where multidisciplinary staff of a local medical school provided feedback on its readability, clarity and contextualization. Participants suggested terms to replace technical jargon and reduced ambiguity in questions. Questions were structured according to domains of the body systems and each question was verified to assess only one domain or concept to the extent permissible (Supplementary Box 1). A glossary of terms (Supplementary Box 2) was also appended to provide explanation of medical terms.

With the collective feedback obtained, Form 1 was finalised and administered as a pen-and-paper survey to a convenience sample of 33 patients in a pilot study, herewith referred to as "Study 1". The aim of this survey was to identify problems that were not addressed or considered during the design of the questionnaire. Inclusion criteria for patient recruitment were: age ≥ 21 years, ability to read and write in English and scheduled for same-day-admission surgery. After written informed consent, all patients were given instructions on the completion of Form 1, with emphasis on unassisted self-assessment. Following that, each patient underwent a semi-structured interview using questions adapted from the QQ-10 questionnaire, [14] an established instrument for measuring face validity, feasibility and utility of healthcare questionnaires. For our purpose, the original QQ-10 questionnaire was modified by amending options of "mostly disagree" to "disagree" and "mostly agree" to "agree". Upon completion of the interview, each patient underwent a nurse-led assessment as per standard of care. Demographic data and time taken to complete Form 1 were recorded. Data from Form 1 was

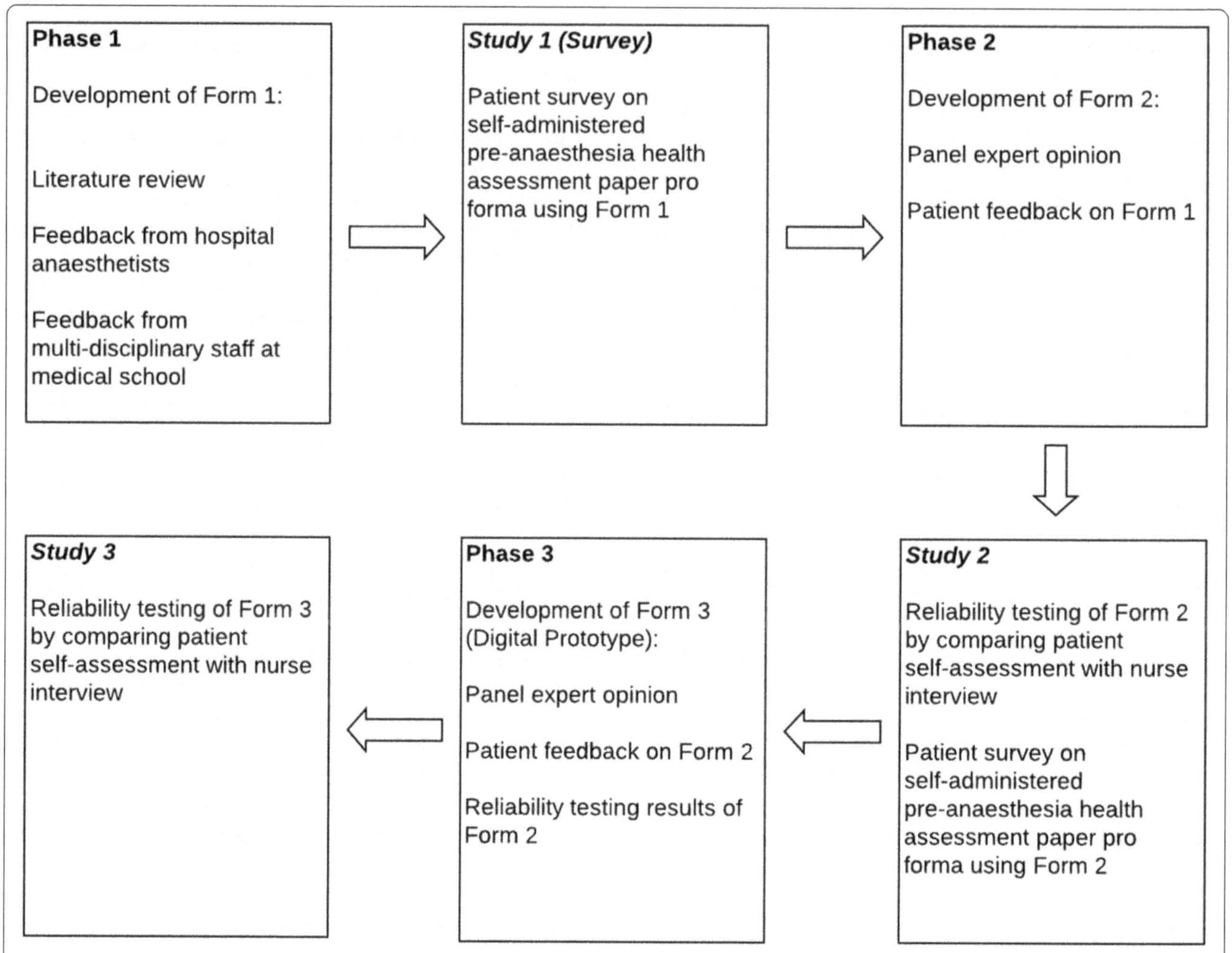

Fig. 1 Mixed-methods approach to the development of PATCH

analyzed using IBM SPSS version 25 (IBM corp. Armonk, NY, USA). Data from the QQ-10 questionnaire was analyzed both quantitatively and qualitatively, using thematic analysis.

Phase 2 – iteration of form 1 to form 2, with validation

Form 2 was an iteration of Form 1, based on the feedback received from participants of Study 1. Improvements included the re-phrasing of questions to improve clarity and insertion of visual illustrations. The explanation of eight terms in the glossary section was also edited to improve ease of understanding (Supplementary Box 3).

A validation study targeting a larger convenience sample size of 104 patients was conducted. Referred as "Study 2", 104 patients scheduled for same-day-admission surgery were recruited on presentation to the preoperative evaluation clinic during the designated study period. The primary aim of the study was to evaluate the criterion validity of Form 2 before its conversion to a digital prototype. The inclusion criteria were similar to those of Study 1.

The sample size was chosen, based on a similar study reported in the literature [15]. Consenting patients first completed Form 2 independently, after which their responses were verified by the nurse via a structured face-to-face interview, guided by Form 2. If a discrepancy of response was noted, the nurse would make annotations upon verification with the patient. Each patient was also interviewed using the modified QQ-10 questionnaire, as described for Study 1.

Criterion validity of the questionnaire was assessed by measuring the agreement between the patient responses and those obtained during nurse assessment. To account for questions with prevalence < 5% or > 95%, we have opted to report percentage agreement (PA), instead of the Kappa coefficient. PA is defined as number of questions with concurring responses divided by the total number of questions. Criterion validity is considered good if PA ≥ 95%, moderate if PA between 90 to < 95% and poor when PA < 90% [10]. The frequency of identical ("Yes/Yes", "No/No" and "Unsure/Unsure"), contradictory ("Yes/No" or "No/Yes"), and non-contradictory ("Unsure/Yes", "Unsure/No," "Yes/Unsure", and "No/Unsure") response pairs were also analysed. Sum of the contradictory and non-contradictory response rates describe the total discrepancy error rate. Data were analyzed using IBM SPSS version 25, as described for Survey 1.

Phase 3 – development and validation of form 3

The iteration of Form 2 to Form 3 (the first digital protoype) was based on findings obtained from Phase 2 and renewed input from the working group (Supplementary Box 4). The digital application, called PreAnaesThesia Computerized Health assessment, or PATCH, was developed on an iOS platform on a tablet, using React Native (JavaScript framework). The server was made using NodeJS, a JavaScript framework. Data was stored on MongoDB database. For the purpose of the study, the server program and database were located on a secure server at the Nanyang Technological University.

Improvements adopted for Form 3 included further rephrasing of questions to reduce ambiguity and deletion of questions deemed to be irrelevant. To facilitate patients in listing their medications and previous surgeries, a drop-down list of common medications and surgeries was developed, using data gathered from participants in Phase 1 and 2. The glossary of terms was configured to appear as pop-up boxes of explanation when activated by screen-touch. In addition, the application was designed to provide a summary page for review and final edit before submission. Screenshots of the digital prototype are shown in Supplementary Figure 1.

As the criterion validity of a paper questionnaire does not necessarily extend to its electronic format [16], validation of the digital prototype, Form 3, was conducted in Study 3. In addition to the inclusion criteria described in the earlier phases, the ability to use a tablet device was added as a criterion for recruitment. One hundred and six patients were recruited at the preoperative evaluation clinic over 8 weeks. Consenting participants completed digital self-assessment on a tablet unaided, then underwent nurse assessment using a provider interface of the digital tool and with the nurse blinded to the patient's responses. PA for each response pair was measured. Time to completion of self-assessment was automatically captured by the application. Data was analysed using IBM SPSS verison 25.

Results

Study 1 (survey)

Of 33 patients recruited, 32 completed the study. One patient was excluded when the nature of admission was converted from same-day-admission to inpatient. Patients identified themselves as Chinese (23/71.9%), Malay (4/12.5%), Indian (1/3.1%), and others (4/12.5%), consistent with the ethnic distribution in the local general population. Median (IQR) age was 37 (32.2, 43) years. Median (IQR) time to complete self-assessment was 4 (3, 5) minutes. None of the patients identified any question as being uncomfortable to answer (Table 1). Table 2 describes the patient perception of selected statements from the QQ-10. Overall, patient perception of self-assessment was favourable.

A total of 48 feedback comments were obtained from 21 patients. They pertained mostly to the clarification of medical terms (13/61.9%) and availability of options to guide entry of medications and past surgeries (8 / 38.1%). These comments were taken into consideration in the iteration of Form 1 to Form 2.

Study 2

Of 104 patients recruited, 98 patients (94.2%) completed the study and 6 were excluded due to incomplete paperwork. The patients identified themselves as Chinese (50/51%), Malay (24/24.5%), Indian (10/10.2%), and others (14/14.3%), with a median (IQR) age of 38.5 (33, 44) years. Patients took 7.3 (5.6, 9.4) [median (IQR)] minutes to complete pre-anaesthesia self-assessment and generally responded favourably to statements measuring value in the QQ-10 questionnaire (Table 3). Among negative perceptions, length of questions emerged as the most frequent reason. Of note, 82 (83.7%) of participants were willing to utilize a digital version of the questionnaire in the future.

Analysis of patient feedback on the design of Form 2 revealed a total of 56 comments from 32 (32.7%) patients. Majority of comments referred to the need for clarification of medical terms (23/71.9%). There were requests to shorten the length of the questionnaire (3/9.4%). Overall QQ-10 value and burden scores were 76% (SD = 13%) and 30% (SD = 12.5%), respectively. Mean score for value questions ranged from 2.9 to 3.3, while the mean score for burden questions ranged from 0.9 to 1.64.

Table 4 shows the inter-rater reliability of Form 2. Good criterion validity was attained for 24 of 37 (65%) questions. Six (16%) questions were classified as having moderate criterion validity while seven (19%) had poor criterion validity. Total number of response pairs was 3626. Of these, 3432 were identical, giving a concordance rate of 94.6%. Sixty-seven (1.8%) were discrepant contradictory responses while 127 (3.5%) were discrepant non-contradictory responses, giving total discrepant responses of 194 (5.4%). Of these, the most common discrepant response pair was "unsure/no" (94/2.6%), followed by "yes/no" (63/1.7%) and "unsure/yes" (32/0.9%).

Study 3

Of 104 patients recruited, 98 (94.2%) patients completed the study. They were predominantly of Chinese (55/55.1%), Malay (18/18.4%) and Indian (6/6.1%) ethnicity. Notably, 88 (89.8%) patients were below 50 years old.

Table 1 Patients' assessment of Form 1 (*n* = 32)

	Yes (n/%)	No (n/%)
Relevance		
Do you understand why we have asked you to complete the questionnaire?	32 (100)	0 (0)
Did the questions seem relevant to you and your medical history?	31 (96.9)	1 (3.1)
Language and content		
Did you understand most of the wording of the questionnaire?	31 (96.9)	1 (3.1)
Were there any medical terms you did not understand?	9 (28.1)	23 (71.9)
Were there any questions you felt were important but missed?	5 (15.6)	27 (84.4)
Did the questions prompt you to remember anything?	3 (9.4)	29 (90.6)
Was there any area that had too many questions on?	2 (6)	30 (94)
Were there any questions you did not feel comfortable/expect answering?	0 (0)	32 (00)

Median (IQR) completion time to self-assessment on the digital application was 6.4 (4.8, 8.6) minutes. Table 5 shows the results of reliability testing of Form 3. Good criterion validity was obtained for 23 of 37 (62%) questions. Eight (22%) questions had moderate criterion validity while 6 (16%) questions had poor criterion validity. Total number of response pairs was 3626. Of these, 3405 were identical, giving a concordance rate of 93.9%. There were 133 (3.7%) discrepant contradictory responses and 88 (2.4%) discrepant non-contradictory responses, giving a total of 221 (6.1%) discrepant responses. The most common discrepant response pair was "yes/no" (89/2.5%), followed by "unsure/no "(76/2.1%), "no/yes" (44/1.2%), "unsure/yes" (11/0.3%) and "yes/unsure" (1/0.03%).

Based on these findings, the working group made further enhancements to the digital application (Supplementary Box 6). In summary, the "unsure" option was deleted to encourage commitment to a definitive response. Probing stems of questions were also added to specific domains to improve qualification of symptoms. Drop-down options of past surgeries, medications and allergies were updated to include more choices. These amendments led to the development of an improved digital version. The feasibility of its implementation was reported in a study published recently [17].

Discussion

Using a robust, mixed-methods approach, the present study describes the development and validation of a patient-administered digital assessment application on a tablet device for the purpose of gathering medical history relevant to preanaesthesia assessment. The PreAnaesthesia Computerized health Assessment (PATCH) application is accepted by patients and reliable when compared with nurse-led assessment.

For health assessment instruments to have practical value, they should have reliability and validity. An example of content validity is face validity – the extent to which items are perceived to be relevant to the intended construct, while criterion validity is a dimension of reliability. Compared to published studies [10], the present study achieved > 90% criterion validity in 84% of questions in the digital prototype. The difference could be related to differences in subject characteristics, such as literacy and social factors, which result in different perception and interpretation of the questions [15].

In the analysis of responses between patient self-assessment and nurse assessment, discrepant contradictory response-pairs, such as ""no/yes" and "unsure/yes", can be concerning as they suggest failure of the digital tool to detect an issue that is eventually uncovered by nurse assessment. Fortunately, these constitute only

Table 2 Patient feedback on Form 1, based on modified QQ-10 questionnaire (n = 32)

	Strongly agree and agree n (%)	Neutral (n/%)	Strongly disagree and disagree (n/%)
The questionnaire was relevant to my condition.	30 (93.8)	0 (0)	2 (6.3)
The questionnaire was easy to complete.	30 (93.8)	0 (0)	2 (6.3)
I would be happy to complete it again in the future as part of my routine care.	25 (78.1)	5 (16)	2 (6)
The questionnaire was too embarrassing.	0 (0)	1 (3)	31 (97)
The questionnaire was too complicated.	3 (9)	4 (13)	25 (78)
The questionnaire was too long.	3 (9)	8 (25)	21 (66)

Table 3 Patient feedback on Form 2, based on modified QQ-10 questionnaire ($n = 98$)

	Strongly agree – agree (n/%)	Neutral (n/%)	Strongly disagree – disagree (n/%)
The questionnaire helped me to communicate about my condition with the nurse.	95 (96.9)	2 (2.04)	1 (1.02)
The questionnaire was easy to complete.	89 (90.8)	8 (8.2)	1 (1.02)
The questionnaire included all the aspects of my condition that I am concerned about.	88 (89.8)	9 (9.2)	1 (1.02)
The questionnaire was relevant to my condition.	85 (86.7)	12 (12.2)	1 (1.02)
I would be happy to complete it again in the future as part of my routine care.	75 (76.5)	16 (16.3)	7 (7.1)
I enjoyed filling in the questionnaire.	56 (57.1)	32 (32.7)	10 (10.2)
The questionnaire was too long.	15 (15.3)	36 (36.7)	47 (48)
The questionnaire was too complicated.	7 (7.1)	19 (19.4)	72 (73.5)
The questionnaire was too embarrassing.	1 (1.02)	9 (9.2)	88 (89.8)
The questionnaire upset me.	2 (2)	6 (6.1)	90 (91.8)
The information sheet was helpful.	89 (90.8)	8 (8.2)	1 (1)
If you had to complete this at home or in the clinic online, do you think you could?	77 (78.6)	16 (16.3)	5 (5.1)
I liked completing the questionnaire while in the waiting area.	65 (66.3)	21 (21.4)	12 (12.2)
I am comfortable answering sensitive questions in the questionnaire first than I would with the nurse.	70 (71.4)	20 (20.4)	8 (8.2)
I answered the questionnaire truthfully to the best of my knowledge.	94 (95.9)	4 (4.1)	0 (0)
I am willing to take an iPad version of this questionnaire in the future.	82 (83.7)	13 (13.3)	3 (3)
I prefer to talk to the nurse/doctor instead completing the questionnaire.	25 (25.5)	43 (43.9)	30 (31)

3.7% of total responses in the validation of the digital prototype. The fact that 93.9% of total response-pairs were concordant strongly supports its reliability in gathering preoperative medical information.

We observed that participants in the present study were mainly English-literate female, with median age < 40 years. Studies suggest that age and literacy can affect a patient's perception and willingness to adopt mobile health technology. In a systematic review to evaluate barriers in adopting telemedicine, age, level of education and computer literacy emerged as key patient-related determinants [18]. The authors speculated that preference for personalised care and lack of training in new technology among older patients could have contributed to this observation. In another study that examined the usage patterns of virtual health services, younger and predominantly female patients were more likely to be early adopters of virtual medical consultations [19]. In driving digital strategies for patient care, healthcare organisations must address the needs of patients and tailor the engagement platform according to patients' prefences and technology know-how. In the present study, 83.7% of participants in Phase 2 of the study had expressed receptiveness to the use of a digital self- assessment tool. This is not surprising, given the young age of our patients and the high internet penetration rate in the local population [20]. Concerns of data breach should be addressed with strict regulation and compliance with Health Level 7 (HL7) standards, through secure networks, data encryption, login controls and auditing.

Positive patient acceptance of digital health assessment has motivated us to re-design our clinical pathways, leveraging on telemedicine to achieve greater value. PATCH could serve as an online triage tool to determine if patients undergo a tele-consultation or in-person consultation for anaesthetic referral. With an average patient wait-time of 24 min at the preoperative evaluation clinic (unpublished data from internal audit), conversion of physical to tele-consultation could improve patient experience and clinic efficiency. The clinic could, in turn, focus its resources on optimizing care for medically-complex patients who present physically for consultation. Reducing physical visits to healthcare facilities could also confer the benefit of reducing the transmission of infectious diseases [21].

There are limitations to the present study. Recruitment of a larger sample would have allowed the use of Kappa coefficient for measurement of criterion validity. As the patients' socio-economic characteristics were not reported, we could not control for bias due to socio-economic factors. The study was conducted in young adult female patients of a local healthcare facility. The study may yield

Table 4 Inter-rater Reliability Testing of Form 2

		PA	Criterion validity
1	Do you have any allergies (to medicines, sticking plaster, iodine, latex, food, etc.)?	94	Moderate
2	As medicines and supplements can affect body functions and interact with anaesthetics, please list all the medicines (including traditional medicines and health supplements) you are currently taking on a regular or daily basis in the last 2 weeks. [a]	–	–
3	Have you ever had an operation?	97	Good
4	Are you ever short of breath after walking up two flights of stairs or an overhead bridge?	88	Poor
5	Was your heart activity ever measured using wires on your chest (an ECG or electrocardiogram)?	76	Poor
6	Has a doctor ever told you, you have high blood pressure, also known as 'hypertension'?	96	Good
7	Do you have, or have you ever had chest pain that you felt tight or heavy (not from coughing)?	88	Poor
8	Have you ever had a heart attack?	100	Good
9	Do you have frequent swelling in feet or ankles?	89	Poor
10	Do you have, or have you ever had treatment for problems with your heartbeat (too low, too fast, irregular)?	91	Moderate
11	Has a doctor ever told you they heard an abnormal sound (e.g. a click or a murmur) whilst listening to your heart?	98	Good
12	Do you have a cardiac pacemaker or an implanted cardioverter-defibrillator?	100	Good
13	Have you ever had heart surgery (valve or stent or bypass operation)?	99	Good
14	Do you have or have you ever had blood clots in legs or lungs?	98	Good
15	Have you ever had a blood transfusion?	99	Good
16	Do you have asthma or have you had asthma as a child?	98	Good
17	Do you currently have a cough lasting more than 8 weeks?	99	Good
18	Do you have a long-term lung disease (such as chronic bronchitis or chronic obstructive pulmonary disease)?	98	Good
19	Do you have or have you had sleep apnoea?	92	Moderate
20	Have you been told that you snore so loud you keep others awake while you are asleep?	91	Moderate
21	Have you ever had an X-ray of your chest?	86	Poor
22	Do you smoke or have you ever smoked?	100	Good
23	Do you have gastric reflux or heartburn?	85	Poor
24	Do you have or have you ever had liver problems (such as hepatitis or cirrhosis)?	98	Good
25	How many days a week do you drink alcohol (on average)? [a]	–	–
26	Do you have or have you ever had abnormal kidney function or kidney disease?	100	Good
27	Have you ever had a (minor) stroke or a brain bleed?	100	Good
28	Do you have or have you ever had fits/seizures/epilepsy?	99	Good
29	Have you ever lost consciousness?	99	Good
30	Do you have or have you ever had diabetes or diabetes related to pregnancy?	98	Good
31	Do you have or have you ever had thyroid problems (e.g. thyroid hormone levels being too high or too low or having an enlarged thyroid)?	93	Moderate
32	Do you have loose/chipped teeth, crowns, bridges, veneers or dentures?	94	Moderate
33	Do you have difficulty swallowing?	98	Good
34	Do you have difficulty opening your mouth wide?	97	Good
35	Do you have or have you ever had pain or stiffness in the lower back, neck or jaw?	82	Poor
36	Have you ever been told that you have had problems with anaesthetics in a previous operation, such as an abnormal reaction to anaesthesia or allergy to anaesthetics?	95	Good
37	Has any of your blood relatives ever had problems with anaesthetics in a previous operation?	96	Good
38	Do you have or have you ever had anxiety, depression or other emotional/psychiatric disorders?	95	Good
39	Do you have any other medical information that we should know about?	98	Good

[a] This question required a free-text response and thus, was excluded from reliability testing

Table 5 Inter-rater Reliability Testing of Form 3

		[a]PA	Criterion validity
1	Do you have any allergies (to medicines, sticking plaster, iodine, latex, food, etc.)?	97	Good
2	As medicines and supplements can affect body functions and interact with anaesthetics, please list all the medicines (including traditional medicines and health supplements) you are currently taking on a regular or daily basis in the last 2 weeks. [b]	–	–
3	Have you ever had an operation (including major dental surgery e.g. wisdom teeth extraction)?	89	Poor
4	Are you ever short of breath after walking up two flights of stairs or an overhead bridge?	76	Poor
5	Have you ever had an ECG (or electrocardiogram) and been told it was not normal?	86	Poor
6	Has a doctor ever told you, you have high blood pressure, also known as 'hypertension'?	95	Good
7	Do you have, or have you ever had chest pain that you felt tight or heavy (not from coughing)?	91	Moderate
8	Have you ever had a heart attack?	100	Good
9	Do you have frequent swelling in both feet or both ankles?	92	Moderate
10	Do you have, or have you ever had treatment for problems with your heartbeat (too low, too fast, irregular)?	97	Good
11	Has a doctor ever told you they heard an abnormal sound (e.g. a click or a murmur) whilst listening to your heart?	97	Good
12	Do you have a cardiac pacemaker or an implanted cardioverter-defibrillator?	98	Good
13	Have you ever had heart surgery (valve or stent or bypass operation)?	100	Good
14	Do you have or have you ever had blood clots in legs or lungs?	98	Good
15	Have you ever had a blood transfusion?	100	Good
16	Do you have asthma or have you had asthma as a child?	95	Good
17	Do you currently have a cough lasting more than 8 weeks?	97	Good
18	Do you have a long-term lung disease (such as chronic bronchitis or chronic obstructive pulmonary disease)?	99	Good
19	Has anyone told you that you stop breathing of choke during your sleep – a condition also known as sleep apnoea?	99	Good
20	Have you been told that you snore so loud you keep others awake while you are asleep?	90	Moderate
21	Do you often feel tired, fatigued or sleepy during the daytime (tired enough that you could fall asleep while performing activities e.g. driving, waking, texting)?	96	Good
22	Do you smoke or have you ever smoked?	90	Moderate
23	Do you have gastric reflux or heartburn?	80	Poor
24	Do you have or have you ever had liver problems (such as hepatitis or cirrhosis)?	97	Good
25	How many days a week do you drink alcohol (on average)? [b]	–	–
26	Do you have or have you ever had abnormal kidney function or kidney disease?	100	Good
27	Have you ever had a (minor) stroke or a brain bleed?	100	Good
28	Do you have or have you ever had fits/seizures/epilepsy?	100	Good
29	Have you ever lost consciousness?	98	Good
30	Do you have or have you ever had diabetes or diabetes related to pregnancy?	98	Good
31	Do you have or have you ever had thyroid problems (e.g. thyroid hormone levels being too high or too low or having an enlarged thyroid)?	95	Good
32	Do you have loose/chipped teeth, crowns, bridges, veneers or dentures?	91	Moderate
33	Do you have difficulty swallowing?	97	Good
34	Do you have difficulty opening your mouth wide?	98	Good
35	Do you have or have you ever had pain or stiffness in the lower back, neck or jaw?	81	Poor
36	Have you ever been told that you have had problems with anaesthetics in a previous operation, such as an abnormal reaction to anaesthesia or allergy to anaesthetics?	94	Moderate
37	Has any of your blood relatives ever had problems with anaesthetics in a previous operation?	91	Moderate
38	Do you have or have you ever had anxiety, depression or other emotional/psychiatric disorders?	94	Moderate
39	Do you have any other medical information that we should know about?	83	Poor

[a] denotes Percentage of Agreement
[b] This question required a free-text response and thus, was excluded from reliability testing

different results in a mixed gender population or another clinical setting. As the application is developed in English, the results may not be extrapolated to questionnaires translated to other languages. Further research is directed at improving validity of the digital application and adapting it for use in other languages. There is also a plan to incorporate decision support tools to aid in risk prediction and clinical decision-making. To maintain the human touch, questions would be developed to simulate human-to-human conversation, incorporating elements of empathy [22] – a technique demonstrated to evoke responses more effectively from subjects during a computerised interview.

Conclusion

Self-administration of digitized preanaesthesia health assessment is acceptable to patients and reliable in eliciting medical history. Further iteration should focus on improving reliability of the digital tool, adapting it for use in other languages and incorporating clinical decision tools.

Abbreviations

PATCH: Preanaesthesia computerized health (assessment); PHA: Preanaesthesia health assessment; SDA: Same-day-admission; PA: Percentage agreement

Acknowledgments

The authors would like to thank: Choy Jin Xiang and Lee King Chuan for helping to develop the software; Teng Han Hong April and Liu Juan for research administrative support; Xu Xuelian, Kee Hwei Min, Noor Haslinda Binte Khamis, Noraidah Binte Mansoor, Yip SeokCheng and Liew Chow Fong for the excellent nursing support at the preoperative clinic; Dr. Thach Thuan Quoc and Dr. Leong Wan Ling for reviewing the draft manuscripts.

Authors' contributions

TO helped with the planning of the study, data collection, compilation of statistics and the constitution of the manuscript. EL helped with the planning of the study and constitution of the manuscript. EPML helped with the planning of the study, feedback workshop for Form 1, research mentoring of TO, and constitution of the manuscript. LG helped with the planning of the study. RD and BLS helped with the planning of the study and constitution of the manuscript. JC helped with the planning of the study and constitution of the manuscript. All authors have read and agreed to the published version of the manuscript.

Author details

[1]Centre for Population Health Sciences, Lee Kong Chian School of Medicine, Nanyang Technological University (Singapore), Singapore, Singapore. [2]Department of Women's Anaesthesia, KK Women's and Children's Hospital (Singapore), 100 Bukit Timah Road, Singapore 229899, Singapore. [3]Present address: Duke-NUS Medical School, 8, College Road, Singapore 169857, Singapore. [4]Present address: Department of Internal Medicine, VU University Medical Center, De Boelelaan 1117, Room ZH 4A58, 1081 HV Amsterdam, Netherlands. [5]Global eHealth Unit, Department of Primary Care and Public Health, School of Public Health, Imperial College London (United Kingdom), London, UK.

References

1. Committee on S, Practice P, Apfelbaum JL, Connis RT, Nickinovich DG, American Society of Anesthesiologists Task Force on Preanesthesia E, Pasternak LR, Arens JF, Caplan RA, Connis RT, et al. Practice advisory for preanesthesia evaluation: an updated report by the American Society of Anesthesiologists Task Force on Preanesthesia Evaluation. Anesthesiology. 2012;116(3):522–38.
2. Ferschl MB, Tung A, Sweitzer BJ, Huo D, Glick DB. Preoperative clinic visits reduce operating room cancellations and delays. Anesthesiology. 2005; 103(4):855–9.
3. Vitkun SA, Gage JS, Anderson DH, Williams SA, Halpern-Lewis JG, Poppers PJ. Computerization of the preoperative anesthesia interview. Int J Clin Monit Comput. 1995;12(2):71–6.
4. VanDenKerkhof EG, Goldstein DH, Blaine WC, Rimmer MJ. A comparison of paper with electronic patient-completed questionnaires in a preoperative clinic. Anesth Analg. 2005;101(4):1075–80.
5. Tompkins BM, Tompkins WJ, Loder E, Noonan AF. A computer-assisted preanesthesia interview: value of a computer-generated summary of patient's historical information in the preanesthesia visit. Anesth Analg. 1980;59(1):3–10.
6. Essin DJ, Dishakjian R, Essin CD, Steen SN. Development and assessment of a computer-based preanesthetic patient evaluation system for obstetrical anesthesia. J Clin Monit Comput. 1998;14(2):95–100.
7. Goodhart IM, Andrzejowski JC, Jones GL, Berthoud M, Dennis A, Mills GH, Radley SC. Patient-completed, preoperative web-based anaesthetic assessment questionnaire (electronic personal assessment questionnaire PreOperative): development and validation. Eur J Anaesthesiol. 2017;34(4):221–8.
8. Beers RA, O'Leary CE, Franklin PD. Comparing the history-taking methods used during a preanesthesia visit: the HealthQuiz versus the written questionnaire. Anesth Analg. 1998;86(1):134–7.
9. Howell M, Hood AJ, Jayne DG. Use of a patient completed iPad questionnaire to improve pre-operative assessment. J Clin Monit Comput. 2017;31(1):221–5.
10. Zuidema X, Leuverink T, Houweling P. Validation of a patient self-administered pre-anaesthetic screening questionnaire. Int J Cover Surg Anaesthesiol Nurs Manag Issues Day Surg. 2014;31:181–5.
11. Vitkun SA, Halpern-Lewis JG, Williams SA, Gage JS, Poppers PJ. Patient's perceptions of an anesthesia preoperative computerized patient interview. J Clin Monit Comput. 1999;15(7):503–7.
12. Zuidema X, Tromp Meesters RC, Siccama I, Houweling PL. Computerized model for preoperative risk assessment. Br J Anaesth. 2011;107(2):180–5.
13. Lew E, Pavlin DJ, Amundsen L. Outpatient preanaesthesia evaluation clinics. Singap Med J. 2004;45(11):509–16.
14. Moores KL, Jones GL, Radley SC. Development of an instrument to measure face validity, feasibility and utility of patient questionnaire use during health care: the QQ-10. Int J Qual Health Care. 2012;24(5):517–24.
15. Hilditch W, Asbury A, Jack E, McGrane S. Validation of a pre-anaesthetic screening questionnaire. Anaesthesia. 2003;58(9):876–7.
16. Juniper EF, Langlands JM, Juniper BA. Patients may respond differently to paper and electronic versions of the same questionnaires. Respir Med. 2009; 103(6):932–4.
17. Osman T, Lew E, Lum E, Chew J, Dabas R, Sng BL, Car J. Effect of PreAnaesThesia computerized health (PATCH) assessment on duration of nurse—patient consultation and patient experience: a pilot trial. Int J Environ Res Pub Health. 2020;17(14):4972.
18. Kruse CS, Karem P, Shifflett K, Vegi L, Ravi K, Brooks M. Evaluating barriers to adopting telemedicine worldwide: a systematic review. J Telemed Telecare. 2018;24(1):4–12.
19. Jung C, Padman R. Virtualized healthcare delivery: understanding users and their usage patterns of online medical consultations. Int J Med Inform. 2014; 83(12):901–14.
20. Digital Influence Lab Pte Ltd. Singapore Digital Marketing Statistics. Availabe online: https://digitalinfluencelab.com/singapore-digital-marketing-stats/ (Accessed on 21 January 2020).
21. Wosik J, Fudim M, Cameron B, Gellad ZF, Cho A, et al. Telehealth transformation: COVID-19 and the rise of virtual care. J Am Med Inform Assoc. 2020;27(6):957–62.
22. Peiris DR, Gregor P, Alm N. The effects of simulating human conversational style in a computer-based interview. Interact Comput. 2000;12(6):635–50.

11

The low fresh gas flow anesthesia and hypothermia in neonates undergoing digestive surgeries

Yu Cui[1*†], Yu Wang[2†], Rong Cao[1†], Gen Li[3], Lingmei Deng[1] and Jia Li[1]

Abstract

Background: Based on the previous investigation in our institution, the incidence of intraoperative hypothermia in neonates was high. Since September 1st, 2019, the recommendation had been launched to utilize ≤1 L/min fresh gas flow during the neonates' surgical procedure. We therefore intended to evaluate the association between low fresh gas flow anesthesia and the occurrence of hypothermia in neonates undergoing digestive surgeries.

Methods: A retrospective chart review, before-after study was conducted for neonates who underwent digestive surgeries. The primary outcomes were the incidence of hypothermia. The secondary outcomes included hospital mortality, the value of lowest temperature, blood loss, mean body temperature during the surgery, the length of hypothermia during the surgery and postoperative hospital length-of- stay.

Results: 249 neonates fulfilled the eligibility criteria. The overall incidence of intraoperative hypothermia was 81.9%. The low fresh gas flow anesthesia significantly reduced the odds of hypothermia [routine group: 149 (87.6%) versus low flow group: 55 (69.6%); $p < 0.01$]. Moreover, the low fresh gas flow anesthesia could reduce the length of hypothermia [routine group: 104 mins (50, 156) versus low flow group: 30 mins (0,100); $p < 0.01$], as well as elevate the value of lowest temperature for neonates [routine group: 35.1 °C (34.5, 35.7) versus low flow group: 35.7 °C (35.3, 36); $p < 0.01$]. After adjustment for confounding, low fresh gas flow anesthesia and the length of surgical time were independently associated with intraoperative hypothermia.

Conclusions: Low fresh gas flow anesthesia is an effective way to alleviate hypothermia in neonates undergoing open digestive surgery.

Keywords: Low fresh gas flow anesthesia, Neonates, Hypothermia

* Correspondence: cuiyu19831001@163.com
†Yu Cui, Yu Wang and Rong Cao contributed equally to this work.
[1]Department of Anesthesiology, The Affiliated Hospital, School of Medicine, UESTC Chengdu Women's & Children's Central Hospital, No.1617, Riyue Avenue, Qingyang District, Chengdu 610091, PR China

Background

Intraoperative hypothermia that is defined as core temperature < 36.0 °C is one of complications faced by anesthesiologists during surgical period, which may exposure patients to acidosis, imbalanced oxygen consumption, delayed anesthesia recovery, coagulopathy, wound infections and bleeding [1, 2]. Available literature has proved that intraoperative hypothermia is an independent risk factor of early perioperative complications and mortality [3].

Among various surgeries, the occurrence of intraoperative hypothermia is high in digestive surgeries due to visceral and peritoneal surface exposure, anesthetic-induced impairment of thermoregulatory control and requirement of intestinal irrigation fluid. Lai et al. reported that patients' age is one of main factors contributed to inadvertent intraoperative hypothermia, and the overall incidence is as high as 83.3% in neonates despite the passive and active temperature management have been conducted [4]. Some congenital intestinal disorders in neonates need urgent surgical intervention, i.e., necrotizing enterocolitis, meconium ileus, and congenital intestinal atresia. This is indeed a challenge for anesthesia providers and scrub nurses because normothermia is hard to be maintained on neonates undergoing digestive surgeries. Compared to adults, the neonates are more susceptible to develop hypothermia since the mechanism of thermoregulation has not yet been well established. This problem is amplified by inadequately warmed operating room and fluid infusion. With increasing awareness of intraoperative hypothermia, emerging evidence has proposed various methods to maintain normothermia [5], while the effectiveness strategies on neonates are limited.

Previous study had demonstrated that low-flow anesthesia technique was accepted by some anesthesiologists due to heat and humidity preservation, as well as decreased gas consumption [6]. Kleemann et al. found that the temperature of inspired gas during low-flow anesthesia was higher when compared to high-flow anesthesia, indicating heat could be well reserved by low-flow anesthesia [7]. However, that low fresh gas flow in sevoflurane anesthesia led to compound A generation was an issue worried by some anesthesia providers, since compound A had a dose-related nephrotoxicity which had been confirmed in laboratory test [8]. Even in the developed country, the target of fresh gas flow was 2 L/min for sevoflurane anesthesia [9]. Some anesthesia providers were reluctant to further reduce fresh gas flow during sevoflurane administration and utilized more than 1 L/min fresh gas flow to achieve desired anesthesia in clinical practice. In fact, as early as in 2000, Obata and colleagues had confirmed that prolonged low-flow sevoflurane anesthesia had the same effects on renal and hepatic functions as high-flow sevoflurane [10].

Based on the previous investigation in our institution, although the active temperature managements had been implemented, such as cotton blankets, mattress, and infusion fluid warming, the incidence of hypothermia in neonates reached up to 90%. To reduce the incidence of hypothermia in neonates, we hypothesized that low fresh gas flow anesthesia was a good way to keep normothermia in neonates. In our institution, till August 2019, the fresh gas flow to perform neonate's anesthesia relied on the practitioner's experience and opinion, and it might exceed 1 L/min. Since September 1st, 2019, the new recommendation had been launched to utilize ≤1 L/min fresh gas flow during the neonates' surgical procedure. Therefore, we intended to evaluate the association of low fresh gas flow anesthesia with the occurrence of intraoperative hypothermia in neonates undergoing digestive surgeries.

Methods

After obtaining Institutional Review Board (IRB) approval [No. 2020(3)], we retrieved patient data from the electrical record system at Chengdu Women's and Children's Central Hospital between June 31, 2018 (from the very beginning of electrical medical record utilization) and April 1, 2020. This study had been registered at http://www.chictr.org.cn/index.aspx with No. ChiCTR2000034242 on June 27, 2020. The necessity of informed consents was waived by the IRB, considering the nature of the retrospective study and the anonymized patient data.

Study population

The inclusion criteria were neonates who were underwent digestive surgeries. The exclusion criteria include as follows: 1. Conversion from laparoscopic surgery to open surgeries; 2. Lacking documentation of temperature; 3. Congenital heart disease patients with clinical symptoms; 4. Digestive surgery were performed concurrently with other procedures.

Data collection

Once the list of the patients was created, the following variables were collected from our electronic patient registration system, i.e., age at surgery, weight at surgery, sex, birth body weight, gestational days, ASA status, comorbidities, the length of surgical time, mean body temperature during the surgery, intraoperative flow of fresh gas, estimated blood loss, blood transfusion, plasma transfusion, fluid infusion during surgery, preoperative hemoglobin, postoperative hemoglobin, the duration of hypothermia, the lowest temperature, postoperative hospital length-of-stay (PLOS) and intraoperative urinary volume. Neonates were defined as patients under the age of 28 days. Mortality data was obtained from a combination of hospital discharge disposition, our death records and the legal guardian or power of attorney who withdrew treatment in the patients with endotracheal tube. Actual PLOS was from surgical date to discharge date. The duration of hypothermia was calculated from the beginning of hypothermia to the beginning of normothermia. As the rule in our institution, only anesthesia providers with 5 years' experience were authorized to perform anesthesia in neonates. Since we had strict standard operative procedure guidelines, the strategies for avoiding hypothermia in our institution, included utilizing anesthesia station with heat and humidity exchanger, warm air circulation, warm infusion fluids, and warm mattress pads and blankets. Forced air warming was routinely used before and after the change in fresh gas flow practice. The temperature of the operating room was usually controlled between 22.0 °C and 24.0 °C. Dräger Primus anesthesia workstation with a heat and moisture exchanger was used for neonates. According to the description in background section, we therefore looked at the results from the patients that were underwent surgery before (Routine group) and after September 2019 (Low flow group).

Intraoperative esophageal temperature

For neonates undergoing surgery under general anesthesia in our institution, an esophageal probe was inserted into esophagus after general anesthesia. Body temperature was automatically recorded at 10-min intervals until the patients left the operating room. Based on definition from several previous studies [1, 2], hypothermia was defined as body temperature < 36.0 °C and normothermia was considered as 36.0 °C ≤ body temperature ≤ 37.4 °C. When <36.0 °C was recorded on the electronic record, the patient was considered to have hypothermia. Intraoperative mean body temperature was defined as the sum of recorded body temperature divided by the total times. The esophageal probe was removed immediately before the patient left the operating room.

Outcome measures

The primary outcome was the incidence of intraoperative hypothermia.

The secondary outcomes included.

1. hospital mortality,
2. the value of lowest temperature,
3. blood loss,
4. mean body temperature during the surgery,
5. the length of hypothermia during the surgery,
6. postoperative hospital length-of-stay (PLOS).

Statistical analysis

The sample size was calculated based on the previous study done by Lo et al. [11] To detect a change in temperature of 0.5 °C with a study power of 90% and an alpha error of 5% the sample size required was 54. Considering 20% dropout because of lacking documentation of temperature, we recruited 65 patients in each group at least. The categorical variables were expressed as percentages. Continuous variables are presented as the mean ± standard deviation [SD] or median and interquartile range [IQR] (25–75%) if nonnormally distributed. The student t test was used to compare normally distribute data, otherwise the Mann Whitney U-test was used to compare two groups. The chi-squared test was used for categorical data. Multivariable logistic regressions were performed to determine the association between potential confounding variables and occurrence of intraoperative hypothermia. To adjust for confounding, analysis was performed using clinically relevant, the variables was selected in advance, including age, sex, weight at surgery, birth body weight, gestation days, the length of surgical time and fresh gas flow rate. These clinically relevant variables were selected based on biologic plausibility and were the most popular reported confounders in cohort on neonates [12]. Variance inflation factors for all predictors in multivariable regression were chosen to 1.0. Patients lacking documentation of temperature was excluded from the study. The analyses were carried out with R studio 3.5.2. The main R packages were listed in the additional file 1. $P < 0.05$ was statistically significant, and all tests were two-sided.

Results

A total of 315 neonates were identified as having digestive surgeries during the study period. Of this group, 66 neonates were excluded from the study as lacking documentation of intraoperative temperature. After screening for inclusion and exclusion criteria, 249 patients enrolled in this retrospective study, including 170 who underwent routine fresh gas flow anesthesia group (routine group) and 79 in the low fresh gas flow anesthesia group (low flow group). All the patients underwent general anesthesia with tracheal intubation. (Fig. 1).

Patient and clinical characteristics

Demographics data for both groups were presented in Table 1. The neonates in the two groups were demographically similar with the routine group composed of 98 boys (57.6%) and low flow group 50 boys (63.3%). At the time of surgery, body weight [2.7 kg (2.1, 3.2) in routine group and 2.9 kg (2.4, 3.2) in low flow group] and age [6 days (4, 13) in routine group and 6 days (3, 9) in low flow group] were comparable between two groups. There was no statistically significant difference detected

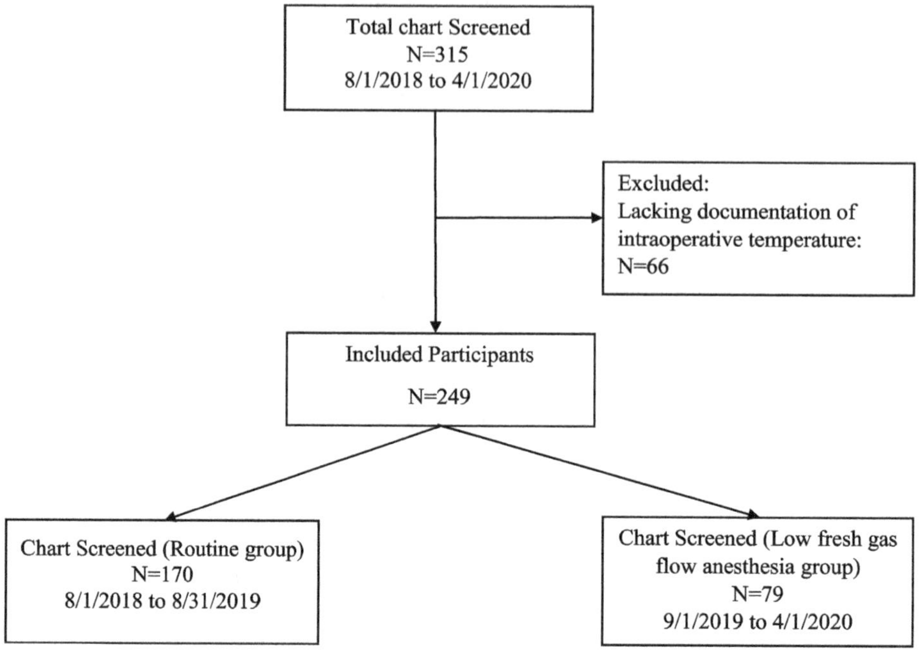

Fig. 1 Study patient flow diagram

between two groups with respect to gestation days, birth weight, ASA status, type of surgery, diagnosis, and surgical service.

Primary and secondary outcomes

Primary and secondary outcomes were reported in Table 2. In intraoperative period, the duration of surgery, blood loss, fluid infusion and pre-/post hemoglobin were comparable in both groups (Table 2). The overall incidence of hypothermia was 81.9%. Of the 249 patients in the cohort, the hypothermia occurred in 149 of 170 neonates (87.6%) allocated to routine group and in 55 of 79 neonates (69.6%) allocated to low flow group. The low fresh gas flow significantly reduced the odds of hypothermia [routine group: 149 (87.6%) versus low flow group: 55 (69.6%); $p<0.01$) and elevated the intraoperative mean temperature [routine group: 35.6 ± 0.8 °C versus low flow group: 36.0 ± 0.6 °C; $p<0.01$) (Table 2, Fig. 2). Moreover, low fresh gas flow could reduce the length of hypothermia [routine group: 104 mins (50, 156) versus low flow group: 30 mins (0,100); $p<0.01$], as well as elevate the value of lowest temperature for neonates [routine group: 35.1 °C (34.5, 35.7) versus low flow group: 35.7 °C (35.3, 36); $p<0.01$] (Table 2). No episodes of hypoxia or cardiac arrest were founded in our patients intraoperatively.

Factors associated with intraoperative hypothermia

Multivariable logistic regression was performed using the presence of intraoperative hypothermia as the dependent variable (Table 3). This complete case analysis included 249 neonates. Among the pre-chosen predictors, the length of surgical time (adjusted odds ratio, 1.01[95% CI, 1.00 to 1.02]; $p = 0.025$) and fresh gas flow (adjusted odds ratio, 3.04 [95% CI, 1.45 to 6.39]; $p = 0.003$) were independently associated with the occurrence of intraoperative hypothermia.

Discussion

In our study, low fresh gas flow anesthesia (≤ 1 L/min) for the neonates undergoing digestive surgery was associated to reduce the incidence of hypothermia. This method could shorten the length of hypothermia, as well as help to alleviate further decreasing of body temperature. Moreover, by multivariable logistic regression performed, we found that low fresh gas flow anesthesia and the length of surgical time were significantly associated with intraoperative hypothermia.

In this study, intraoperative hypothermia was defined as a core temperature (nasopharyngeal temperature) < 36 °C, in accordance with the definition of the National guideline in UK [13]. The overall incidence of hypothermia was about 81.9% in our study, which was like the result (83.3%) from a study by Lai [4]. Lai et al. also pointed that the incidence of hypothermia was higher in neonates, compared with infants, toddlers and children [4]. From above evidence, we confirmed that compared to other population, neonates had a faster body heat loss during the intraoperative period due to their physiological characteristics. To our knowledge, hypothermia should be prevented rather than treated after its occurrence. With the increasing awareness of

Table 1 Baseline demographic characteristics of each group

	Overall patients ($n = 249$)	Routine ($n = 170$)	Low flow ($n = 79$)	*P value*
Age at surgery (days) (Median, IQR)	6.0 (4.0, 11.0)	6.0 (4.0, 13.0)	6.0 (3.0, 9.0)	*0.35*
Weight at surgery (kg) (Median, IQR)	2.8 (2.2, 3.2)	2.7 (2.1, 3.2)	2.9 (2.4, 3.2)	*0.27*
Sex (male, %)	148 (59.4)	98 (57.6)	50 (63.3)	*0.48*
Birth body weight (kg) (Median, IQR)	2.8 (2.1, 3.3)	2.8 (2.1, 3.3)	2.9 (2.2, 3.4)	*0.20*
Gestation days (Median, IQR)	264 (245, 274)	263 (242, 274)	265 (248, 274)	*0.83*
ASA, n (%)				*0.20*
I	1 (0.4)	0 (0)	1 (1.3)	
II	70 (28.1)	49 (28.8)	21 (26.6)	
III	159 (63.9)	111 (65.3)	48 (60.8)	
IV	19 (7.6)	10 (5.9)	9 (11.4)	
Type of surgery				*0.38*
Elective, n (%)	77 (30.9)	56 (32.9)	21 (26.6)	
Emergency, n (%)	172 (69.1)	114 (67.1)	58 (73.4)	
Diagnosis				*0.11*
Congenital anorectal malformation, n (%)	51 (20.5)	30 (17.6)	21 (26.6)	
Gastric perforation, n (%)	9 (3.6)	5 (2.9)	4 (5.1)	
Ileus, n (%)	10 (4.0)	7 (4.1)	3 (3.8)	
Intestinal atresia, n (%)	37 (14.9)	23 (13.5)	14 (17.7)	
Neonatal necrotizing enterocolitis (NEC), n (%)	117 (47.0)	90 (52.9)	27 (34.2)	
Pyloric hypertrophy, n (%)	5 (2.0)	2 (1.2)	3 (3.8)	
Umbilical bulge, n (%)	9 (3.6)	6 (3.5)	3 (3.8)	
Hernia, n (%)	1 (0.4)	1 (0.6)	0 (0)	
Diaphragmatic hernia, n (%)	3 (1.2)	2 (1.2)	1 (1.3)	
Appendicitis, n (%)	1 (0.4)	1 (0.6)	0 (0)	
Intestinal malrotation, n (%)	3 (1.2)	3 (1.8)	0 (0)	
Others, n (%)	3 (1.2)	0 (0)	3	
Surgical service				*0.08*
Anoplasty, n (%)	51 (20.5)	30 (17.6)	21 (26.6)	
Enterectomy, n (%)	164 (65.9)	120 (70.6)	44 (55.7)	
Gastric perforation repair, n (%)	9 (3.6)	5 (2.9)	4 (5.1)	
Pyloric myotomy, n (%)	5 (2.0)	2 (1.2)	3 (3.8)	
Umbilical bulge repair, n (%)	9 (3.6)	6 (3.5)	3 (3.8)	
Hernia repair, n (%)	1 (0.4)	1 (0.6)	0 (0)	
Others, n (%)	10 (4.0)	6 (3.5)	4 (5.1)	

the harms of intraoperative hypothermia, many ways had been proposed to prevent it from happening. In our institution, the strategies for avoiding hypothermia included utilizing anesthesia station with heat and humidity exchanger, warm air circulation, warm infusion fluids, and warm mattress pads and blankets, but the incidence of hypothermia was still high before September 2019 (87.6%), which indicated the available strategies were not enough. To date, some anesthesia providers attributed it to patients' age, weight and different surgical procedures. Actually, in 2017, Engorn et al. did a retrospective research in neonates and revealed that gestation days, weight, type of surgery, sex, and length of surgery were not the risk factors for hypothermia except the thermoregulation interventions, which pointed that active and passive warming strategies played the pivotal role in maintaining normothermia [12]. A study with multiple logistic regression in Thailand showed that the following risk factors for core hypothermia included high ASA physical status and open surgery. Significant

Table 2 Intraoperative and postoperative data

	Overall patients ($n = 249$)	Routine ($n = 170$)	Low flow ($n = 79$)	P value
Fresh gas flow rate (L/min) (Median, IQR)	2.0 (1.0, 2.0)	2.0 (2.0, 2.0)	1.0 (1.0, 1.0)	< 0.01*
Mean temperature during surgery (Mean ± SD)	35.7 ± 0.8	35.6 ± 0.8	36.0 ± 0.6	< 0.01*
Hospital mortality, n (%)	25 (10.0)	20 (11.8)	6 (7.6)	0.43
Hypothermia, n (%)	204 (81.9)	149 (87.6)	55 (69.6)	< 0.01*
Length of hypothermia (mins) (Median, IQR)	90 (20, 148)	104 (50, 156)	30 (0, 100)	< 0.01*
The lowest temperature (°C) (Median, IQR)	35.4 (34.7, 35.8)	35.1 (34.5, 35.7)	35.7 (35.3, 36.0)	< 0.01*
Duration of surgery (mins) (Mean ± SD)	92.0 ± 45.0	91.8 ± 45.9	92.6 ± 43.4	0.81
Transfusion (ml)				
Blood (Mean ± SD)	7.1 ± 12.7	7.7 ± 13.8	5.7 ± 10.4	0.52
Plasma (Mean ± SD)	0.9 ± 1.8	1.4 ± 2.7	0 ± 0	0.17
Blood loss during surgery (ml) (Mean ± SD)	4.4 ± 4.0	4.3 ± 4.0	4.4 ± 4.1	0.94
Fluid infusion during surgery (mL) (Mean ± SD)	98.9 ± 50.8	99.9 ± 53.4	97.1 ± 44.8	0.72
Urine (ml) (Mean ± SD)	13.6 ± 11.0	13.2 ± 10.4	14.3 ± 12.2	0.85
Preoperative Hemoglobin (g/dL) (Mean ± SD)	146.3 ± 47.2	141.4 ± 41.3	156.9 ± 60.0	0.39
Postoperative Hemoglobin (g/dL) (Mean ± SD)	125.4 ± 34.2	124.8 ± 35.5	126.7 ± 31.2	0.30
Postoperative hospital length-of- stay (PLOS), days (Mean ± SD)	22.9 ± 18.6	23.9 ± 19.6	20.8 ± 16.6	0.13

Note: Sample (n), Standard deviation (SD), Interquartile Range (IQR), *$P<0.05$

protective factor against core hypothermia was heavier body weight [14]. In our study, the enrolled patients were neonates who underwent digestive surgeries, all of whom had the above risk factors rather than the protective factor, which demonstrated the importance of this study.

Our study proved that the length of hypothermia in low fresh gas flow (≤ 1 L/min) group was less than in routine group and the value of lowest body temperature was higher. As far as we know, inhaled air was warmed and humidified in upper air ways in spontaneous breathing. During mechanical ventilation with tracheal tube, this mechanism was disturbed, and the air was inhaled to lower airway directly without being warmed and humidified. Ventilation with dry and cold gases would lead to a considerable loss of heat from airway. In the Dräger Primus breathing system, to reduce the loss of heat, the exhaled gases moved through the hotplate once before mixing with cold and dry fresh air [15]. In 2011, Castro et al. reported that insertion of a heat and moisture exchanger increased the temperatures of inhaled gas in adults [15]. Moreover, by comparing 1 L/min and 3 L/min fresh gas flow in a Dräger Primus anesthesia workstation, Bicalho et al. revealed that 1 L/min fresh gas flow provided better inhaled gas temperature conservation in children [16], which implied that different gas

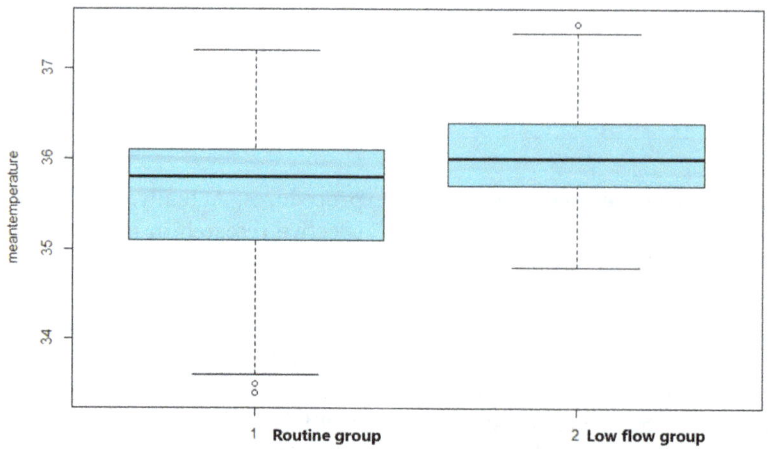

Fig. 2 The meantemperature in Routine group and Low flow group. 1 = Routine group; 2 = Low flow group

Table 3 Results of Multivariable Logistic Regression with Occurrence of Intraoperative Hypothermia

Variable	Adjusted Odds Ratios	95%CI	*P* value
Age (days)	0.99	0.94, 1.05	*0.95*
Male sex (vs. Female)	1.11	0.54, 2.29	*0.77*
Weight at the surgery time (kg)	0.52	0.09, 2.9	*0.46*
Birth body weight (kg)	1.42	0.26, 7.83	*0.69*
Gestation days (days)	0.99	0.96, 1.02	*0.56*
The length of surgical time (min)	1.01	1, 1.02	*0.025**
Fresh gas flow (L/min)	3.04	1.45, 6.39	*0.003**

Note: Results of multivariable logistic regression using pre-chosen predictors forced into the model 95%; Confidence Intervals (95% CI)
*$P<0.05$ is statistically significant

flow was potentially influence body temperature. However, this theory had not been proven in neonates. In our institution, Dräger Primus anesthesia workstation was used for neonates, but the incidence of hypothermia was still high. Two factors might explain the difficulties to sustain normothermia in neonate even though some active and passive tactics had been applied. First, neonates had a large body face ratio, thin skin, low fat content, which was inconducive to temperature preservation. Of course, this problem was compounded by the effects of anesthetic agents that inhibited central thermoregulation by interfering with these hypothalamic reflex responses. Moreover, non-shivering thermogenesis by metabolism of brown fat was limited in premature or critical neonates who were deficient in fat store. Second, the maintenance of body temperature depended on the balance of heat production and loss. According to our results, we had enough evidence to doubt that compared to other resource, the heat loss from respiratory tract due to high fresh gas flow might occupy a large proportion and 1 L/min fresh gas flow might be the critical value. The body temperature was hard to be maintained when the fresh gas flow exceeded 1 L/min since heat loss was beyond production, but this was only our suspicion and further studies were needed to verify it.

Previous studies had revealed that hypothermia was correlated with increased perioperative blood loss and rates of surgical wound infection, which might result in prolonged hospitalization and increased incidence of postoperative adverse events [17, 18]. In neonates, the literature about the relationship between hypothermia and prognosis was limited. Our study demonstrated that compared to routine group, the value of lowest temperature was higher, and the duration was less in low flow group, which indicated that low fresh gas flow could alleviate the severity of hypothermia. However, we did not find that fresh gas flow had a relationship with PLOS. The result should be interpreted cautiously because of the shortage of medical resources and insufficient economic development in our region. The guardians might withdraw the treatment because of heavy economic burden, which could artificially shorten length of hospital stay. Besides, other potentially relevant clinical outcomes should be examined in our study—like wound infections, but we could not collect the data about wound infections from our electronic patient registration system. Some surgeons might be reluctant to admit the fact that the wound was infected. Thus, the wound infections were not recorded properly in the chart, especially in the patients with mild wound infections.

Limitations

There were some limitations that should be noted. (1) This was a retrospective study which was at risk of patient selection bias and measurement bias. To reduce the effect of those bias, multivariable regression was conducted to determine the independent association between exposure and outcome. (2) Baseline and preoperative temperature were unknown. When the patients had pre-existed hypothermia, the outcome might be biased. (3) The confidence interval for the "treatment effect" of fresh gas flow was wide, and that a larger sample size would be needed to better delineate the true impact. (4) Because of the shortage of medical resources and insufficient economic development in developing countries like China, most neonates did not have medical-insurance, or the health insurance did not cover newborns. Some critically ill neonates with surgical indications might not be able to receive surgical treatment due to family poverty. Even the patients underwent the surgery, the guardians might withdraw the treatment because of heavy economic burden. In our study, the result of postoperative mortality and PLOS, therefore, might be biased. (5) One potential limitation of the investigation was limited generalizability to other settings.

Conclusions

In summary, we concluded that low fresh gas flow (≤ 1 L/min) could be considered as an effective way to alleviate hypothermia for the neonates undergoing digestive surgery. Intraoperatively low fresh gas flow was

independently associated with the occurrence of hypothermia.

Abbreviations

PLOS: Postoperative hospital length-of- stay; IRB: Institutional Review Board; SD: Standard deviation; IQR: Interquartile range

Authors' contributions

YC: Data collection, original draft writing, conceptualization, and draft writing. YW: Conceptualization and original draft writing. RC: Original draft writing, conceptualization, and draft writing. GL: Statistical analysis. LMD: Data collection. JL: Data collection. All authors read and approved the final manuscript.

Author details

[1]Department of Anesthesiology, The Affiliated Hospital, School of Medicine, UESTC Chengdu Women's & Children's Central Hospital, No.1617, Riyue Avenue, Qingyang District, Chengdu 610091, PR China. [2]Department of Anesthesilogy, No.363 hospital, Chengdu 610041, China. [3]Department of Anesthesiology, Vanderbilt University Medical Center, Nashville, TN 37232, USA.

References

1. Blum R, Cote C. Pediatric equipment. In: Blum R, Cote C, editors. A practice of Anaesthesia for infants and children. Philadelphia: Saunders Elsevier; 2009. p. 1099–101.
2. Sessler D. Temperature disturbances. In: Sessler D, editor. Pediatric anesthesia. Philadelphia: Churchill Livingstone; 2002. p. 53–84.
3. Moslemi-Kebria M, El-Nashar SA, Aletti GD, Cliby WA. Intraoperative hypothermia during cytoreductive surgery for ovarian cancer and perioperative morbidity. Obstet Gynecol. 2012;119:590–6.
4. Lai LL, See MH, Rampal S, Ng KS, Chan L. Significant factors influencing inadvertent hypothermia in pediatric anesthesia. J Clin Monit Comput. 2019; 33:1105–12.
5. Horosz B, Malec-Milewska M. Methods to prevent intraoperative hypothermia. Anaesthesiol Intensive Ther. 2014;46:96–100.
6. Bilgi M, Goksu S, Mizrak A, Cevik C, Gul R, Koruk S, Sahin L. Comparison of the effects of low-flow and high flow inhalational anaesthesia with nitrous oxide and desflurane on mucociliary activity and pulmonary function tests. Eur J Anaesthesiol. 2011;28:279–83.
7. Kleemann PP. Humidity of anaesthetic gases with respect to low flow anaesthesia. Anaesth Intensive Care. 1994;22:396–408.
8. Keller KA, Callan C, Prokocimer P, Delgado-Herrera L, Friedman MB, Hoffman GM, Wooding WL, Cusick PK, Krasula RW. Inhalation toxicity study of a haloalkene degradant of sevoflurane, compound a (PIFE), in Sprague-Dawley rats. Anesthesiology. 1995;83:1220–32.
9. Patel N, Maguire D, Dexter F, Epstein RH. Reduction of fresh gas flow during administration of volatile anesthetic agents via monthly individualized e-mail feedback: Annual Meeting of the Society for Technology in Anesthesia; 2014. Available at: http://www.stahq.org/files/7013/9171/8017/13_ Abstract_ Epstein.pdf. Accessed January 3, 2015.
10. Obata R, Bito H, Ohmura M, Moriwaki G, Ikeuchi Y, Katoh T, Sato S. The effects of prolonged low-flow sevoflurane anesthesia on renal and hepatic function. Anesth Analg. 2000;91:1262–8.
11. Lo C, Ormond G, McDougall R, Sheppard SJ, Davidson AJ. Effect of magnetic resonance imaging on core body temperature in anaesthetised children. Anaesth Intensive Care. 2014;42:333–9.
12. Engorn BM, Kahntroff SL, Frank KM, Singh S, Harvey HA, Barkulis CT, Barnett AM, Olambiwonnu OO, Heitmiller ES, Greenberg RS. Perioperative hypothermia in neonatal intensive care unit patients: effectiveness of a thermoregulation intervention and associated risk factors. Paediatr Anaesth. 2017;27:196–204.
13. National Institute for Health and Care Excellence. Inadvertent perioperative hypothermia: the management of inadvertent perioperative hypothermia in adults [CG65]. London: National Institute for Health and Care Excellence [UK]; 2016. https ://www. nice.org.uk/guida nce/cg65.
14. Kongsayreepong S, Chaibundit C, Chadpaibool J, Komoltri C, Suraseranivongse S, Suwannanonda P, Raksamanee EO, Noocharoen P, Silapadech A, Parakkamodom S, Pum-In C, Sojeoyya L. Predictor of core hypothermia and the surgical intensive care unit. Anesth Analg. 2003;96: 826–33.
15. de Castro J Jr, Bolfi F, de Carvalho LR, Braz JR. The temperature and humidity in a low-flow anesthesia workstation with and without a heat and moisture exchanger. Anesth Analg. 2011;113:534–8.
16. Bicalho GP, Braz LG, de Jesus LS, Pedigone CM, de Carvalho LR, Módolo NS, Braz JR. The humidity in a Dräger primus anesthesia workstation using low or high fresh gas flow and with or without a heat and moisture exchanger in pediatric patients. Anesth Analg. 2014;119:926–31.
17. Frank SM, Fleisher LA, Breslow MJ, Higgins MS, Olson KF, Kelly S, Beattie C. Perioperative maintenance of normothermia reduces the incidence of morbid cardiac events. A randomized clinical trial. JAMA. 1997;277:1127–34.
18. Kurz A, Sessler DI, Lenhardt R. Perioperative normothermia to reduce the incidence of surgical-wound infection and shorten hospitalization. Study of wound infection and temperature group. N Engl J Med. 1996;334:1209–15.

12

Sevoflurane versus PRopofol combined with remifentanil anesthesia impact on postoperative neurologic function in supratentorial gliomas (SPRING)

Yan Xing[1†], Nan Lin[1*†], Ruquan Han[1*], John F. Bebawy[2], Yuming Peng[1], Jiaxin Li[1], Xiaoyuan Liu[1], Yan Li[1], Jia Dong[1], Min Zeng[1], Manyu Zhang[1] and Lanyi Nie[1]

Abstract

Background: Patients with intracranial tumors are more sensitive to anesthetics than the general population and are therefore more susceptible to postoperative neurologic and neurocognitive dysfunction. Sevoflurane or propofol combined with remifentanil are widely used general anesthetic regimens for craniotomy, with neither regimen shown to be superior to the other in terms of neuroprotective efficacy and anesthesia quality. There is no evidence regarding the variable effects on postoperative neurologic and neurocognitive functional outcome under these two general anesthetic regimens. This trial will compare inhalational sevoflurane or intravenous propofol combined with remifentanil anesthesia in patients with supratentorial gliomas and test the hypothesis that postoperative neurologic function is equally affected between the two regimens.

(Continued on next page)

* Correspondence: linnan127@gmail.com; Hanrq666@aliyun.com
†Yan Xing and Nan Lin are co-first authors who equally contributed to this trial.
[1]Department of Anesthesiology, Beijing Tiantan Hospital, Capital Medical University, No.119, West Road 4th ring South, Fengtai District, Beijing 100070, China

(Continued from previous page)

Methods: This is a prospective, single-center, randomized parallel arm equivalent clinical trial, which is approved by China Ethics Committee of Registering Clinical Trials (ChiECRCT-20,160,051). Patients with supratentorial gliomas diagnosed by magnetic resonance imaging will be eligible for the trial. Written informed consent will be obtained before randomly assigning each subject to either the sevoflurane-remifentanil or propofol-remifentanil group for anesthesia maintenance to achieve an equal-desired depth of anesthesia. Intraoperative intervention and monitoring will follow a standard anesthetic management protocol. All of the physiological parameters and other medications administered during the intervention will be recorded. The primary outcome will be neurologic function change assessed by National Institute of Health Stroke Scale (NIHSS) within 4 h after general anesthesia when observer's assessment of alertness/sedation (OAA/S) reaches 4. Secondary outcomes will include NIHSS and modified NIHSS change 1 and 2 days after general anesthesia, hemodynamic stability, intraoperative brain relaxation, quality of anesthesia emergence, quality of anesthesia recovery, postoperative cognitive function, postoperative pain, postoperative neurologic complications, as well as perioperative medical expense.

Discussion: This randomized equivalency trial will primarily compare the impacts of sevoflurane-remifentanil and propofol-remifentanil anesthesia on short-term postoperative neurologic function in patients with supratentorial gliomas undergoing craniotomy. The exclusion criteria are strict to ensure that the groups are comparable in all aspects. Repeated and routine neurologic evaluations after operation are always important to evaluate neurosurgical patients' recovery and any newly presenting complications. The results of this trial would help specifically to interpret anesthetic residual effects on postoperative outcomes, and perhaps would help the anesthesiologist to select the optimal anesthetic regimen to minimize its impact on neurologic function in this specific patient population.

Keywords: (3–10): propofol, Sevoflurane, General anesthesia, Total intravenous anesthesia, Supratentorial glioma, Craniotomy, Neurologic function

Background

According to the statistical report released from Primary Brain and Central Nervous System Tumors Diagnosed in the United States in 2015, thirty out of every 100,000 people in the general population suffered from a primary intracranial tumor requiring craniotomy for tumor resection. Glioma accounted for 60.8% of all primary intracranial tumors [1], of which most of these operations require general anesthesia. These patients have vulnerable central nervous systems because of their intracranial tumors (e.g., gliomas are aggressive lesions that invade central neuronal structures anatomically, and at the neuropathologocial level disturb neuronal connections to impair neural function). Compared to intact brains, neuronal network connection disruptions from intracranial lesions and central nervous system inhibition by anesthetics yield a "double insult" to neurosurgical patients, so to speak, and may make them more sensitive to general anesthesia and surgery, leading to both short and long-term neurologic and neurocognitive dysfunction. Anesthesiologists attempt to choose the anesthetic regimen cautiously, taking into account anesthetics' effects on cerebral physiology (e.g., intracranial pressure and cerebral perfusion pressure), as well as to minimize the seeming disturbance to neuronal function by facilitating rapid emergence and orientation during recovery. The less postoperative neuronal function is affected by anesthetics, the more accurately the patient's intracranial disease-related status is reflected, and this is beneficial to neurosurgeons so as to correctly evaluate neural function. The optimal postoperative treatment based on neurological evaluation contributes to reduction of neurologic complications and is critical for long-term quality of life. Therefore, it is important to investigate how different mechanisms of general anesthesia affect postoperative neural function and anesthesia recovery in patients with supratentorial (frontal-parietal-temporal) gliomas in both a qualitative and quantitative (over time) manner, as this may guide anesthetic choice in supratentorial craniotomies for gliomas to ensure a reasonable, safe, and economical perioperative anesthetic regimen.

Inhalational anesthesia and intravenous anesthesia are widely used in current neurosurgical anesthesiology [2], and sevoflurane combined with remifentanil or propofol combined with remifentanil are both accepted as general anesthesia strategies. Comparative studies have been done to investigate the effects of different anesthetics on craniotomies [3], both primary and secondary outcomes focused on the changes in intraoperative physiological parameters [3, 4], laboratory results [3], and anesthesia recovery indices during emergence [5, 6]; however, neuronal disease-specific study is lacking, and there is no evidence related to how postoperative neurological function and neurocognitive outcomes are affected by different general anesthesia strategies [7]. Patients with neurological diseases, e.g., brain tumors, are usually excluded in studies examining the correlation between anesthesia and neural function [8], as those diseases are major confounders leading to nervous system dysfunction, however, anesthetic effects on neural function cannot be ignored in neurosurgical patients, let alone the previously mentioned "vulnerable" brain tumor patient who is even more susceptible to anesthetics [9]. Recent findings have reported patients with supplementary motor area (SMA) lesions presenting with intraoperative neurological deficits for awake craniotomy which could not be explained anatomically by their intact corticospinal tracts as detected by cortical stimulation or cortical mapping [10, 11], and these deficits were reversible after operations over time without further intervention. Although this finding may have been related to lesion location, which is called "SMA symptom", this phenomenon cannot exclude the possibility of residual anesthetic-induced neurological deficits in both the intraoperative and early postoperative periods.

It has been reported that in some supratentorial brain mass patients, a small plasma concentration of sedative could significantly worsen neurologic deficits before any operative intervention [9], but there is no evidence related to how residual anesthetics affect neurologic deficits after operations. Repeated neurological evaluations after neurosurgeries can help to assess whether surgical interventions are successful and whether long-term neurologic outcomes are primarily related to diseases and surgeries, while short-term neurologic outcomes are subject to perioperative care beyond the above factors; despite only a few hours of surgical intervention for brain tumor, the overlap of general anesthesia and its effects, after surgery is completed, can linger for hours to days, which may worsen neurologic function and confuse providers. However, in the early postoperative stage, it is unknown whether sevoflurane combined with remifentanil and/or propofol combined with remifentanil could result in unexpected neurologic function deterioration, and whether one strategy is inferior or superior to another.

In this study, we will use sevoflurane combined with remifentanil or propofol combined with remifentanil to maintain anesthesia during craniotomy in patients with supratentorial gliomas to determine whether they have comparable effects on neurologic function and neurocognition in the early postoperative period. Since both sevoflurane and propofol are GABAergic anesthetics, we hypothesize that these two general anesthesia methods equivalently affect early postoperative neural function in this group of patients.

Methods

Study purpose

(1) Primary purpose: To investigate neurologic function in the early postoperative period for patients with supratentorial intracranial gliomas under inhalational general anesthesia compared to intravenous general anesthesia. The hypothesis is that the difference in postoperative National Institute of Health Stroke Scale (NIHSS or modified NIHSS) score changes under the two general anesthesia methods are not different, with the score difference within − 1 to 1.

(2) Secondary purpose: To compare the effects of inhalational general anesthesia versus intravenous general anesthesia on neurocognition, hemodynamics, cerebral physiology, anesthesia recovery quality, pain scores, anesthesia expenses, and stress responses in patients with supratentorial intracranial gliomas undergoing elective craniotomy.

Trial design

The study is a prospective, single-center, open label, randomized parallel arm equivalent clinical trial comparing sevoflurane and propofol, both combined with remifentanil, general anesthesia (Sevoflurane-remifentanil versus Propofol-remifentanil group) in patients with supratentorial gliomas; it will be carried out in the neurosurgical operation room in Beijing Tiantan Hospital (a large city), Capital Medical University, Beijing, China.

Populations

Adult male and female patients scheduled for elective craniotomy under general anesthesia with supratentorial (frontal-parietal-temporal) gliomas diagnosed by magnetic resonance imaging (MRI) are eligible for the study. All patients must sign institutional approval and informed consent before enrollment, the written informed consent will be obtained 1 day or a few days before operation, when patients are seen by anesthesiologists in the ward. The information and reasons why eligible patients are not recruited to the trial will be documented. The inclusion and exclusion criteria are listed in Table 1.

Patients will be recruited in Beijing Tiantan Hospital, Beijing, China. The potentially eligible patient will be screened and contacted by a trial team member who explains the study and ascertains the patient's interest 1 or 2 days before the scheduled operation day. If interested in enrolment, the patient will receive the detailed trial explanation and written consent form.

Table 1 Inclusion and exclusion criteria

Inclusion Criteria	
Patients aged between 18 to 65 years old with American Society of Anesthesiology (ASA) status I ~ II who are scheduled for elective craniotomy for the treatment of supratentorial gliomas must fulfill the following:	
1	Frontal-Parietal-Temporal glioma diagnosed by preoperative MRI
2	Glasgow score of 15 without preoperative symptomatic elevated intracranial pressure
3	New and/or recurrent intracranial gliomas are allowed
Exclusion Criteria	
1	Unable to comprehend and cooperate with the neurologic examination
2	Emergency craniotomy or changed to emergency from elective craniotomy
3	Insular lobe is invaded by glioma
4	Scheduled intraoperative motor evoked potential monitoring
5	Patients with traumatic brain injury, intracerebral hemorrhage, or cerebral vascular diseases
6	Patients with prolonged emergence, postoperative mechanical ventilation, and/or sedation dependence due to a definite reason (e.g., surgery itself or tumor location)
7	Hypothalamic dysfunction
8	Radiotherapy and/or chemotherapy before surgery
9	Uncontrolled hypertension or severe heart disease that impairs cardiac function (New York Heart Association Functional Classification ≥ III)
10	History of related anesthetic allergy
11	Severe endocrine system dysfunction that impair metabolic index
12	Impaired mental status
13	Drug and/or alcohol abuse
14	Pregnant and/or lactation period patients
15	Neuromuscular diseases
16	Infectious and/or immune diseases with positive biomarker(s)
17	Body mass index > = 35

Randomization and blinding

Permuted-block randomization will be used with a block size of 4 and an allocation ratio of 1:1 to either sevoflurane-remifentanil group or propofol-remifentanil group. Random allocation sequence will be based on a computer-generated random digits table. One investigator who will not participate in anesthetic management or follow-up will implement the randomization and enroll patients, and allocation will be concealed in a sealed opaque envelope until patient enters the operating room. Randomization will occur for patients conforming to the above criteria, and written informed consent will then be obtained from themselves or their next-of-kin. Since the two general anesthetic administration routes are distinct (inhalational versus intravenous), patients and anesthesiologists cannot be blinded. An independent team who is not involved in the intraoperative management will be in charge of postoperative follow-up and is blinded to the intervention.

Interventions

Standard anesthetic management

On the day of operation, patients will be admitted into the operating room to be randomly assigned into either the sevoflurane-remifentanil or propofol-remifentanil group. Vital signs including electrocardiography (ECG), blood pressure (BP), heart rate (HR), pulse oxygen saturation (SpO2), end-tidal carbon dioxide ($ETCO_2$), body temperature, and urine output will be monitored throughout the study. 100% fraction of oxygen will be provided by mask to the patients for preoxygenation for 5 min prior to anesthetic induction. No premedication will be given.

All patients will be induced with 0.3 μg/kg sufentanil, 2–2.5 mg/kg propofol, and 0.7–0.8 mg/kg rocuronium or cisatracurium. After tracheal intubation, mechanical ventilation will be established, at a tidal volume of 8-10 ml/kg, respiratory rate of 12–15/min, inspiratory:expiratory ratio of 1:2, fraction of inhaled fresh oxygen as 60%, and flow rate of fresh gas as 1.5 L/min. After induction, anesthesia will be maintained according to one of the two group allocations: (1) 6-8 mg/kg propofol with 0.05–0.2 μg/kg remifentanil for the propofol group or (2) 1.3–1.5 Minimum Alveolar Concentration (MAC) sevoflurane with 0.05–0.2 μg/kg remifentanil for the sevoflurane group. The dosage of anesthetic will be adjusted according to the bispectral index (BIS) value, which will be maintained between 40 and 60. 0.5% ropivacaine 1 to 2 mL for each injection point will be used for scalp nerves block before the start of surgeries. Sufentanil 5–10 mcg can be given, by anesthesiologist discretion, to alleviate potent stress responses when head pins are placed or scalp incision is performed, based on the hemodynamic parameters. Additional sufentanil bolus at the dose of 5-10mcg during operation is allowed, the last bolus should be given ahead of at least 60 min before expected end of surgery. The muscle relaxant cisatracurium will be infused at 0.1 mg/kg/h during the operation for all patients and stopped once the bone flap is secured. Propofol and sevoflurane will be reduced according to BIS and hemodynamic parameters once the bone flap is fixed and stopped at skin dressing.

At the end of the operation, ondansetron 4 mg will be prophylactically administered to all patients to prevent nausea and vomiting, and tramadol 1.5-2 mg/kg will be given if patients are experiencing rigors/chills. Neostigmine 20-40mcg/kg and atropine 0.5-1 mg will be available to antagonize residual muscle relaxation when deemed necessary by train-of-four (TOF) twitch monitoring. Peripheral nerve stimulator will be performed for TOF monitoring, achieving TOF ratio of 1.0 at the ulnar nerve/adductor pollicis is considered an adequate sign of recovery from muscle relaxant.

Adverse hemodynamic responses will be recorded and classified as hypertension, hypotension, tachycardia, or bradycardia, which require standard treatment according to the protocol (Table 2). These episodes of blood pressure and heart rate changes and the medication administered during their treatment will be recorded as "hypertension" (MAP > 20% above preoperative baseline value) or "hypotension" (MAP < 20% below preoperative baseline value), Tachycardia and bradycardia are defined as HR > 100 bpm and HR < 45 bpm, respectively. Standard treatment for hemodynamic disturbances are shown in Table 2.

Patient-controlled intravenous analgesia (PCIA) will be used for postoperative pain control with 100mcg sufentanil and 16 mg ondansetron diluted to a total volume of 100 ml within normal saline being prepared, with a bolus dose set at 0.5 ml, a lockout time set at 15 min, and a background infusion of 2 ml/h. PCIA will be started after the patient is discharged from the operating room.

Anesthesia monitoring

Anesthesia management will aim to achieve targeted physiological parameters. The blood pressure will be monitored by radial artery catheter placement, and the target value is defined as the range of ±20% of the baseline MAP value, which is defined as the average MAP of the first three values measured after the patient enters the operating room and before induction. When the blood pressure is out of this range, measures will be taken such as changing the infusion rate of crystalloid or colloid and remifentanil, or giving bolus injection of sufentanil or vasoactive agent (such as 0.5 μg/kg/min phenylephrine or 0.01 μg/kg/min norepinephrine). Heart rate will be maintained between 50 and 90 beats per minute. SpO2 will be kept ≥98% during the operation. End-tidal CO_2 will be maintained between 30 and 35 mmHg by adjusting ventilation parameters. Core body temperature will be kept between 36 and 37 degree Celsius. Plasma glucose concentration will be maintained between 5.0–7.8 mmol/L.

Discontinuation criteria

Massive hemorrhage or massive transfusion

Massive intraoperative bleeding can occur, and this study defines massive bleeding as blood loss exceeding the entire blood volume within 24 h from the start of operation or 50% of circulating blood volume loss within 3 h during operation requiring emergency intervention. Intraoperative massive transfusion (transfusion of more than 10 units of packed red blood cells) may be needed if massive hemorrhage is encountered. If bleeding occurs to this extent and meets either or both of the above criteria, the trial will be discontinued for this particular patient.

Anaphylaxis during the operation

Anaphylaxis rarely but occasionally occurs intraoperatively, especially in the setting of antibiotic and muscle relaxant administration, but also with the administration of other medications, and normally can be treated quickly. If such a reaction occurs and is severe, necessitating discontinuation of the operation, the patient will be withdrawn from the trial. Anaphylaxis will be reported as an adverse event.

Venous air embolism

Significant venous air embolism has been observed in rare cases, but neurosurgery carries the potential risk for this sometimes intractable complication, especially when the operative intervention occurs near venous sinuses or in the sitting position [12–14]. Venous air embolism may result in severe hypoxia and hypotension which can impair cerebral perfusion and oxygenation. If this happens, timely intervention and resuscitation needs to be

Table 2 Treatment for hemodynamic disturbances

Hemodynamic Fluctuation	Definition (if any of the below changes are sustained for equal and/or longer than 5 min)	Standard Treatment Algorithm
Hypertension Episode	MAP > 20% above preoperative baseline	Increase propofol or sevoflurane concentration according to BIS, increase remifentanil infusion rate, or administer 5mcg sufentanil; if correction still not achieved, nicardipine will be given as bolus and/or infusion
Hypotension Episode	MAP < 20% below preoperative baseline	Decrease propofol or sevoflurane concentration according to BIS, give adequate volume loading; if correction still not achieved, vasoactive agent administration (dopamine, norepinephrine, or phenylephrine) will be given with the dose and infusion rate adjusted according to the blood pressure response
Tachycardia Episode	HR > 100 bpm	Esmolol bolus and/or infusion according to heart rate response
Bradycardia Episode	HR < 45 bpm	Atropine administration

MAP mean arterial pressure, *HR* heart rate, *bpm* beat per minute carried out and the patient will be withdrawn from the trial. This will be reported as an adverse event.

Postoperative coma

If the patient is in a coma (nonresponsive) after operation for any reason, the subject will not be able to cooperate with any neurological assessment, the subsequent follow-up will need to be discontinued, and this will be noted in the neurologic complication section. The patient will be withdrawn from the trial.

Outcomes

Patients will have been screened 1 to 2 days before operation, and the demographic characteristics, clinical manifestations, and past history obtained at this time. Detailed descriptions of the lesion in MRI will be obtained. The lesions' pathologic diagnoses will be obtained 2 weeks after the tumor removal. Neurologic function will be assessed using the National Institute of Health Stroke Scale (NIHSS/mNIHSS) at baseline and in the postoperative period. NIHSS scores 15 items including consciousness, visual function, facial and motor function, ataxia, sensory and language function, and attention, and the total score ranges from 0 (no deficit) to a maximum of 42. A modified version of the NIHSS (mNIHSS) abridges to 11 items by deleting level of consciousness, facial palsy, limb ataxia, and dysarthria; the sensory item is collapsed from 3 to 2 choices [15]. Since there is no reliability and validity evidence comparing NIHSS and mNIHSS use in the intracranial tumor population, we will score both as primary outcomes in this study. The scoring system is shown in appendix. Mini-mental state examination (MMSE) will be used to assess the cognitive performance of patients at baseline and after operation. During anesthesia recovery, Anesthesia Recovery Quality and the modified Aldrete scale will be used to assess the recovery condition of patients. Visual Analog Scale (VAS) will be used to assess postoperative pain. QoR-40 (Quality of Recovery from Anesthesia) will be used at 2 days after operation to assess the recovery condition and the satisfaction of the patient related to anesthesia. All adverse events will be recorded. The schedule of data collection is shown in Fig. 1.

Study endpoint

The primary endpoint will be NIHSS score change within 4 h after general anesthesia by sevoflurane-remifentanil or propofol-remifentanil when observer's assessment of alertness/sedation (OAA/S) reaches 4. The time to reach OAA/S score of 4 at the first time point will be recorded.

Secondary endpoints will be as follows:

1) The NIHSS score change at postoperative day 1 and postoperative day 2 from the baseline, the level of OAA/S in these two time points will be recorded.

	STUDY PERIOD									
	Enrolment	Allocation	Post-allocation							Close-out
					Post-operation					
TIMEPOINT	Preoperative Assessment $-T_1$	Allocation 0	Intra-operation T_1	Recovery T_2	within 4 hours after operation when OAA/S=4 F_1	1-day after operation F_2	2-day after operation F_3	3-day after operation F_4	7-day after operation F_5	Before discharge F_6
ENROLMENT:										
Eligibility screen	X									
Informed consent	X									
Allocation		X								
INTERVENTIONS:										
Sevoflurane-Remifentanil			X							
Propofol-Remifentanil			X							
ASSESSMENTS:										
Hemodynamic stability			◆———	———◆						
Brain relaxation			X							
NIHSS	X				X	X	X			
mNIHSS	X				X	X	X			
MMSE	X						X			
Quality of emergence (Aldrete score)				X						
Intraoperative awareness						X				
VAS					X	X	X			
QoR-40							X			
Stress response biomarkers								X	X	
Postoperative neurologic complications										X
Medical expenses										X

Fig. 1 Schedule of enrollment, interventions and assessments for the SPRING trial

2) Hemodynamic stability including blood pressure, heart rate, episodes of hypertension, hypotension, tachycardia, and bradycardia;
3) Intraoperative brain relaxation (Brain relaxation assessed immediately after opening of the dura on a scale ranging from 1 to 4 (1 = perfectly relaxed, 2 = satisfactorily relaxed, 3 = firm brain, 4 = bulging brain);
4) Quality of anesthesia emergence including time of eye opening, time of emergence, coughing during extubation, postoperative nausea and vomiting (PONV), shivering, and agitation;
5) Quality of anesthesia recovery assessed by QoR-40 at postoperative day 2;
6) Changes of cognitive function at postoperative day 2 assessed by MMSE;
7) Postoperative pain at PACU, 1, and 2 days after surgery evaluated by VAS;
8) Postoperative neurological complications (e.g., intracranial hematoma, infection, seizure etc.);
9) Anesthesia expenses and in-hospital total expenses;

Data collection and management

Anesthesiologists on the follow-up team are all trained and received certification from the NIHSS official training program website (www.nihstrokescale.org). Data collection ends when patients are discharged from the hospital. All the information will be recorded on a Case Report Form (CRF), and raw, non-numerical data are coded for data storage, review, tabulation and analysis. Data will be entered at our medical center and stored and monitored securely in an electronic databases. Each of the data collection forms and the detailed information will be discussed on an item-by-item basis. Double data entry will be used, different data entering individuals will use standardized terminology and abbreviations, training will be performed regarding entering data on forms, and we will respond promptly to data discrepancy queries and general concerns about overall quality. Any missing data or errors in the data will be summarized along with detailed descriptions, and will be queried by checking the original forms. Data safety and monitoring inspectors will evaluate the trial safety, efficacy, and any ethical issues. The data to be collected and the procedures to be conducted at each visit will be reviewed in detail. There will not be a formal data monitoring committee (DMC) in this study, because the intraoperative anesthesia management is standard with minimal risks and the follow-up duration is short for this trial.

Paper case report forms are stored in numerical order and kept in locked cabinets. The electronic data will be saved in a database with password protection, and the passwords will be changed on a regular basis. Database backup will be performed once a month. All the original files will be maintained in storage for a period of 5 years after completion of the study.

Participant retention

Once a patient is enrolled in the study, the team will make every effort to follow the patient for the entire study period. For patients whose consent is withdrawn, who are lost to follow-up, or discontinue for any reason, the reason will be recorded in the CRF in order to better interpret the results. The strategies that are used to improve participant retention are:

1) provide letters regarding the evaluation time schedule prior to data collection to remind patients and relatives of each assessment and test;
2) provide adequate communication when visiting patients in the ward to let them be informed of upcoming data collection;
3) limit patient burden related to follow-up visits to the greatest extent possible;
4) patients who withdraw for follow-up assessment for one of the primary or secondary outcomes can continue with assessments for the other outcomes.

Sample size calculation

Sample size calculation was conducted by PASS software (NCSS, LLC, USA). The mean difference of NIHSS change between the two types of anesthetics was estimated as 0.5, the estimated within group standard deviation was 1.5, and 1.0 was set as the equivalent margin based on clinical significance. Z-test was used as power analysis of equivalence tests of two independent proportions to detect equivalence. The minimum number of cases was 160 per group to achieve 80% power to detect a possible equivalence between the two groups. Considering the possibility of early termination during the study and allowing for a 10% drop-out rate, this number was raised to 176 subjects for each group. As two groups were to be studied, we aim to enroll 352 subjects.

Statistical analysis plan

Kolmogorov-Smirnov testing will be used for evaluating if the continuous variables have a normal distribution or not. Descriptive statistics will be reported as means with standard deviation for normally distributed data; medians with interquartile range will be described for non-normally distributed data; for categorical variables, count (percentage) will be described. The difference in postoperative NIHSS scores at certain time points between the propofol and sevoflurance groups will be analyzed by t-test or Mann-

Whitney U test depending on normal or non-normal distribution, respectively, and 95% confident interval will be determined for the NIHSS score change and difference between the two groups. The changes in VAS scores, intraoperative parameters, and stress response biomarkers over the observation time will be compared using repeated measurement, and post hoc analysis will be used for sensitivity analysis. For other secondary outcomes such as brain relaxation, MMSE score, anesthesia quality score and medical expense, the difference between the two groups will be analyzed by t-test or Mann-Whitney U test. All the categorical variables will be analyzed by chi-square testing. Missing data will be adjusted using inverse probability weighting and worst-case imputation scenarios. Statistical significance is defined as a type I error of 0.05, and the nature of the testing is two-tailed. Analyses will be conducted using Statistical Package for the Social Sciences (SPSS) version 17.0 (Chicago, IL, USA).

All data will be analyzed according to an intent-to-treat, such that all randomized patients originally allocated to the propofol or sevoflurane anesthesia arm at the time of randomization will be used for efficacy analysis. No interim analysis is planned. Worst observation carried forward method will be used to handle missing data.

Reporting of adverse events

All adverse events associated with this trial will be closely monitored until the adverse events are resolved, stable, or confirmed as having no relation to the trial. Once adverse events occur, they will be immediately reported to the research department and to the principal investigator to determine the severity of the adverse events and the consequences of the injury. All adverse events associated with this study will be recorded and reported to the Ethics Committee within 1 week, which will be part of the annual report. The principal investigator will be responsible for all reported adverse events.

Protocol amendment

The principle investigator of the SPRING trial will be responsible for any decision to amend the protocol. If there is any modification that impacts the conduct of the study and affects potential safety or benefit to the patient, such as trial objectives, design, patient population, sample sizes or study procedures in the protocol, the principle investigator will notify and gain approval from the China Ethics Committee of Registering Clinical Trials prior to implementation, and the related trial registration information will be updated in the Chinese Clinical Trial Registry.

Trial results and publication

Publications and presentations related to this trial will always maintain and protect the integrity of the major objectives of this study. Each paper or abstract will be reviewed and approved by the principle investigator before being submitted. The SPRING trial may terminate at a planned target of 6 months after the last patient has been randomized. We expect to take about 4 to 6 months to compile the final results for publication in an appropriate medical journal. The results will be reported and disseminated to the public regardless of the magnitude or direction of effect. The principle investigator of the study should be considered as the lead author. All professionals that have participated in the SPRING trial for a minimum of 3 months will be listed in the authorship, and those who do not fulfill such criteria will be acknowledged in the publication.

Discussion

In current neurosurgical anesthesia practice for elective craniotomy for brain tumor resection, either an inhalational agent or intravenous propofol in combination with a short-acting opioid and muscle relaxant may be used. For patients with normal intracranial pressure and those without need of intraoperative neurophysiological monitoring, there does not appear to be one technique that is deemed superior to another in terms of neuroprotective efficacy, anesthesia maintenance efficacy, or postoperative recovery quality. With respect to neurofunctional outcome, so far, no clinical evidence exists to elucidate whether there is a difference or equivalence between these two general anesthetics. Since both sevoflurane and propofol are GABAergic general anesthetic that have similar mechanism, we hypothesize that these two general anesthesia methods equivalently affect early postoperative neural function in patients with supratentorial gliomas.

We chose sevoflurane in one arm of this study as it is one of the most frequently used inhalational agents in our medical center, and worldwide. Compared to isoflurane and desflurane, it has the least vasoactive (vasodilatory) effect and can preserve cerebral blood flow best up to 1–1.5 MAC, while maintaining cerebral autoregulation [16–19]. Propofol is the only available intravenous general anesthetic for maintenance in both TIVA and combined inhaled-intravenous anesthesia. It is pharmacologically difficult to use only a single anesthetic agent to maintain general anesthesia during surgery, as usually an intraoperative analgesic is necessary as well, and so we selected an ultra short-acting opioid (remifentanil), which has a very short elimination half-life, so as to avoid respiratory depression postoperatively, which is especially important for neurosurgical patients.

The 15-item National Institutes of Health Stroke Scale (NIHSS) was developed for and is widely used to evaluate neurologic function [20]. Although the modified NIHSS (mNIHSS) appears to be a more easily-used measure that is identical with the original NIHSS in its validation and reliability when evaluating the severity of stroke [21, 22], the deletion of limb ataxia in the mNIHSS has significance in patients with intracranial tumors based on our previous study [9], and there is no evidence showing the superiority of one to another in the intracranial tumor population. We therefore will choose to calculate both the NIHSS and the mNIHSS for comprehensive neurologic function evaluation. The Chinese version of NIHSS has been validated in a previous study [23].

Motor evoked potential (MEP) monitoring is very important for some supratentorial craniotomies if the tumor is located in or near the motor strip or descending motor pathways near the prefrontal cortex. Clinical evidence shows that sevoflurane suppresses MEP amplitudes in a dose-dependent manner [24, 25]. When using a sevoflurane-propofol combination in clinical practice, sevoflurane concentration is usually maintained below 0.4 MAC; while in this study, sevoflurane will be the only general anesthetic to maintain the desired anesthetic depth in the sevoflurane arm, the concentration will be much higher and vary among individual patients, resulting in failure of MEP monitoring. Therefore, patients who require intraoperative neurophysiological monitoring will be excluded from the study.

The current study aims primarily to elucidate the possible differential effect of inhalational sevoflurane versus intravenous propofol anesthesia on the short period of post-operative neurologic function in patients receiving supratentorial tumor resection in a randomized controlled trial. As the repeated neurologic function assessments are important to evaluate the patients' recovery from surgical intervention and the presence of any complications, the results of this trial would help to interpret anesthetic residual effects on postoperative outcomes, and perhaps help to determine the intraoperative general anesthetic that affects neurologic function with the least detriment and therefore optimizes anesthetic management in this specific patient population.

Trial status

This registered study (ChiCTR-IOR-16009177) started recruiting on May 28th, 2018, and is planned to complete recruiting on December 31st, 2020. The protocol version number is 01 (September 1, 2016).

Appendix

Table 3 NIHSS and mNIHSS score system

Item	NIHSS	mNIHSS	Score
1a	LOC	[deleted]	0 = Alert 1 = Arousable by minor stimulation 2 = Arousable by strong/repeated stimulation 3 = Unresponsive
1b	LOC questions		0 = Answers both correctly 1 = Answers one correctly 2 = Answers neither correctly
1c	LOC Commands		0 = Performs both tasks correctly 1 = Performs one task correctly 2 = Performs neither task
2	Gaze		0 = Normal 1 = Parial gaze pulsy 2 = Forced deviation
3	Visual		0 = Normal 1 = Partial hemianopia 2 = Complete hemianopia 3 = Bilateral hemianopia
4	Facial Palsy	[deleted]	0 = Normal 1 = Minor 2 = Parial 3 = Complete
5a 5b 6a 6b	Motor Arm (left) Motor Arm (right) Motor Leg (left) Motor Leg (right)		0 = No drift 1 = Drift before 10s 2 = Falls before 10s 3 = No effort against gravity 4 = No movement UN = Amputation or joint fusion explain:
7	Limb Ataxia	[deleted]	0 = Absent 1 = In one limb 2 = In two Limb UN = Amputation or joint fusion
8	Sensory		In NIHSS: 0 = Normal 1 = Mild-to-Moderate loss 2 = Severe to total loss In mNIHSS: 0 = Normal 1 = Abnormal
9	Language		0 = Normal 1 = Mild-to-Moderate aphasia 2 = Severe aphasia 3 = Mute or global aphasia
10	Dysarthria	[deleted]	0 = Normal 1 = Mild-to-Moderate 2 = Severe UN=Intubated
11	Extinction and Inattention		0 = Normal 1 = Visual, tactile, auditory, spatial, or personal inattention 2 = Profound hemi-inattention or extinction to more than one modality

NIHSS National Institute of Health stroke scale, *mNIHSS* modified National Institute of Health stroke scale, *LOC* Level of Consciousness
The total score in NIHSS and mNIHSS are 42 and 31 respectively

Abbreviations

BP: Blood pressure; BIS: Bispectral index; ECG: Electrocardiography; $ETCO_2$: End-tidal carbon dioxide; GABA: Gamma-aminobutyric acid; HR: Heart rate; LOC: Level of consciousness; MAC: Minimum alveolar concentration (the concentration of an inhalational anesthetic in the alveoli of the lungs that is needed to prevent movement in 50% of subjects in response to surgical stimulus.); MAP: Mean arterial pressure; MEP: Motor evoked potential; MMSE: Mini-mental state examination; MRI: Magnetic resonance imaging; NIHSS: National Institute of Health stroke scale; mNIHSS: Modified National Institute of Health stroke scale; OAA/S: Observer's assessment of alertness/ sedation; PCIA: Patient-controlled intravenous analgesia; SMA: Supplementary motor area; SpO_2: Pulse oxygen saturation; VAS: Visual analog scale

Acknowledgements

Not applicable.

Authors' contributions

NL contributed to the study design and concept, conduct, as well as being involved in the statistical analysis planning, writing the protocol draft, and revising it critically and approving the final version. YX contributed to the study design and conduct, data collection, and writing the protocol draft. YP was involved in the data collection coordination and contributing to the statistical plan. RH was involved in coordination and supervision of data collection and reviewing the protocol. JFB contributed to the protocol writing, reviewing, and revising. XL, YL, JD and MZ were involved in data collection and protocol writing. JL, MZ, and LN were involved in follow-up data collection. All authors have read and approved the manuscript as submitted.

*Yan Xing and Nan Lin are co-first authors who equally contributed to this trial. Nan Lin and Ruquan Han are co-corresponding authors who are equally responsible for this protocol.

Author details

[1]Department of Anesthesiology, Beijing Tiantan Hospital, Capital Medical University, No.119, West Road 4th ring South, Fengtai District, Beijing 100070, China. [2]Departments of Anesthesiology & Neurological Surgery, Northwestern University Feinberg School of Medicine, 251 E. Huron St., F5-704, Chicago, IL 60611, USA.

References

1. Ostrom QT, Gittleman H, Fulop J, Liu M, Blanda R, Kromer C, et al. CBTRUS Statistical Report: Primary Brain and Central Nervous System Tumors Diagnosed in the United States in 2008–2012. Neuro-oncol. 2015;17(Suppl 4):iv1–iv62.
2. Engelhard K, Werner C. Inhalational or intravenous anesthetics for craniotomies? Pro inhalational. Curr Opin Anaesthesiol. 2006;19(5):504–8.
3. Citerio G, Pesenti A, Latini R, Masson S, Barlera S, Gaspari F, et al. A multicentre, randomised, open-label, controlled trial evaluating equivalence of inhalational and intravenous anaesthesia during elective craniotomy. Eur J Anaesthesiol. 2012;29(8):371–9.
4. Fukui K, Morioka T, Hashiguchi K, Kawamura T, Irita K, Hoka S, et al. Relationship between regional cerebral blood flow and electrocorticographic activities under sevoflurane and isoflurane anesthesia. J Clin Neurophysiol. 2010;27(2):110–5.
5. Lauta E, Abbinante C, Del Gaudio A, Aloj F, Fanelli M, de Vivo P, et al. Emergence times are similar with sevoflurane and total intravenous anesthesia: results of a multicenter RCT of patients scheduled for elective supratentorial craniotomy. J Neurosurg Anesthesiol. 2010;22(2):110–8.
6. Necib S, Tubach F, Peuch C, LeBihan E, Samain E, Mantz J, et al. Recovery from anesthesia after craniotomy for supratentorial tumors: comparison of propofol-remifentanil and sevoflurane-sufentanil (the PROMIFLUNIL trial). J Neurosurg Anesthesiol. 2014;26(1):37–44.
7. Flexman AM, Meng L, Gelb AW. Outcomes in neuroanesthesia: what matters most? Can J Anaesth. 2016;63(2):205–11.
8. Rohm KD, Piper SN, Suttner S, Schuler S, Boldt J. Early recovery, cognitive function and costs of a desflurane inhalational vs. a total intravenous anaesthesia regimen in long-term surgery. Acta Anaesthesiol Scand. 2006; 50(1):14–8.
9. Lin N, Han R, Zhou J, Gelb AW. Mild sedation exacerbates or unmasks focal neurologic dysfunction in neurosurgical patients with Supratentorial brain mass lesions in a drug-specific manner. Anesthesiology. 2016;124(3):598–607.
10. Sundararaj MS, Singh G, Prabhu K. Supplementary motor area (SMA) syndrome: an enigma to anesthesiologists. J Neurosurg Anesthesiol. 2016; 28(4):438–9.
11. Nakajima R, Nakada M, Miyashita K, Kinoshita M, Okita H, Yahata T, et al. Intraoperative motor symptoms during brain tumor resection in the supplementary motor area (SMA) without positive mapping during awake surgery. Neurol Med Chir. 2015;55(5):442–50.
12. Balki M, Manninen PH, McGuire GP, El-Beheiry H, Bernstein M. Venous air embolism during awake craniotomy in a supine patient. Can J Anaesth. 2003;50(8):835–8.
13. Spence NZ, Faloba K, Sonabend AM, Bruce JN, Anastasian ZH. Venous air embolus during scalp incision. J Clin Neurosci. 2016;28:170–1.
14. Kapurch CJ, Abcejo AS, Pasternak JJ. The relationship between end-expired carbon dioxide tension and severity of venous air embolism during sitting neurosurgical procedures - a contemporary analysis. J Clin Anesth. 2018;51: 49–54.
15. Meyer BC, Lyden PD. The modified National Institutes of Health stroke scale: its time has come. Int J Stroke. 2009;4(4):267–73.
16. Gupta S, Heath K, Matta BF. Effect of incremental doses of sevoflurane on cerebral pressure autoregulation in humans. Br J Anaesth. 1997;79(4):469–72.
17. Matta BF, Heath KJ, Tipping K, Summors AC. Direct cerebral vasodilatory effects of sevoflurane and isoflurane. Anesthesiology. 1999;91(3):677–80.
18. Summors AC, Gupta AK, Matta BF. Dynamic cerebral autoregulation during sevoflurane anesthesia: a comparison with isoflurane. Anesth Analg. 1999; 88(2):341–5.
19. Bedforth NM, Hardman JG, Nathanson MH. Cerebral hemodynamic response to the introduction of desflurane: a comparison with sevoflurane. Anesth Analg. 2000;91(1):152–5.
20. Goldstein LB, Samsa GP. Reliability of the National Institutes of Health stroke scale. Extension to non-neurologists in the context of a clinical trial. Stroke. 1997;28(2):307–10.
21. Meyer BC, Hemmen TM, Jackson CM, Lyden PD. Modified National Institutes of Health stroke scale for use in stroke clinical trials: prospective reliability and validity. Stroke. 2002;33(5):1261–6.
22. Kasner SE, Cucchiara BL, McGarvey ML, Luciano JM, Liebeskind DS, Chalela JA. Modified National Institutes of Health stroke scale can be estimated from medical records. Stroke. 2003;34(2):568–70.
23. Cheung PLP, Tsoi Y, Huang M, Liu S, Hon R, Raman, Liu L. Production and validation of Putonghua- and Cantonese-Chinese language National Institutes of Health Stroke Scale Training and Certification Videos. Int J Stroke. 2010;5:6.
24. Chong CT, Manninen P, Sivanaser V, Subramanyam R, Lu N, Venkatraghavan L. Direct comparison of the effect of desflurane and sevoflurane on intraoperative motor-evoked potentials monitoring. J Neurosurg Anesthesiol. 2014;26(4):306–12.
25. Reinacher PC, Priebe HJ, Blumrich W, Zentner J, Scheufler KM. The effects of stimulation pattern and sevoflurane concentration on intraoperative motor-evoked potentials. Anesth Analg. 2006;102(3):888–95.

13

Anesthetic management of gigantic pheochromocytoma resection with inferior vena cava and right atrium tumor thrombosis

Jingli Chen†, Caihua Liu†, Chang Liu, Quanyuan Fu, Dingwei Pei, Linyun Ren and Hong Yan*

Abstract

Background: This report describes one case of anesthetic management about surgical resection of a malignant phaeochromocytoma with tumor extension into vena cava and right atrium in a patient. Report for anesthetic management is limited in these patients under surgical resection until now.

Case presentation: In September 2015, a 24-year-old male presented to the department of cardiology with right flank pain and hypertensive urgency in our hospital. Contrast-enhanced CT abdomen and MRI abdomen revealed a mass phaeochromocytoma in right adrenal, which invaded the right inferior vena cava(IVC)wall along with IVC thrombus. Echocardiography shown no abnormal detection. Finally, this patient gave up the surgical resection of phaeochromocytoma and chose the expectant treatment. In April 2018, this patient once again presented to the emergence department in our hospital, he had experienced persistent cough and intermittent wheezing for 5 h. Contrast-enhanced CT and echocardiography shown existing IVC thrombus had extended into the right atrium. After the careful preoperative preparation, adrenalectomy with complete thrombus excision by inferior vena cava exploration and right atriotomy were performed successfully by a multidisciplinary team. After one month post-operation care, this patient healthily left our hospital.

Conclusion: To the best of our knowledge, the occurrence of pheochromocytoma with IVC and right atrium thrombosis has not been reported in mainland China so far. This clinical case may supply a rare reference experience for surgical treatment and anesthetic management in the group of phaeochromocytoma patient with distance vascular extension.

Keywords: Adrenal tumor, Malignant phaeochromocytoma, Inferior vena cava, Right atrium, Tumor thrombus

Background

Pheochromocytoma is a rare tumor, which produce catecholamine in the adrenal medulla. Prevalence of the disease may vary but approximately 1 to 2 per 100,000 individuals are diagnosed annually [1]. The classic hallmark of the disease is headache, sudden perspiration, and tachycardia [2]. The disease is commonly diagnosed biochemically by plasma-free metanephrines or 24-h urine fractionated metanephrines and localized by imaging modalities like contrast-enhanced CT, MRI, or metaiodobenzylguanidine scintigraphy [3, 4].

Thrombosis of inferior vena cava (IVC) is common pathological phenomena in clinical diagnosis, which normally has comparable etiological factors to lower limb deep venous thrombosis [5]. The hypercoagulable state of blood or inflammatory processes, neoplastic abnormalities, and vessel injury have all been implicated as primary mechanism in the pathophysiology of IVC thrombosis. Based on recently studies report, intravenous extension is a potential mechanism in the evolution of IVC thrombosis. Actually, it is not well-known that endocrine tumor exhibits the ability to extend into vein

* Correspondence: yhmzk1@126.com
†Jingli Chen and Caihua Liu are contributed equally to this work.
Department of Anaesthesia, The Central Hospital of Wuhan, Tongji Medical College, Huazhong University of Science and Technology, Wuhan 430014, Hubei, China

[6]. However, few rare studies have reported that pheochromocytoma really infiltrates to IVC in patients [7]. Two major mechanism of intravenous extension of pheochromocytoma have been presented, including propagation within the veins and directly invasion through the vessel wall [8].

At present, pheochromocytoma associated with IVC thrombosis have been reported [9–12]. However, the vascular extension of pheochromocytoma into right atrium through IVC has never been reported in main china. We describe a successful perioperative anesthetic management of a rare case of pheochromocytoma associated with IVC and right atrium thrombosis for tumor excision.

Case presentation

In September 2015, a 24-year-young man was admitted to our hospital with complaints of headache, sweating, anxiety, dizziness. It was confirmed that he had a history of hypertension and type 2 diabetes by clinical syndromes and examination. He was a smoker with no significant family history. His resting pulse rate was 100 beats/min. The patient's blood pressure was 163/100 mmHg. Physical examination revealed mild lower abdominal tenderness, both edema of lower extremity and collateral formation over abdomen were unremarkable. Hepatomegaly and abdominis hydrops were also absent in the young man.

Abdominal CT revealed a well defined, heterogenous mass lesion of size 11.1 × 10.5 × 11.1 cm at the upper pole of right kidney, which was rooted in right adrenal gland. Vena cava area exhibited filling defect, which indicated the possibility of tumor thrombosis extension from localized tumor. Magnetic resonance imaging (MRI) reveal the proximal part of inferior vena cava was widened (Fig. 1a), and confirmed that intraluminal thrombus is inferior to the right atrium, the distance of extended tumor thrombosis was 6.5 cm approximately (Fig. 1b). Echocardiography indicated this patient had atrial septal defect, the defect size was 0.2 cm, and only showed mild tricuspid regurgitation with 63% EF. Surgical treatment was been suggested. However, the patient gave up the surgical treatment and left hospital.

In April 2018, this young man once again presented to the emergence department with persistent cough and intermittent wheezing character for 5 h. At this time, his blood pressure was 160/120 mmHg with a heart rate of 142 beats per minute and SpO2 was 95% on room air. Bilateral lower limb arterial and venous examination was normal. Contrast-enhance CT showed a 12-cm right adrenal mass with tumor thrombosis in IVC, which dubiously extended into right atrium (Fig. 2a), the distance of extended tumor thrombosis was 13.5 cm approximately (Fig. 2b). Echocardiography conformed that existing IVC tumor thrombus had extended into the right atrium (Fig. 3), EF was only 42%. The biochemical evaluation revealed elevated of dopamine 6.03 nmol/L (normal range: 2.09–3.91 nmol/L), adrenaline 15.15 nmol/L (normal range:1.31–2.51 nmol/L), noradrenline 33.17 nmol/L (normal range:1.31–2.30 nmol/L). Preoperative electrocardiography showed supraventricular tachycardia and 24 h Holter monitoring showed no significant cardiac arrhythmia except intermittent junctional rhythm. A primary diagnosis of pheochromocytoma with IVC and right atrium tumor thrombosis was established. The patient finally agreed to receive a surgical treatment. Before receiving the surgical treatment, the patient recurrently presented heart failure in intensive care unit, a combination of alpha-adrenergic and beta-adrenergic blockade and calcium channel blockers were routinely used to maintain the blood pressure and stabilize heart function. In order to avoid the occurrence of hypotension after resecting the phaeochromocytoma, phentolamine was discontinued on the day before the operation. In addition, the

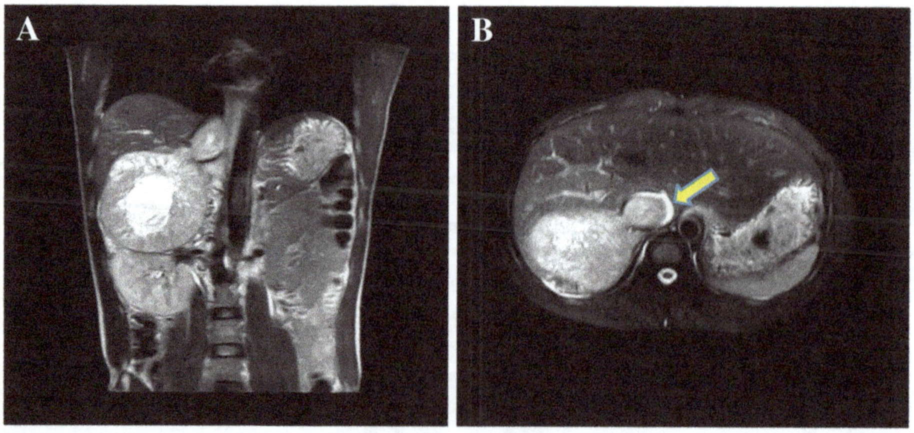

Fig. 1 a. Magnetic resonance image of the abdomen shows the proximal part of inferior vena cava was widened on longitudinal scan. **b**. Magnetic resonance image of the abdomen indicated tumor thrombus in the inferior vena cava next to the large adrenal phaeochromocytoma on horizontal scan

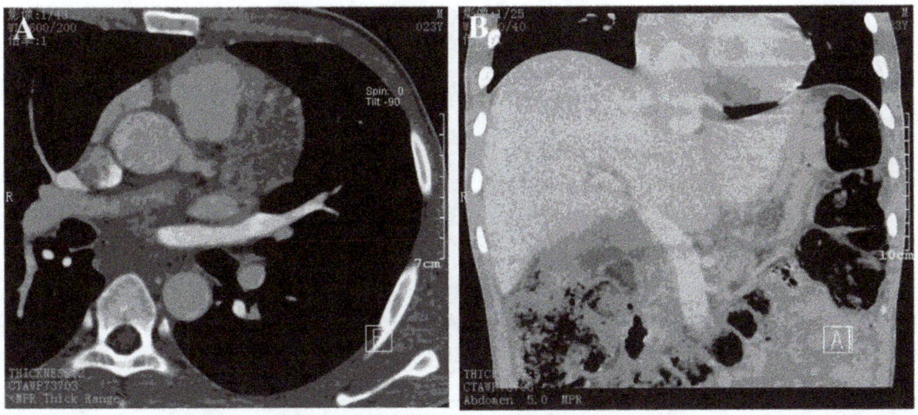

Fig. 2 a. Contrast-enhanced CT revealed tumor thrombus extended into right atrium on horizontal scan of heart. **b**. Contrast-enhanced CT revealed the distance of tumor thrombus was 13.5 cm on longitudinal scan

beta-adrenergic blockade was continued until the day of operation.

Nearly two months later, our anesthetist team finally evaluated the cardiac system of the patient. And we considered that it was an appropriate time to perform the operation based on the relatively favorable physical condition. After being administered intravenous midazolam (1.5 mg), the patient was brought to the operating room. The initial SBP and HR were 144 mmHg and 110 beats/min, respectively, Spo2 was 98% under room air. Two peripheral venous access were established by nurse immediately. After intravenous midazolam (2 mg) and sufentanil (5μg), the left radial artery was cannulated for continuous arterial blood pressure monitoring. Meanwhile, FloTrac system was employed to monitor the cardio output (CO), stroke volume (SV), stroke volume variation (SVV), systemic vascular resistance (SVR). Midazolam (4 mg), sufentanil (70 μg), rocuronium (70 mg) and etomidate (20 mg) were injected via peripheral venous access in sequence. After 2 min of mask positive pressure ventilation, reinforced tracheal tube was intubated. Intravenous infusion of propofol and remifentanil were induced to maintain the anesthesia during the surgery, which were combined with 1–2 MAC of sevoflurane and 100% O_2. Internal jugular vein puncture was performed to place the central venous catheter and monitor central venous pressure (CVP). Subsequently, transesophageal echocardiography (TEE) probe was inserted to evaluate the ventricular function. Before incising the skin, methylprednisolone (80 mg) and Ulinastatin (7×10^5 unit) were used to resist systematic inflammation reaction. Pantolazole (80 mg) was induced to protect stomach. Subsequently, a midline xiphoid to pubic symphysis incision was induced. Because of the tumor thrombosis in the inferior vena cava and the right atrium, the liver was enlarged and congested secondary to the Budd-Chiari syndrome. A large and well-circumscribed right adrenal phaeochromocytoma was observered clearly, which actually extended through the adrenal vein and lateral wall of inferior vena cava into the right atrium. After the carefully dissociation of tissue, the tumor was successfully dissected from the kidney, liver, and retroperitoneum until it was only attached to the lateral wall of the vena cava at the area of tumor invasion, the resected tumor was shown in Fig. 4a. During the exploration of abdominal, the circulation was extremely unstable. Sodium nitroprusside (0.5-3μg/kg/min) and phentolamine (0.5-3μg/kg/min) were induced to control the SPB in 60-160 mmHg and the DPB in 50–100 mmHg. Nicardipine (1 mg) and phentolamine (1 mg) were also discontinuously intravenous injected to control the blood press cooperatively. Esmolol (50-300μg/kg/min) was induced to revolt tachycardia, but the control of heat rate was unsatisfactory, the heat rate was maintained in 90–140 beats/min. During the resection, the cardiac function and hemodynamic parameters were not relative stable (CO: 3.3–4.5 L/min, SV: 60-82 ml, SVV: 8–26%, SVR: 1023–1368 dynes-s/cm ^{5}). Blood gas analysis was

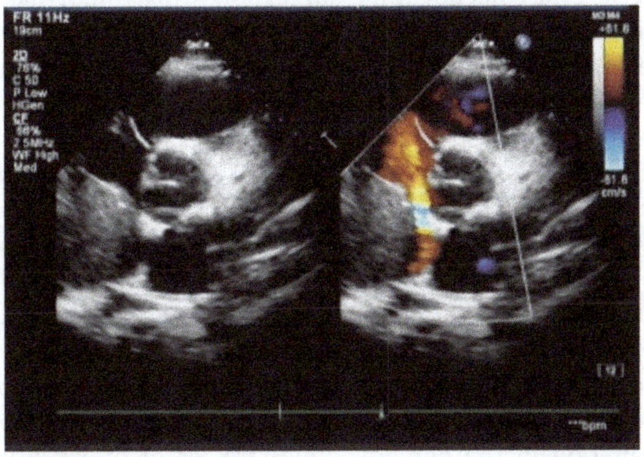

Fig. 3 Echocardiography shown existing IVC thrombus had extended into the right atrium

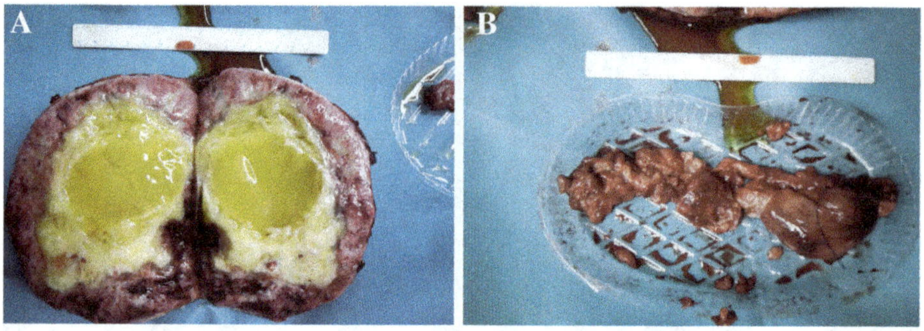

Fig. 4 a. The image of resected gigantic pheochromocytoma. **b**. The image of removed inferior vena cava and right atrium thrombosis after the operation

performed hourly (PH: 7.34–7.23, PaO_2:345-222 mmHg, $PaCO_2$:37–41 mmHg, SaO_2:97.9–100% ctHb: 8.1–13.4 g/L, cK^+: 3.1–5.1 mmol/L, cNa^+: 135–141 mmol/L, cCa^+: 0.97–1.23 mmol/L, cLac: 0.8–5.7 mmol/L), these related parameters was modulated to approach the normal range. Subsequently, the cardiac surgeon continued to perform median sternotomy. After systemic heparinisation, the right femoral vein, superior vena cava, and the aorta were cannulated to establish cardiopulmonary bypass. Before the aorta was cross-clamped, the patient was gradually cooled to 32 °C. After the infusion of cold cardioplegia into aortic root, cardiac arrest was achieved. Meanwhile, cardiopulmonary bypass was induced to support the circulation system. By cutting open the right atrium, tumor thrombosis at the right atrium was then resected, the elimination of tumor thrombosis in the vena cava was performed subsequently. The removal tumor thrombosis form IVC and right atrium was shown in Fig. 4b. After repairment of right atrium and vene cava, The patient was weaned off from cardiopulmonary bypass after full re-warming. During the cardiopulmonary bypass, the blood pressure remained relatively stable with any severe hemodynamic disorder. In summarize, the operating time of this patient was totally 11.5 h, the blood loss was approximately 10,000 mL. The diagnosis of phaeochromocytoma was finally confirmed by immunohistochemical method. After one month post-operation care, the patient healthily left our hospital.

Discussion and conclusion

Pheochromocytoma represents very significant challenges to the anesthetist, which are not uncommon in anesthetic practice. Generally, the laparoscopic approach is preferred for most pheochromocytoma resections [13]. The anesthetic management of the surgical approach has improved remarkably over the years, in conjunction with the evolution of surgical techniques. However, the pheochromocytoma combined with cardiovascular extension was rare. The perioperative anesthetic management will be very hard because of the vascular obstruction induced severe hemodynamic disturbance. In this case, the patient presented gigantic pheochromocytoma with inferior vena cava and right atrium thrombosis. Actually, limited number of case reports on malignant phaeochromocytoma with extension into the right atrium were been reported in the literature. This present report is believed to be the first case of a malignant phaeochromocytoma extending into the right atrium in mainland china.

Surgical resection has been proved to the efficient treatment option for phaeochromocytoma patients [14]. Up to now, various techniques of tumor resection have been applied to limit blood loss and eliminate the tumor completely. However, complexity of anesthetic management is largely depended on surgical approach. In this case, the mass of phaeochromocytomas was nearly 12 cm diameter, and tumor thrombus extended into the right atrium. The radical surgery with the use of cardiopulmonary bypass with hypothermic circulatory arrest is recommended based on previous case report [15]. This surgical approach was highly risky, and anesthetic management was sufficiently challenging.

In the case, the primary anesthesic goal is the delivery of an anesthetic which provides stable hemodynamics in the face of catecholamine surges following tumor handling and opposite scenario following tumor ligation. It is necessary to prepare careful planning with surgical team. Relief from anxiety prior to anesthetic induction is a key component, as apprehension can predispose to catecholamine surges. We made a judicious dose of IV midazolam (1.5 mg) prior to transfer to the operating suite creates a calm patient less prone to hypertensive crises at induction. Traditional vasodilator set up includes nitroglycerin, sodium nitroprusside, nicardipine, diltiazem as indicated, esmolol infusion for heart rate control, magnesium sulfate, and vasoconstrictors such as norepinephrine and vasopressin. For anesthetic induction, limitation of the hemodynamic stresses of direct laryngoscopy should be considered. Propofol and etomidate were recommended. Propofol has been documented to be safe in these patients [16]. Etomidate has the advantage of conferring cardiovascular stability, especially in volume-depleted patients [17]. All agents that cause histamine release should be avoided. During the operation, we also employed TEE to monitor the heart function and confirm the removal of thrombus after surgery. Importantly, intraoperative TEE has the added advantage of real-time monitoring of intravascular volume status, as well as the earlier detection of myocardial wall motion abnormalities aiding the diagnosis of intraoperative myocardial ischemia. Fortunately, the patient did not show significantly myocardial ischemia and heart failure in the presence of unstable circulation during the operation.

In this case, the successful anesthetic management is mainly due to the positive circulation regulation. In generally, tumor manipulation usually generates a far more dramatic pressor response, which is related to increases in plasma levels of norepinephrine and epinephrine [18]. Significant reductions in cardiac output, and associated left ventricular systolic and diastolic dysfunction may be observed in this situation. Acute hemodynamic crises during resection are not uncommon and must be immediately treated. During the process of tumor resection, severe bradycardia accompanied by hypertension and tachyarrhythmias are the common hemodynamic disorder. Deepening the depth of anesthesia and rapidly administering direct arterial vasodilators are the efficient response to control unstable hemodynamics in this condition. Traditionally, sodium nitroprusside is the key drug in conjunction with nitroglycerin, to reduce preload of heart. In addition, the ligation of the tumor bleeding by surgeon and anesthetic-induced persistent vasodilation normally induced the sudden hypotension. The administration of large-volume fluid prior to tumor ligation will be useful to avoid the occurrence of sudden hypotension, as well as stopping the infusion of all vasodilators in due course. In addition, it had been suggested that massive fluid treatment was more effective strategy than vasopressor treatment to reverse the hypotension in these situations.

In conclusion, understanding of the physiology of this type of patients is essential to perform a successful anesthetic management. Meanwhile, we recommend that all this type of patients should be optimized preoperatively and intraoperative precautions taken, including drug intervene and hemodynamic monitoring, which may ensure a stable perioperative course and life safety.

Abbreviations

CO: Cardio output; CVP: Central venous pressure; IVC: Inferior vena cava; MRI: Magnetic resonance imaging; SV: Stroke volume; SVR: Systemic vascular resistance; SVV: Stroke volume variation; TEE: Transesophageal echocardiography

Acknowledgements

Not applicable.

Authors' contributions

YH, CJL, LCH and RLY were major contributors in performing the anesthesia management. FQY and PDW performed the cardiovascular on-pump manual. LC mainly wrote the manuscript. All authors read and approved the final manuscript.

References

1. Lenders JW, Eisenhofer G, Mannelli M, Pacak K. Phaeochromocytoma. Lancet. 2005;366:665–75.
2. Tsirlin A, Oo Y, Sharma R, Kansara A, Gliwa A, Banerji MA. Pheochromocytoma: a review. Maturitas. 2014;77:229–38.
3. Lenders JW, Pacak K, Walther MM, Linehan WM, Mannelli M, Friberg P, Keiser HR, Goldstein DS, Eisenhofer G. Biochemical diagnosis of pheochromocytoma: which test is best? Jama. 2002;287:1427–34.
4. Szolar DH, Korobkin M, Reittner P, Berghold A, Bauernhofer T, Trummer H, Schoellnast H, Preidler KW, Samonigg H. Adrenocortical carcinomas and adrenal pheochromocytomas: mass and enhancement loss evaluation at delayed contrast-enhanced CT. Radiology. 2005;234:479–85.
5. Giordano P, Weber K, Davis M, Carter E. Acute thrombosis of the inferior vena cava. Am J Emerg Med. 2006;24:640–2.
6. Geelhoed GW, Dunnick NR, Doppman JL. Management of intravenous extensions of endocrine tumors and prognosis after surgical treatment. Am J Surg. 1980;139:844–8.
7. Kota SK, Kota SK, Jammula S, Meher LK, Modi KD. Pheochromocytoma with inferior vena cava thrombosis: an unusual association. Journal of cardiovascular disease research. 2012;3:160–4.
8. Lau TN, Goddard P, Vaidya M, Calloway M, Bullimore J. Involvement of the inferior vena cava by adrenal phaeochromocytoma--MRI findings. Br J Radiol. 1997;70:303–5.
9. Lucon AM, Falci R Jr, Praxedes JN, Machado MC, Saldanha LB, Machado MM, Arap S. Multicentric pheochromocytoma and involvement of the inferior vena cava. *Sao Paulo medical journal = Revista paulista de medicina*, vol. 119; 2001. p. 86–8.
10. Rotker J, Oberpennig F, Scheld HH, Hertle L, Knichwitz G, Hammel D. Pheochromocytomas with extension into central vascular structures. Ann Thorac Surg. 1996;61:222–4.
11. Dunn CW, Snyder WH, Ring WS, Latson TW. Pheochromocytoma with extension into the inferior vena cava: a case report. Surgery. 1992;111:472–4.
12. Shigemura K, Tanaka K, Arakawa S, Hara I, Kawabata G, Fujisawa M. Malignant pheochromocytoma with IVC thrombus. Int Urol Nephrol. 2007; 39:103–6.
13. Conzo G, Musella M, Corcione F, De Palma M, Ferraro F, Palazzo A, Napolitano S, Milone M, Pasquali D, Sinisi AA, et al. Laparoscopic adrenalectomy, a safe procedure for pheochromocytoma. A retrospective review of clinical series. Int J Surg. 2013;11:152–6.
14. Assalia A, Gagner M. Laparoscopic adrenalectomy. Br J Surg. 2004;91:1259–74.
15. Ku CF, Lo CY, Chan WF, Chiu SW, Fan ST, Lam KS. Resection of phaeochromocytoma extending into the right atrium in a patient with multiple endocrine neoplasia type 2A. Hong Kong medical journal = Xianggang yi xue za zhi. 2005;11:59–62.
16. Strebel S, Scheidegger D. Propofol-fentanyl anesthesia for pheochromocytoma resection. Acta Anaesthesiol Scand. 1991;35:275–7.
17. Hull CJ. Phaeochromocytoma. Diagnosis, preoperative preparation and anaesthetic management. Br J Anaesth. 1986;58:1453–68.
18. Vater M, Achola K, Smith G. Catecholamine responses during anaesthesia for phaeochromocytoma. Br J Anaesth. 1983;55:357–60.

14

Improved haemodynamic stability and cerebral tissue oxygenation after induction of anaesthesia with sufentanil compared to remifentanil

Marieke Poterman[1*], Alain F. Kalmar[1,2], Pieter L. Buisman[1], Michel M. R. F. Struys[1] and Thomas W. L. Scheeren[1]

Abstract

Background: Balanced anaesthesia with propofol and remifentanil, compared to sufentanil, often decreases mean arterial pressure (MAP), heart rate (HR) and cardiac index (CI), raising concerns on tissue-oxygenation. This distinct haemodynamic suppression might be attenuated by atropine. This double blinded RCT, investigates if induction with propofol-sufentanil results in higher CI and tissue-oxygenation than with propofol-remifentanil and if atropine has more pronounced beneficial effects on CI and tissue-oxygenation in a remifentanil-based anaesthesia.

Methods: In seventy patients scheduled for coronary bypass grafting (CABG), anaesthesia was induced and maintained with propofol target controlled infusion (TCI) with a target effect-site concentration (Cet) of 2.0 μg ml^{-1} and either sufentanil (TCI Cet 0.48 ng ml^{-1}) or remifentanil (TCI Cet 8 ng ml^{-1}). If HR dropped below 60 bpm, methylatropine (1 mg) was administered intravenously. Relative changes (Δ) in MAP, HR, stroke volume (SV), CI and cerebral ($SctO_2$) and peripheral ($SptO_2$) tissue-oxygenation during induction of anaesthesia and after atropine administration were analysed.

Results: The sufentanil group compared to the remifentanil group showed significantly less decrease in MAP ($\Delta = -23 \pm 13$ vs. -36 ± 13 mmHg), HR ($\Delta = -5 \pm 7$ vs. -10 ± 10 bpm), SV ($\Delta = -23 \pm 18$ vs. -35 ± 19 ml) and CI ($\Delta = -0.8$ (-1.5 to -0.5) vs. -1.5 (-2.0 to -1.1) l min^{-1} m^{-2}), while $SctO_2$ ($\Delta = 9 \pm 5$ vs. 6 ± 4%) showed more increase with no difference in $\Delta SptO_2$ ($\Delta = 8 \pm 7$ vs. 8 ± 8%). Atropine caused higher ΔHR (13 (9 to 19) vs. 10 ± 6 bpm) and ΔCI (0.4 ± 0.4 vs. 0.2 ± 0.3 l min^{-1} m^{-2}) in sufentanil vs. remifentanil-based anaesthesia, with no difference in ΔMAP, ΔSV and $\Delta SctO_2$ and $\Delta SptO_2$.

Conclusion: Induction of anaesthesia with propofol and sufentanil results in improved haemodynamic stability and higher $SctO_2$ compared to propofol and remifentanil in patients having CABG. Administration of atropine might be useful to counteract or prevent the haemodynamic suppression associated with these opioids.

Keywords: Induction of anaesthesia, Sufentanil, Remifentanil, Atropine, Haemodynamics, Tissue oxygenation

* Correspondence: mpoterman@gmail.com
[1]Department of Anaesthesiology, University Medical Center Groningen, Hanzeplein 1, PO Box 30 001, 9700, RB, Groningen, The Netherlands

Background

Balanced general anaesthesia with a combination of propofol and remifentanil, as compared to propofol with other opioids like sufentanil, provides some beneficial pharmacological properties, such as a fast and reliable induction and reversal of anaesthesia, swift postoperative recovery and avoidance of postoperative nausea and vomiting [1, 2]. However, vasodilation and cardiac depression caused by this type of anaesthesia often induces a decrease in mean arterial pressure (MAP), heart rate (HR) and cardiac index (CI), raising concerns on maintaining an adequate tissue oxygenation [3–5].

Haemodynamic suppression is often observed after induction of general anaesthesia with any combination of hypnotics and opioids. Because of the distinct pharmacodynamic differences of remifentanil compared to other opioids such as sufentanil or fentanyl, different haemodynamic side effects may occur with differential effects on tissue oxygenation [6–8]. In addition to a strong suppressive effect on the heart rate, remifentanil dose-dependently depresses the sinus and AV node function, and significantly prolongates the sinus node recovery time, sino-atrial conduction time and Wenckebach cycle length, resulting in an inhibition of both the intra-atrial conduction and sinus node automaticity [7, 8]. This distinct effect of remifentanil on cardiac conduction might have a particularly significant negative impact on the cardiac index compared to sufentanil.

Perioperative maintenance of adequate tissue oxygenation has been associated with less postoperative complications, such as reduction in surgical wound infections and length of hospital stay, and is specifically important for high-risk surgical patients, including patients scheduled for coronary artery bypass grafting surgery [9–11].

Beneficial effects of atropine, not only on MAP and HR, but also on CI during propofol-remifentanil anaesthesia in patients undergoing non-cardiac surgery have been reported [12]. However, this may not be equally valid during anaesthesia with propofol combined with other opioids, such as sufentanil, and in patients undergoing cardiac surgery. Positive inotropic agents such as dopamine, dobutamine or ephedrine are in general preferably used in cardiac surgery. However, the prominent effect of remifentanil on the cardiac conduction suggests that it has a direct parasympathicomimetic effect, thereby making a beneficial effect of atropine more likely. In these circumstances, atropine may not only mitigate bradycardia and increase the arterial blood pressure, but also increase CI and tissue oxygenation.

We therefore hypothesised that induction of anaesthesia with propofol and sufentanil results in different haemodynamic suppression and tissue oxygenation values compared to anaesthesia with propofol and remifentanil in calculated equipotent dosages. Also, we expected that atropine will have different effects on the haemodynamic suppression and tissue oxygenation in both groups.

Methods

Ethical approval for this study was provided by the Ethical Committee of University Medical Center Groningen, Groningen, The Netherlands. After registration at ClinicalTrials.gov (Ref: NCT01871935), all patients ≥18 years scheduled for elective off-pump performed Coronary Artery Bypass Grafting (CABG) surgery between 17 June 2013 and 1 October 2013 were assessed for eligibility for this interventional, prospective randomised controlled trial according to the CONSORT group statement (Fig. 1) [13]. Patients undergoing emergency surgery or with a contraindication for atropine administration, such as severe aortic valve stenosis, were excluded. In addition, morbidly obese patients (body mass index > 35 $kg\,m^{-2}$) were excluded, since anaesthesia with target controlled infusion (described below) in this patient category is not reliable [14]. There was no selection made based on age, gender, co-morbidity or ethnic background. Following written informed consent, all included patients were randomly assigned to the sufentanil or remifentanil group using the sealed opaque envelope technique. Randomisation was unblinded only after finishing the full data collection. The complete study adhered to CONSORT guidelines [13].

Study protocol

Based on theoretical drug interaction pharmacodynamic models [15], for propofol/sufentanil and propofol/remifentanil, equipotent opioid targeted effect site concentrations (Cet) were calculated to be 0.48 $ng\,ml^{-1}$ (Gepts model) and 8 $ng\,ml^{-1}$ (Minto model) respectively.

Before induction of anaesthesia, adequate pre-oxygenation of the patient's lungs was performed via a face mask. Anaesthesia was induced as follows: according to randomisation, a syringe pump with sufentanil (target-controlled infusion (TCI), targeted effect site concentration (Cet) 0.48 $ng\,ml^{-1}$, Gepts model) or dose of remifentanil (TCI Cet 8 $ng\,ml^{-1}$, Minto model) was started, followed in both cases by a syringe pump containing propofol (TCI Cet 2.0 $\mu g\,ml^{-1}$, Schnider model) [16–18].

Doses were left unchanged throughout the study period. Maximal reproducibility of the anaesthetic pharmacological condition was pursued by using these propofol and opioids effect site concentrations to obtain a tolerance of laryngoscopy in 95% of patients as predicted by a hierarchical interaction model [3, 19, 20]. After loss of consciousness and achievement of a bispectral index value between 40 and 60, rocuronium (0.6 mg kg^{-1}) was administered and the patient's trachea was intubated. Mechanical ventilation was started in the volume control mode (tidal volume: 8 $ml\,kg^{-1}$) with an O_2/

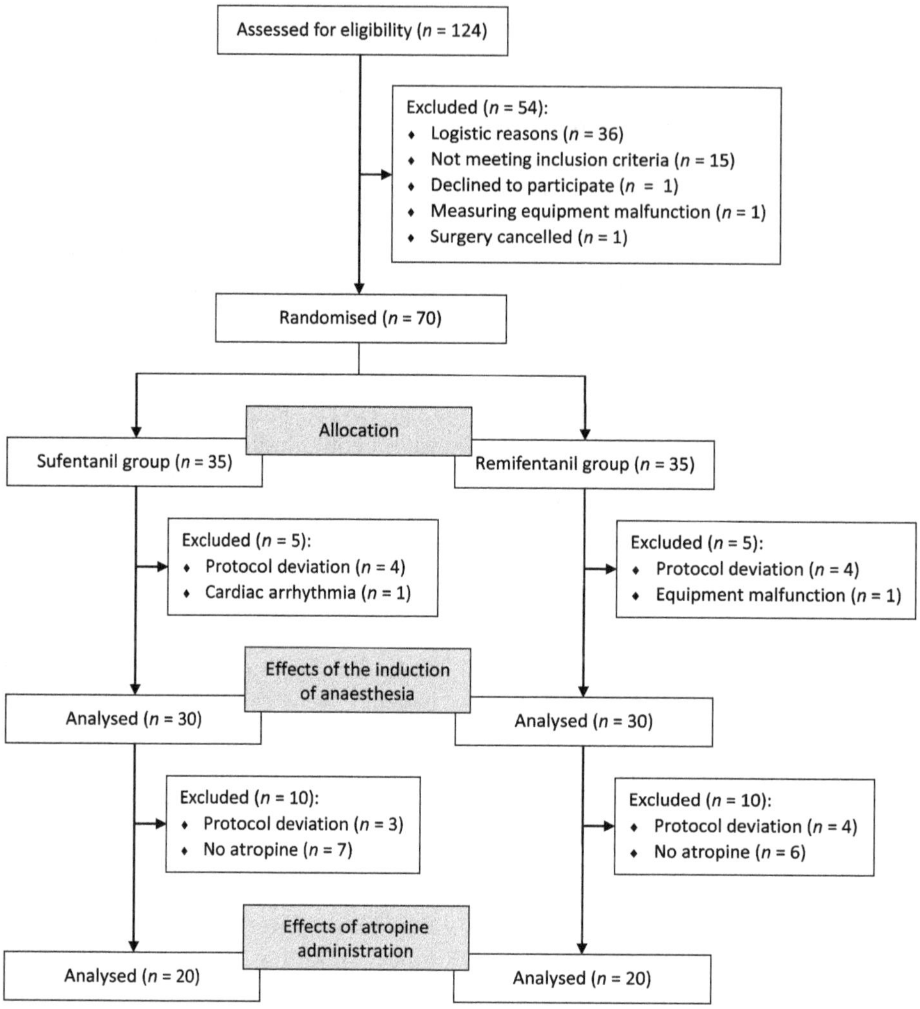

Fig. 1 CONSORT flow diagram

air mixture (F_iO_2 0.4) and a positive end-expiratory pressure of 5 cmH_2O. The respiratory rate was adjusted to keep end-tidal carbon dioxide partial pressure between 4.5 kPa (34 mmHg) and 5.5 kPa (42 mmHg).

If the HR dropped below 60 beats per minute (bpm), methylatropine (1 mg) was administered intravenously. In those cases where the patient had a baseline HR < 60 bpm prior to the induction of anaesthesia, methylatropine (1 mg) was administered when HR dropped more than 10% below the awake HR value.

If the MAP dropped below 80% of the baseline value, without the above-mentioned indications for administration of atropine or from 3 min after the administration of atropine, other appropriate measures (e.g. fluid or vasopressor administration) were taken.

Haemodynamic monitoring

Upon arrival in the operating theatre standard monitoring equipment was connected to the patient: ECG, pulse oximetry and non-invasive blood pressure monitoring (Philips IntelliVue MX800, Philips, Eindhoven, The Netherlands) and routine physiological measurements and monitoring was started. Subsequently two large peripheral intravenous cannulas and an invasive arterial catheter were inserted for invasive blood pressure monitoring, as is usual practice in cardiothoracic anaesthesia.

In addition, a FloTrac sensor (Edwards Lifesciences, Irvine, United States) was connected to the arterial line and subsequently to the Vigileo monitor (Edwards Lifesciences). The FloTrac-Vigileo system analysis the arterial pressure waveform for calculation of the stroke volume (SV) and CI [21]. Two INVOS™ Cerebral Oximeter (Medtronic, Minneapolis, United States) sensors were placed on the patients' forehead to record cerebral tissue oxygenation ($SctO_2$) [22] and an InSpectra™ (Hutchinson Technology Inc., Hutchinson, United States) probe was positioned on the thenar eminence to measure the peripheral tissue oxygenation ($SptO_2$) [23].

Both devices rely on near-infrared spectroscopy technology [24]. Briefly, the sensors positioned on the patient's skin emit light in several device-specific wavelengths from the near infrared spectrum. Based on the ratio of oxygenated and deoxygenated haemoglobin in the underlying tissue, these light signals are partially absorbed and partially reflected to the sensors [25]. Changes relative to baseline tissue oxygenation are significantly correlated with oxygen delivery and perfusion deficits [26].

Data registration and analysis

All data from routine physiological measurements and from the additional study devices were recorded continuously (sampling rate of 1 Hz) on the central hospital server using a cardiothoracic specific data management system (Carola, University Medical Center Groningen, Groningen, The Netherlands).

The electronic data were imported into Microsoft Excel 2016® (Microsoft, Redmond, United States) for synchronization and analysis. After graphical representation, absent values caused by artifacts were corrected by interpolation during a visual inspection of the data plots. Subsequently, we calculated the rate pressure product (RPP) by multiplying the systolic arterial pressure and heart rate. RPP is a surrogate measure of myocardial oxygen uptake [27, 28].

Additionally, a 30 s running median with 15 s steps was calculated for all studied variables. The evolution of the absolute values and of the changes relative to baseline was plotted from 1 min before the induction of anaesthesia until 6 min afterwards, and from 1 min before the administration of atropine until 4 min afterwards. This covers the time to achieve relative steady state for all study variables.

Statistical analysis

The primary outcome measure was the change in CI around the moment of atropine administration. Secondary outcome measures were the changes in MAP, $SctO_2$ and $SptO_2$.The sample size calculation was based on the primary endpoint, CI. A mean difference in CI of 10% between sufentanil and remifentanil was considered clinically relevant. We expected the standard deviation to be 10% in both groups. A type I error probability of 0.05 and a power of 0.95 delivers a total sample size of 54 [29]. A supplemental 25% of patients were included in each group to anticipate invalid data recordings and patients not meeting the criteria for atropine administration, making a total of 70 patients (35 patients in each group).

Statistical analysis was performed in SPSS version 23 (IBM Corporation, Armonk, United States). Categorical variables are given as number of patients and analysed with the Chi-square test or the Fisher's exact test. Continuous data are expressed as mean ± SD or median (IQR), depending on the Kolmogorov-Smirnov tested normality. Differences between groups were tested on absolute values during the induction of anaesthesia and during atropine administration, Time = 0 min (T_0), and at the moment of steady state (after the time to peak of propofol, sufentanil and remifentanil or atropine [30, 31], Time = 6 min (T_6) for the induction of anaesthesia and Time = 4 min (T_4) for the administration of atropine, and on relative changes (Δ = value (T_6 or T_4) − value (T_0)). To compare continuous variables of the different groups, the unpaired student t-test was used for parametric variables, and the Mann-Whitney U test for non-parametric variables. Comparison of the values of the haemodynamic variables from the same group between T_0 and T_6 (for the induction of anaesthesia) or T_4 (for the administration of atropine) was performed using a paired t-test and Wilcoxon signed rank test for parametric and non-parametric variables, respectively. Two-tailed tests were performed and statistical significance was defined as $P < 0.05$ (after Bonferroni correction for multiple comparisons) in all cases.

Results

A total of 70 patients were included in this double blind, randomised controlled trial and subsequently allocated to the sufentanil or remifentanil group (Fig. 1). From these, we had to exclude 10 patients before the analysis of the haemodynamic effects of the induction of anaesthesia due to deviation from the study protocol (n = 8), cardiac arrhythmia (n = 1) or measuring equipment malfunction (n = 1). An additional 20 patients were excluded from the analysis of the effects of atropine administration by reason of study protocol deviation (n = 7) and not meeting the criteria for atropine administration (n = 13). Protocol deviations comprises usage of a different dose of hypnotics and/or opioids than described in the protocol, additions to anaesthesia (e.g. volatile anaesthesia) or the use of additional haemodynamic support (fluid or vasopressor administration) during the measurement periods (from 1 min before induction of anaesthesia or administration of atropine until respectively 6 or 4 min thereafter). Table 1 shows the baseline characteristics of the patients per analysis in both groups. American Society of Anaesthesiologists classification of Physical Health was not included in this table, because all patients belong to American Society of Anaesthesiologists class III. There were no significant between-group differences for both analyses.

Haemodynamic effects after the induction of anaesthesia

The course over time of the investigated variables after the induction of anaesthesia is shown in Figs. 2 and 3.

Table 1 Baseline characteristics of the patients per analysis in the sufentanil and remifentanil group

	Induction of anaesthesia		Atropine administration	
	Sufentanil (n = 30)	Remifentanil (n = 30)	Sufentanil (n = 20)	Remifentanil (n = 20)
Age (years)	64 ± 8	67 ± 8	66 ± 9	70 ± 7
Sex, male	23	23	18	16
Height (cm)	174 ± 10	174 ± 11	175 ± 8	175 ± 11
Weight (kg)	81 ± 16	78 ± 11	82 ± 14	83 ± 11
BMI (kg m^{-2})	27 ± 4	26 ± 3	27 ± 4	27 ± 3
Medical history				
Arterial hypertension	20	21	13	15
Peripheral vascular disease	4	2	4	0
Diabetes mellitus	11	7	8	5
Chronic obstructive pulmonary disease	8	8	6	4
Relevant medication				
Beta blocking agents	27	29	18	18
Angiotensin receptor blockers	7	4	6	1
Angiotensin-converting enzyme inhibitors	14	19	9	13

Continuous variables are reported as mean ± SD and categorical data as numbers

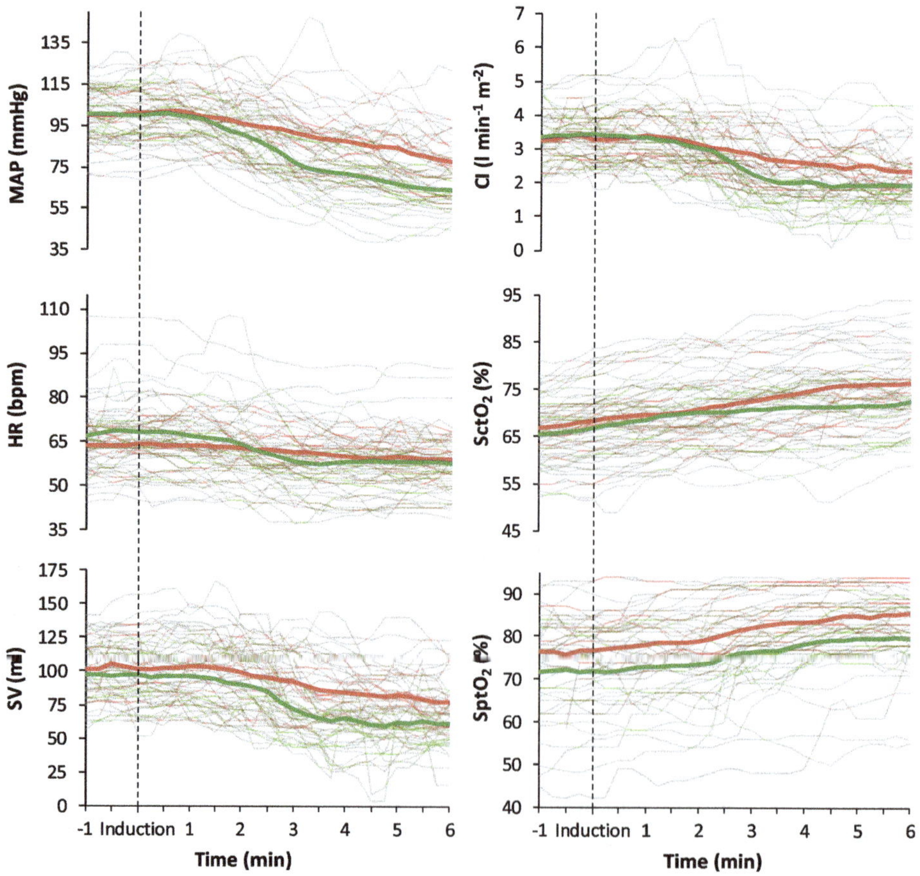

Fig. 2 Mean values (thick lines) and individual patient data (thin lines) of the investigated haemodynamic variables: mean arterial pressure (MAP), heart rate (HR), stroke volume (SV), cardiac index (CI), cerebral tissue oxygen saturation ($SctO_2$) and peripheral tissue oxygen saturation ($SptO_2$). Red lines represent the sufentanil group and green lines the remifentanil group. Graphs are shown from 1 min before until 6 min after the induction of anaesthesia

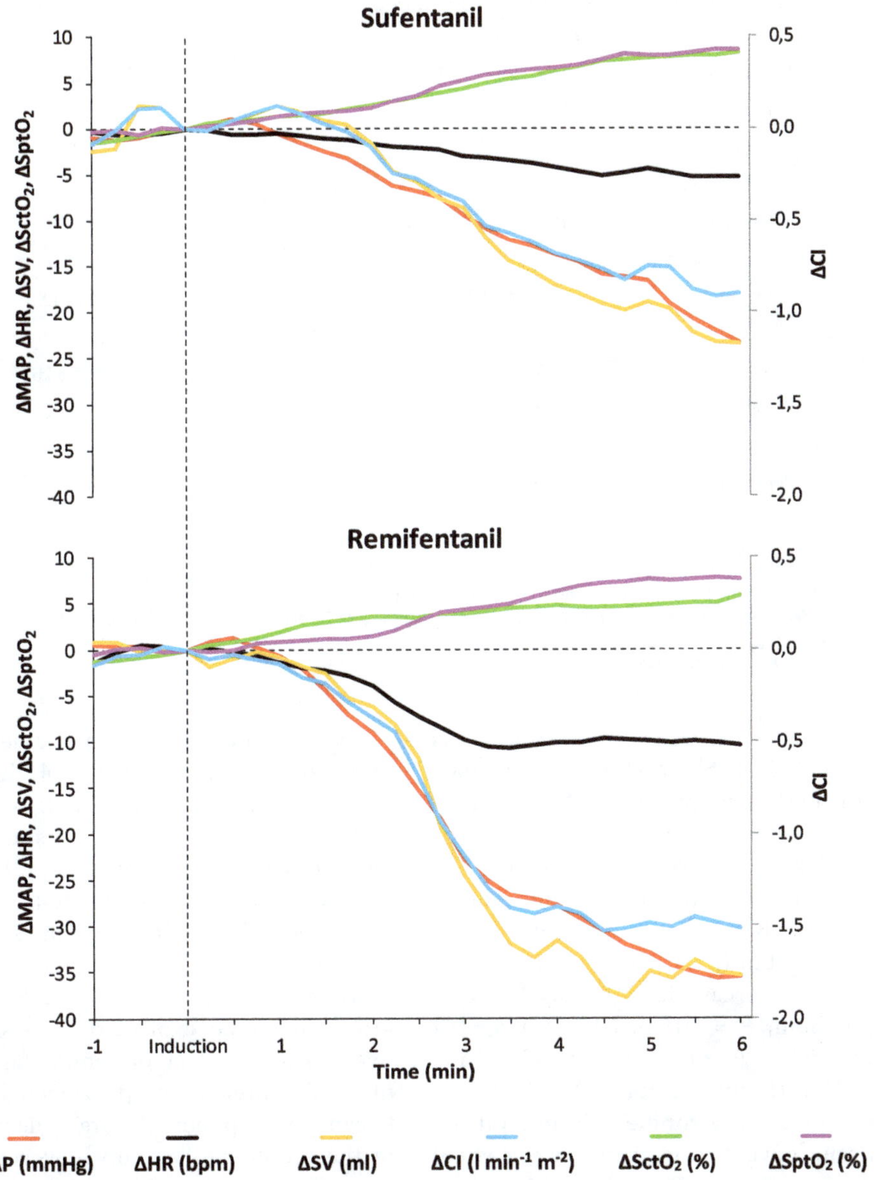

Fig. 3 Mean relative changes of the investigated haemodynamic variables during the induction of anaesthesia (from 1 min before until 6 min after). Mean arterial pressure (ΔMAP), heart rate (ΔHR), stroke volume (ΔSV), cardiac index (ΔCI), cerebral tissue oxygen saturation ($\Delta SctO_2$) and peripheral tissue oxygen saturation ($\Delta SptO_2$)

Table 2 shows all haemodynamic data. Both in the sufentanil group and in the remifentanil group MAP, HR, SV, CI, and RPP were significantly decreased 6 min after induction (T_6) as compared to baseline (T_0). In contrast, $SctO_2$ and $SptO_2$ were significantly increased between T_0 and T_6. Between-groups comparison (sufentanil vs. remifentanil) of the mean relative changes showed less decrease in: MAP ($\Delta = -23 \pm 13$ vs. -36 ± 13 mmHg; $P < 0.001$), HR ($\Delta = -5 \pm 7$ vs. -10 ± 10 bpm; $P = 0.025$), SV ($\Delta = -23 \pm 18$ vs. -35 ± 19 ml; $P = 0.017$), CI ($\Delta = -0.8$ (-1.5 to -0.5) vs. -1.5 (-2.0 to -1.1) l $min^{-1} m^{-2}$; $P = 0.002$) and RPP ($\Delta = -3077 \pm 2010$ vs. -5002 ± 2369 mmHg bpm; $P = 0.001$) and a larger increase in $SctO_2$ ($\Delta = 9 \pm 5$ vs. $6 \pm 4\%$; $P = 0.040$) in the sufentanil group compared to the remifentanil group. The mean relative changes in $SptO_2$ ($\Delta = 8 \pm 7$ vs. $8 \pm 8\%$; $P = 0.641$) did not differ significantly between groups.

Haemodynamic effects after the administration of atropine

Seventy-seven percent of the patients in the sufentanil group and 80 % in the remifentanil group received atropine. The course of the investigated

Table 2 Haemodynamic data in the sufentanil and remifentanil group after the induction of anaesthesia

		T_0	T_6	Δ	*P* - value*
MAP (mmHg)	Sufentanil	101 ± 15	78 ± 15	− 23 ± 13	< 0.001
	Remifentanil	100 ± 11	65 ± 11	−36 ± 13	< 0.001
HR (bpm)	Sufentanil	64 ± 9	59 ± 8	−5 ± 7	< 0.001
	Remifentanil	68 ± 14	58 ± 12	− 10 ± 10	0.001
SV (ml)	Sufentanil	101 ± 25	78 ± 21	− 23 ± 18	< 0.001
	Remifentanil	97 ± 21	62 ± 21	− 35 ± 19	< 0.001
CI ($l\ min^{-1}\ m^{-2}$)	Sufentanil	3.2 (2.7 to 3.9)	2.3 (1.8 to 2.8)	−0.8 (− 1.5 to − 0.5)	< 0.001
	Remifentanil	3.5 (2.7 to 3.9)	1.8 (1.4 to 2.3)	−1.5 (− 2.0 to − 1.1)	< 0.001
RPP (mmHg bpm)	Sufentanil	10,004 ± 2200	6928 ± 1893	−3077 ± 2010	< 0.001
	Remifentanil	10,730 ± 2444	5728 ± 1845	−5002 ± 2369	< 0.001
$SctO_2$ (%)	Sufentanil	68 ± 8	77 ± 7	9 ± 5	< 0.001
	Remifentanil	67 ± 7	73 ± 8	6 ± 4	< 0.001
$SptO_2$ (%)	Sufentanil	77 ± 10	85 ± 7	8 ± 7	< 0.001
	Remifentanil	72 ± 11	80 ± 9	8 ± 8	< 0.001

Variables are reported as mean ± SD or median (IQR), according to data distribution
Δ: value (T_6) − value (T_0); *MAP* Mean Arterial Pressure; *HR* Heart Rate; *SV* Stroke Volume; *CO* Cardiac Output; *$SctO_2$* Cerebral Tissue Oxygen Saturation; *$SptO_2$* Peripheral Tissue Oxygen Saturation
* (T_6 vs. T_0), paired *t*-test or Wilcoxon signed rank test

variables after the administration of atropine is shown in Figs. 4 and 5. Table 3 shows all haemodynamic data. In both groups HR, CI, and RPP were significantly increased compared to baseline (T_0). $SctO_2$ significantly decreased compared to baseline (T_0) in the remifentanil group, but not in the sufentanil group. Between-groups comparison (sufentanil vs. remifentanil) of the mean relative changes showed more increase in: HR (Δ = 13 (9 to 19) vs. 9 (6 to 14) bpm; P = 0.016), CI (Δ = 0.4 ± 0.4 vs. 0.2 ± 0.3 $l\ min^{-1}\ m^{-2}$; P = 0.023) and RPP (Δ = 1584 ± 1413 vs. 810 ± 917 mmHg bpm; P = 0.027) in the sufentanil group after atropine administration. MAP, SV and tissue oxygenation values were equal in both groups during measurements. Maximum RPP during the measurement period was 12,556 mmHg bpm.

Discussion

This prospective double-blind randomised controlled trial demonstrates that induction of anaesthesia with propofol and sufentanil results in less haemodynamic suppression than induction of anaesthesia with propofol and a calculated equivalent dosage of remifentanil, combined with more pronounced positive effect on $SctO_2$ values in the sufentanil group. Administration of atropine reversed bradycardia and thus maintained haemodynamics and tissue oxygenation with no (clinically) relevant between-groups differences.

After the induction of anaesthesia with comparable doses of opioids, remifentanil did not only cause a more evident decrease in HR, but also in SV. Remifentanil is well known for its direct bradycardic effects, especially compared to other opioids, but not for the negative effect on SV [6, 12]. As a result of a decreased HR, an increase in SV would typically be expected, due to a longer diastolic filling time. This more pronounced decrease in SV in the remifentanil group might be explained by a stronger direct negative inotropic effect of remifentanil, different changes in cardiac preload, or pharmacokinetic differences between both opioids. A larger decrease in HR and SV in the remifentanil group however resulted in a much larger decrease in MAP and CI, and thereby overall more haemodynamic suppression than in the sufentanil group. Furthermore, patients in the remifentanil group demonstrated lower $SctO_2$ values. During induction of anaesthesia, a raised inspired oxygen fraction combined with general vasodilation results in an overall increased tissue oxygenation [12]. Despite this, the more pronounced haemodynamic suppression in the remifentanil group led to lower $SctO_2$ values than in the sufentanil group. This difference could only be demonstrated in terms of absolute $SptO_2$ values, but not in the mean relative values. Also, anaesthesia with more stable haemodynamics, like with sufentanil, will clinically lead to less use of vasoactive medication, e.g. norepinephrine, and thereby less additional haemodynamic suppression and possibly higher tissue oxygenation values [5].

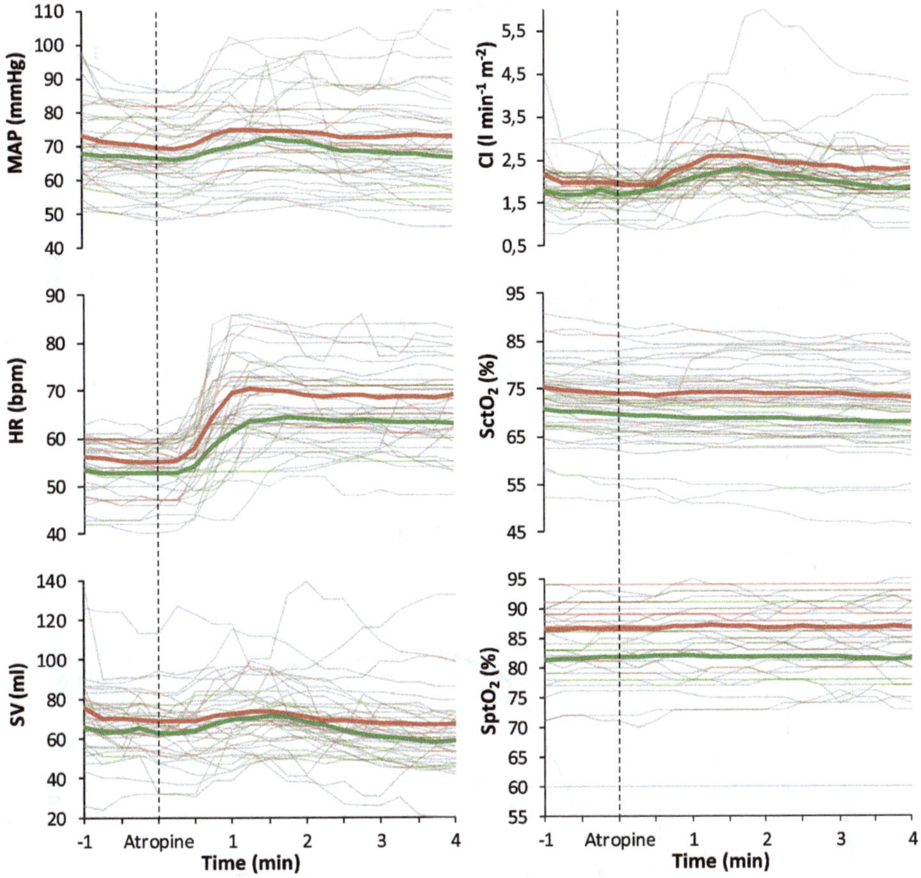

Fig. 4 Mean values (thick lines) and individual patient data (thin lines) of the investigated haemodynamic variables: mean arterial pressure (MAP), heart rate (HR), stroke volume (SV), cardiac index (CI), cerebral tissue oxygen saturation ($SctO_2$) and peripheral tissue oxygen saturation ($SptO_2$). Red lines represent the sufentanil group and green lines the remifentanil group. Graphs are shown from 1 min before until 4 min after the administration of atropine

Contrary to our hypothesis, administration of atropine did not result in better attenuation of the haemodynamic suppression caused by remifentanil or higher tissue oxygenation values compared to anaesthesia with sufentanil. Although only demonstrated in absolute values, the sufentanil group showed higher HR and remarkably higher CI values than the remifentanil group. Compared to other opioids, remifentanil evokes a dose dependent prolongation of the cardiac conduction times (by influencing the sinus and atrioventricular node and intra-atrial conduction), inhibition of sinoatrial automaticity and vagally mediated inotropic effects [7, 32]. In accordance with previous observations, we expected more distinct positive effects of atropine on the haemodynamic variables and tissue oxygenation during remifentanil based anaesthesia [12]. However, in our previous study from non-cardiac surgery, none of the patients were on beta-blocking agents, as opposed to the 90% in both of the groups of the current study, which exclusively included patients with ischemic heart disease. Our results show that, not only in patients with extreme bradycardia, atropine significantly improves cardiac index and blood pressure in many cases, which may in clinical practice often obviate the necessity for further interventions such as starting a syringe pump with vasopressive medication. Unfortunately, the methodology of this study did not permit to show any outcome improvement. This was, however not the purpose of the study; the objective was to demonstrate that atropine (especially in remifentanil-based anaesthesia) can induce a significant increase in blood pressure and cardiac output (CO), allegedly by counteracting the parasympathicomimetic effects of the opiates.

Administering atropine in patients undergoing CABG could lead to certain objections, since all of the patients suffer from coronary artery disease. An unwanted increase in HR can result in an increase

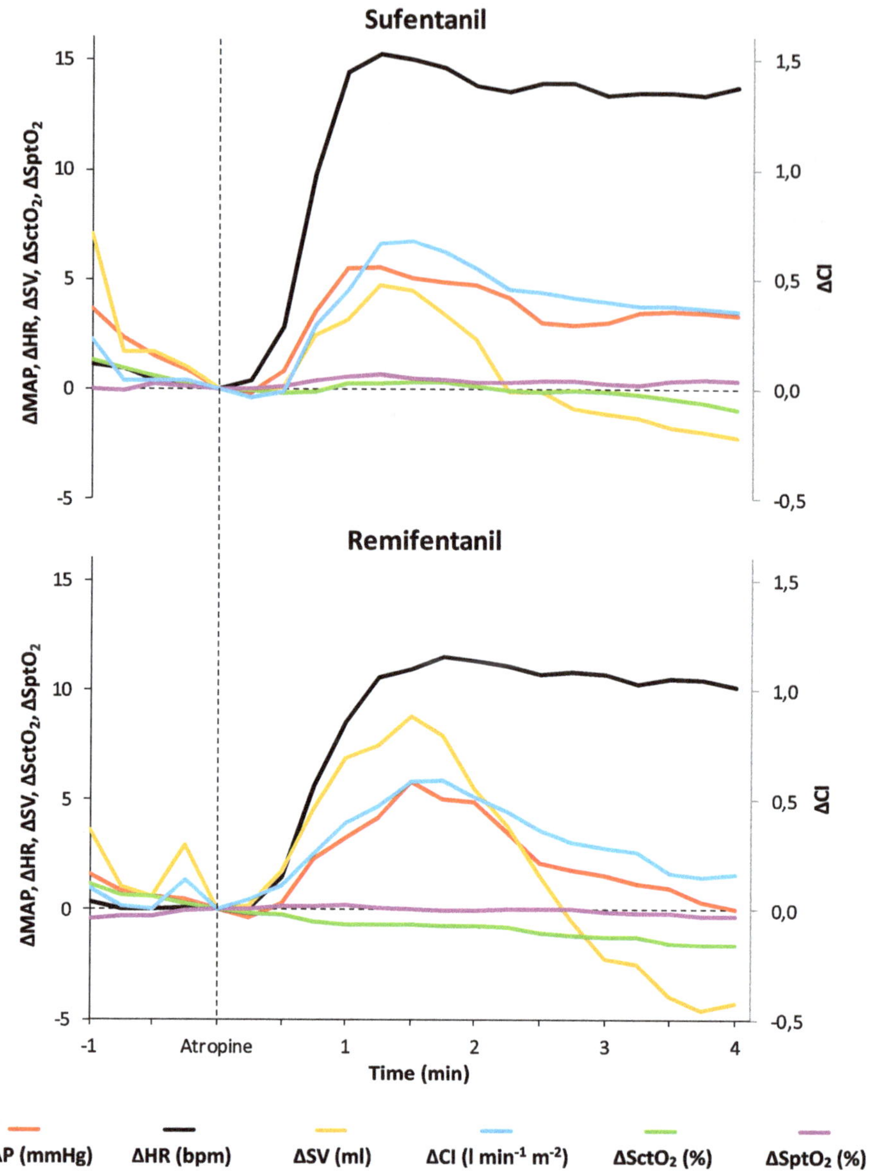

Fig. 5 Mean relative changes of the investigated haemodynamic variables during the administration of atropine (from 1 min before until 4 min after). Mean arterial pressure (ΔMAP), heart rate (ΔHR), stroke volume (ΔSV), cardiac index (ΔCI), cerebral tissue oxygen saturation ($\Delta SctO_2$) and peripheral tissue oxygen saturation ($\Delta SptO_2$)

in the RPP, which is a measure of the internal workload of the heart and a direct indication of the myocardial oxygen demand. However, maximum RPP during the measurement period after the atropine administration was 12,556 mmHg bpm. This value corresponds with a low internal workload and thus indicates a low myocardial oxygen consumption, probably owing to the patients being under anaesthesia [26, 27]. Also, none of the closely monitored patients showed signs of cardiac ischemia. Other contraindications for the use of atropine, like severe aortic valve stenosis, were covered in the exclusion criteria.

There are certain study limitations that need to be addressed. Firstly, equipotent doses of the used opiates are so far not reliably determined in the literature and consequently, we were limited to calculated equipotent doses based on interaction models. Although we consider that these values sufficiently reliably represent clinical reality, different observations may occur depending on opiate doses. Secondly, we used the FloTrac-Vigileo system for the recording of the course of the SV and CI after the induction of anaesthesia and after atropine administration. These variables are calculated via arterial pressure waveform analysis, which leads to a certain inevitable

Table 3 Haemodynamic data in the sufentanil and remifentanil group after atropine administration

		T_0	T_4	Δ	*P* - value*
MAP (mmHg)	Sufentanil	69 (63 to 81)	72 (67 to 80)	4 (−2 to 9)	0.101
	Remifentanil	67 (56 to 78)	64 (57 to 77)	1 (−2 to 6)	0.942
HR (bpm)	Sufentanil	57 (49 to 59)	70 (63 to 74)	13 (9 to 19)	< 0.001
	Remifentanil	53 (50 to 58)	64 (56 to 70)	9 (6 to 14)	< 0.001
SV (ml)	Sufentanil	69 ± 17	67 ± 23	−3 ± 10	0.253
	Remifentanil	63 ± 14	59 ± 12	−4 ± 11	0.110
CI ($l\ min^{-1}\ m^{-2}$)	Sufentanil	2.0 ± 0.5	2.3 ± 0.8	0.4 ± 0.4	0.001
	Remifentanil	1.7 ± 0.3	1.9 ± 0.4	0.2 ± 0.3	0.032
RPP (mmHg bpm)	Sufentanil	5590 ± 918	7173 ± 1589	1584 ± 1413	< 0.001
	Remifentanil	5204 ± 1053	6014 ± 1590	810 ± 917	0.001
$SctO_2$ (%)	Sufentanil	73 (68 to 79)	73 (65 to 78)	−2 (−3 to 1)	0.120
	Remifentanil	72 (66 to 75)	69 (65 to 74)	-2 (−2 to −1)	0.005
$SptO_2$ (%)	Sufentanil	88 (81 to 91)	88 (83 to 91)	1 (−1 to 2)	0.582
	Remifentanil	83 (78 to 86)	81 (77 to 86)	0 (−1 to 0)	0.471

Variables are reported as mean ± SD or median (IQR), according to data distribution
Δ: value (T_4) − value (T_0); *MAP* Mean Arterial Pressure; *HR* Heart Rate; *SV* Stroke Volume; *CO* Cardiac Output; *$SctO_2$* Cerebral Tissue Oxygen Saturation; *$SptO_2$* Peripheral Tissue Oxygen Saturation
* (T_4 vs. T_0), paired *t*-test or Wilcoxon signed rank test

inaccuracy. Previous studies show varying outcomes in agreement and trending ability when FloTrac-Vigileo calculated CO is compared with CO derived from the widely accepted reference method, i.e. thermodilution [19]. Consequently, to minimize measurement bias, we used relative (Δ) values instead of absolute values for the comparisons [33, 34].

Also, tissue oxygenation values based on near-infrared spectroscopy and measured during haemodynamic changes, like after induction of anaesthesia, should be interpreted with caution. Reduced skin blood flow and oxygenation, caused by vasoconstrictive medication, hyperventilation and hypoxia, has shown to influence measurement values to some extent [35, 36]. These results however could not be reproduced when norepinephrine was administered to treat postspinal hypotension [37]. Moreover, reduction in $SctO_2$ after vasoconstrictive medication has previously been correlated with a decrease in oxygen saturation measured at the level of the jugular venous bulb [38]. As a consequence, we have to assume that the changes in $SctO_2$ and $SptO_2$ we demonstrated are at least partially caused by changes in skin perfusion. Nevertheless, our data showed a much more evident increase in tissue oxygenation after induction of anaesthesia (6–9% increase), than reported as influence by a change in skin oxygen saturation (2–3% change) [35, 36].

Lastly, for the analysis of the effects of atropine on haemodynamics and tissue oxygenation we used a fixed dose of 1 mg. This could partially account for the (inter-individual) differences in the response of haemodynamic variables to the administration of atropine.

Conclusions

Induction of anaesthesia with propofol and sufentanil results in improved haemodynamic stability and higher cerebral tissue oxygenation compared to propofol and remifentanil in CABG patients. Administration of atropine might be useful to counteract or prevent the bradycardic action and thus haemodynamic suppression associated with these opioids.

Abbreviations

bpm: Beats per minute; CABG: Coronary artery bypass grafting; Cet: Effect-site concentration; CI: Cardiac index; CO: Cardiac output; HR: Heart rate; MAP: Mean arterial pressure; RCT: Randomised controlled trial; RPP: Rate pressure product; $SctO_2$: Cerebral tissue-oxygenation; $SptO_2$: Peripheral tissue-oxygenation; SV: Stroke volume; T_0: Time = 0 min; T_4: Time = 4 min; T_6: Time = 6 min; TCI: Target controlled infusion

Acknowledgements

Not applicable.

Authors' contributions

MP, AFK and TWLS were responsible for the study design. MP and PLB managed the inclusion of the participants. Together with TWLS they conducted all measurements. MP and PLB were responsible for data collection and analysis. MP and AFK interpreted the data and wrote the first draft of the manuscript. TWLS and MMRFS made substantial contributions to the final version of the manuscript and all revisions. All authors read and approved the final manuscript.

Author details

[1]Department of Anaesthesiology, University Medical Center Groningen, Hanzeplein 1, PO Box 30 001, 9700, RB, Groningen, The Netherlands. [2]Department of Anaesthesiology, AZ Maria Middelares Gent Buitenring Sint-Denijs 30, 9000 Ghent, Belgium.

References

1. Beers R, Camporesi E. Remifentanil update: clinical science and utility. CNS Drugs. 2004;18:1085–104.
2. Hogue CW, Bowdle TA, O'Leary C, Duncalf D, Miguel R, Pitts M, Streisand J, Kirvassilis G, Jamerson B, McNeal S, Batenhorst R. A multicenter evaluation of total intravenous anesthesia with remifentanil and propofol for elective inpatient surgery. Anesth Analg. 1996;83:279–85.
3. Vos JJ, Poterman M, Hannivoort LN, Renardel De Lavalette VW, Struys MM, Scheeren TW, Kalmar AF. Hemodynamics and tissue oxygenation during balanced anesthesia with a high antinociceptive contribution: an observational study. Perioper Med. 2014;3:9.
4. Elliott P, O'Hare R, Bill KM, Phillips AS, Gibson FM, Mirakhur RK. Severe cardiovascular depression with remifentanil. Anesth Analg. 2000;91:58–61.
5. Poterman M, Vos JJ, Vereecke HE, Struys MM, Vanoverschelde H, Scheeren TW, Kalmar AF. Differential effects of phenylephrine and norepinephrine on peripheral tissue oxygenation during general anaesthesia: a randomised controlled trial. Eur J Anaesthesiol. 2015;32:571–80.
6. Wilhelm W, Biedler A, Huppert A, Kreuer S, Bücheler O, Ziegenfuss T, Larsen R. Comparison of the effects of remifentanil or fentanyl on anaesthetic induction characteristics of propofol, thiopental or etomidate. Eur J Anaesthesiol. 2002;19:350–6.
7. Fujii K, Iranami H, Nakamura Y, Hatano Y. High-dose remifentanil suppresses sinoatrial conduction and sinus node automaticity in pediatric patients under propofol-based anesthesia. Anesth Analg. 2011;112:1169–73.
8. Del Blanco Narciso BB, Jimeno Fernandez C, Almendral Garrote J, Anadon Baselga MJ, Zaballos GM. Effects of remifentanil on the cardiac conduction system. Our experience in the study of remifentanil electrophysiological properties. Curr Pharm Des. 2014;20:5489–96.
9. Jhanji S, Lee C, Watson D, Hinds C, Pearse RM. Microvascular flow and tissue oxygenation after major abdominal surgery: association with post-operative complications. Intensive Care Med. 2009;35:671–7.
10. Belda FJ, Aguilera L, García de la Asunción J, Alberti J, Vicente R, Ferrándiz L, Rodríguez R, Company R, Sessler DI, Aguilar G, Botello SG, Ortí R. Supplemental perioperative oxygen and the risk of surgical wound infection: a randomized controlled trial. JAMA. 2005;294:2035–42.
11. Pearse RM, Harrison DA, James P, Watson D, Hinds C, Rhodes A, Grounds RM, Bennett ED. Identification and characterisation of the high-risk surgical population in the United Kingdom. Crit Care. 2006;10:R81.
12. Poterman M, Scheeren TWL, van der Velde MI, Buisman PL, Allaert S, Struys MMRF, Kalmar AF. Prophylactic atropine administration attenuates the negative haemodynamic effects of induction of anaesthesia with propofol and high-dose remifentanil: a randomised controlled trial. Eur J Anaesthesiol. 2017;34:695–701.
13. Schulz KF, Altman DG, Moher D, CONSORT Group. CONSORT 2010 Statement: updated guidelines for reporting parallel group randomised trials. BMC Med. 2010;8:18.
14. La Colla L, Albertin A, La Colla G, Porta A, Aldegheri G, Di Candia D, Gigli F. Predictive performance of the 'Minto' remifentanil pharmacokinetic parameter set in morbidly obese patients ensuing from a new method for calculating lean body mass. Clin Pharmacokinet. 2010;49:131–9.
15. Hannivoort LN, Vereecke HEM, Proost JH, Heyse BEK, Eleveld DJ, Bouillon TW, Struys MMRF, Luginbühl M. Probability to tolerate laryngoscopy and noxious stimulation response index as general indicators of the anaesthetic potency of sevoflurane, propofol, and remifentanil. Br J Anaesth. 2016;116:624–31.
16. Gepts E, Shafer SL, Camu F, Stanski DR, Woestenborghs R, Van Peer A, Heykants JJ. Linearity of pharmacokinetics and model estimation of sufentanil. Anesthesiology. 1995;83:1194–204.
17. Minto CF, Schnider TW, Shafer SL. Pharmacokinetics and pharmacodynamics of remifentanil. II Model application. Anesthesiology. 1997;86:24–33.
18. Schnider TW, Minto CF, Shafer SL, Gambus PL, Andresen C, Goodale DB, Young EJ. The influence of age on propofol pharmacodynamics. Anesthesiology. 1999;90:1502–16.
19. Bouillon TW, Bruhn J, Radulescu L, Andresen C, Shafer TJ, Cohane C, Shafer SL. Pharmacodynamic interaction between propofol and remifentanil regarding hypnosis, tolerance of laryngoscopy, bispectral index, and electroencephalographic approximate entropy. Anesthesiology. 2004;100:1353–72.
20. Bouillon TW. Hypnotic and opioid anesthetic drug interaction on the CNS, focus on response surface modelling. In: Schüttler J, Schwilden H, editors. Modern Anesthetics. Handbook of Experimental Pharmacology. Berlin: Springer; 2008. p. 471–87.
21. Schlöglhofer T, Gilly H, Schima H. Semi-invasive measurement of cardiac output based on pulse contour: a review and analysis. Can J Anaesth. 2014;61:452–79.
22. Fischer GW. Recent advances in application of cerebral oximetry in adult cardiovascular surgery. Semin Cardiothorac Vasc Anesth. 2008;12:60–9.
23. Santora RJ, Moore FA. Monitoring trauma and intensive care unit resuscitation with tissue hemoglobin oxygen saturation. Crit Care. 2009;13:S10.
24. Scheeren TWL, Schober P, Schwarte LA. Monitoring tissue oxygenation by near infrared spectroscopy (NIRS): background and current applications. J Clin Monit Comput. 2012;26:279–87.
25. Scheeren TWL, Kuizenga MH, Maurer H, Struys M, Heringlake M. Electroencephalography and brain oxygenation monitoring in the perioperative period. Anesth Analg. 2019;128(2):265–77.
26. Putnam B, Bricker S, Fedorka P, Zelada J, Shebrain S, Omari B, Bongard F. The correlation of near-infrared spectroscopy with changes in oxygen delivery in a controlled model of altered perfusion. Am Surg. 2007;73:1017–22.
27. Fletcher GF, Balady GJ, Amsterdam EA, Chaitman B, Eckel R, Fleg J, Froelicher VF, Leon AS, Piña IL, Rodney R, Simons-Morton DA, Williams MA, Bazzarre T. Exercise standards for testing and training: a statement for healthcare professionals from the American Heart Association. Circulation. 2001;104:1694–740.
28. Gobel FL, Norstrom LA, Nelson RR, Jorgensen CR, Wang Y. The rate-pressure product as an index of myocardial oxygen consumption during exercise in patients with angina pectoris. Circulation. 1978;57:549–56.
29. Faul F, Erdfelder E, Buchner A, Lang AG. Statistical power analysis using G*power 3.1: tests for correlation and regression analyses. Behav Res Methods. 2009;41:1149–60.
30. Servin FS, Billard V. Remifentanil and Other Opioids. In Schüttler J, Schwilden, editors. Modern Anesthetics. Handbook of Experimental Pharmacology. Berlin: Springer-Verlag; 2008. p. 283–312.
31. Al-Rifai Z, Pharm M, Mulvey D. Principles of total intravenous anaesthesia: basic pharmacokinetics and model descriptions. BJA Educ. 2016;16:92–7.
32. Fattorini F, Romano R, Ciccaglioni A, Pascarella MA, Rocco A, Mariani V, Pietropaoli P. Effects of remifentanil on human heart electrical system. A transesophageal pacing electrophysiological study. Minerva Anestesiol. 2003;69:673–9.
33. Critchley LA, Lee A, Ho AM. A critical review of the ability of continuous cardiac output monitors to measure trends in cardiac output. Anesth Analg. 2010;111:1180–92.
34. Saugel B, Wagner JY, Scheeren TW. Cardiac output monitoring: less invasiveness, less accuracy? J Clin Monit Comput. 2016;30:753–5.
35. Sørensen H, Secher NH, Siebenmann C, Nielsen HB, Kohl-Bareis M, Lundby C, Rasmussen P. Cutaneous vasoconstriction affects near-infrared spectroscopy determined cerebral oxygen saturation during administration of norepinephrine. Anesthesiology. 2012;117:263–70.
36. Sørensen H, Rasmussen P, Sato K, Persson S, Olesen ND, Nielsen HB, Olsen NV, Ogoh S, Secher NH. External carotid artery flow maintains near infrared spectroscopy-determined frontal lobe oxygenation during ephedrine administration. Br J Anaesth. 2014;113:452–8.
37. Lecoq JP, Brichant JF, Lamy ML, Joris JL. Norepinephrine and ephedrine do not counteract the increase in cutaneous microcirculation induced by spinal anaesthesia. Br J Anaesth. 2010;105:214–9.
38. Cho SY, Kim SJ, Jeong CW, Jeong CY, Chung SS, Lee J, Yoo KY. Under general anesthesia arginine vasopressin prevents hypotension but impairs cerebral oxygenation during arthroscopic shoulder surgery in the beach chair position. Anesth Analg. 2013;117:1436–43.

15

Anesthesia management in neonatal congenital bronchobiliary fistula

Hong Yin, Guangyi Zhao, Yingjie Du and Ping Zhao*

Abstract

Background: There is very little published literature and none that discussed care in a neonate regarding anesthetic risk and management of neonate with congenital bronchobiliary fistula during thoracoscopy and thoracotomy. This article analyzes related risk factors and literature review from perioperative ventilation, circulation and other aspects of management.

Case presentation: A neonate diagnosed as congenital bronchobiliary fistula combined with severe chemical pneumonia, consolidation of the lungs, and infection was facing the risk of anaesthesia under thoracoscopy exploration surgery, who experiened more than 20 days diagnostic period before operation. Many risk factors have led to conversion from minimally invasive surgery to thoracotomy, including persistent hypoxemia, hypercapnia, difficult surgical exposure and extremly difficulty of intraoperative ventilation management. Anesthesia maintenance after conversion to open access remained problematic. Fortunately the patient showed no sign of any adverse CNS effects after 4 months of follow-up.

Conclusions: The most prominent anesthesia challenges are hypoxemia, increased airway resistance, impaired ventilation, and the risk of metabolic acidosis. Close cooperation among the entire neonatal medical team is the key factors in successful management of this rare case.

Keywords: Congenital bronchobiliary fistula, CBBF, Neonate, Anesthesia, Chemical pneumonia, Hypoxemia, Hypercapnia

Background

Congenital bronchialbiliary fistula (CBBF) is a rare anomaly with low morbidity and very high mortality. CBBF is characterized by an abnormal communication between the respiratory tract (trachea or bronchi) and the biliary tract [1]. According to literatures, Only 45 cases of CBBF have been reported [2]. Surgical treatment is the only way to complete recovery. Because of the rarity of CBBF, there is very little published on anesthesia management other than a single case report but that this was in a 3 years old rather than neonate [3].

* Correspondence: 1261703452@qq.com
Department of Anesthesiology, Shengjing Hospital of China Medical University, Shenyang 110004, China

Case presentation

A 5-day old full-term female baby, delivered by cesarean section, 2880 g of birth weight, was referred to our hospital because of intermittent cyanosis. She had frequent choking with an excessive volume of yellowish-green saliva at the third day of born. Airway examination showed normal mouth opening and neck movements with no facial anomalies. After admission, her respiratory function continued to deteriorate and endotracheal intubation and ventilator assistance became necessary. Tracheal secretion of a large volume of yellowish-green fluid persisted and three-dimensional computed tomography (3D-CT) of the chest showed a fistula originating from the right bronchus, running distally along the esophagus, and passing through the diaphragm and into the intrahepatic biliary tract at the site of the esophageal hiatus. There was air in the intrahepatic biliary tract and in the common hepatic duct, along with a bilateral, mainly lower-lobe, pneumonia (Fig. 1). CBBF was diagnosed accordingly. Ultrasonography and bronchoscopy confirmed the CT findings. The flexible fiberoptic bronchoscopy identified the opening of the fistula in the right main bronchus. A contrast x-ray examination of the fistula was performed during bronchoscopy. Contrast flowed from the opening in the bronchus through the fistula and into the biliary tract, the gall bladder, and the duodenum (Fig. 2). So the preoperative diagnosis was: 1. bronchobiliary fistula; 2. neonatal pneumonia; 3. gastroduodenal reflux; and 4. congential heart disease.

Preoperative treatment measures included CPAP ventilation (see Table 1 for blood gas results), gastrointestinal decompression and fasting, inhibition of gastric acid secretion, promotion of gastric peristalsis, antibiotics, parenteral nutrition, myocardial nutrition, sedation analgesia, and precise fluid management and keep elevation position to encourage consolidation of the biliary contents to distal lung. Due to the rarity of the disease, it was spent in the preoperative diagnosis process for a relatively long time after hospitalization. And the baby was scheduled for endoscopic cholangiography and thoracoscopic right bronchobiliary fistulectomy under general anesthesia on the second day after the diagnosis.

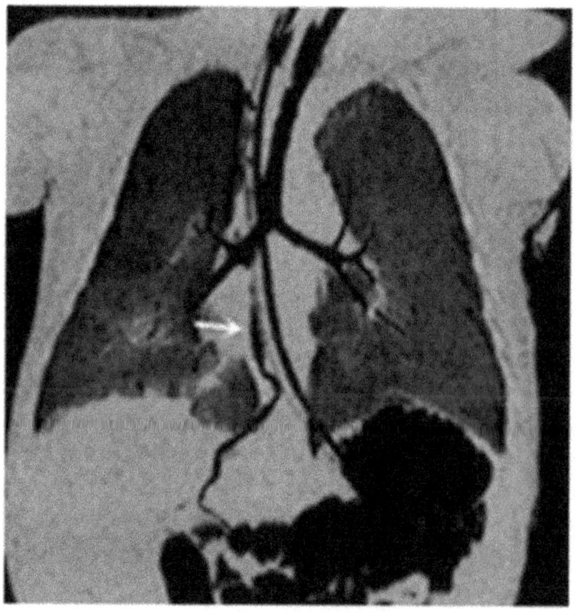

Fig. 1 Three-dimensional chest computed tomogram showing the fistula originating from the right bronchus, travelling along the esophagus, and passing through the diaphragm and into intrahepatic biliary tract at the site of the esophageal hiatus

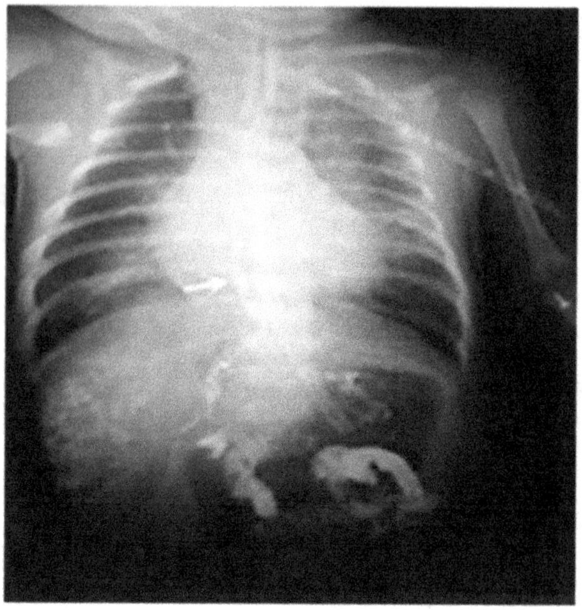

Fig. 2 Bedside x-ray showing contrast flowing from the abnormal opening in the right main bronchus through the fistula and into the biliary tract, the gall bladder, and the duodenum. Contrast study via fiberoptic bronchoscope: contrast is seen in the fistula, the biliary tract, and the duodenum. The white arrow shows the fistula

Anesthesia

Anesthesia: The patient was 16 days old on the day of surgery with 2.2 kg of body weight, and golden-yellow lung secretions persisted (Fig. 3). Taking into account the preoperative examination confirmed that the fistula is away from the tracheal carina, and the fact that CPAP had no obvious abdominal distension symptoms before surgery, the tracheal intubation catheter is placed in the main airway, away from the fistula. In view of the tracheal intubation when entering the operating room, we take more safer method of inhalation anesthesia induction. During anesthetic maintenance, sevoflurane combined with intravenous remifentanil was adopted. In addition to regular monitoring, invasive arterial pressure monitoring, intermittent blood gas analysis, and continuous cerebral oxygen saturation (ScO_2%) monitoring were also performed. Due to the lack of neonatal bronchial obstruction at the time, we did not perform lung isolation techniques and respiratory management as planned [4, 5]. The lungs, particularly the left lung, were infiltrated with iodinated contrast agent during contrast examination of the biliary tree (5 mL intrahepatic iodine tracer), and this was mostly cleared by immediate endotracheal suction. The contrast examination confirmed the right-sided bronchobiliary fistula and showed a

Table 1 Arterial blood gas analysis at different time points

Time Point	PH	PCO2 (mmHg)	PO2 (mmHg)	HCT (%)	tHb (g/dl)	GLU (mmol/l)	LAC (mmol/l)	HCO3- (mmol/l)	BE (mmol/l)
Preoperation	7.37	46.3	55.9	33.1	10.6	5.2	1.5	26.3	2.9
During thoracoscopy	7.37	41.1	45.8	37.3	11.8	4.6	1.1	2.3	−2.26
During open surgery	7.21	39.3	55.6	41.7	13.6	8.2	4.5	15.3	−10.4
End of operation	7.36	32.8	97.6	34.3	11.4	5.8	2.0	19.3	−6.27
Entering NICU	7.38	45.7	64.2	43.9	15.0	5.6	1.5	21.1	−2.15

normal extrahepatic biliary tract (Fig. 4). Bilateral lung sounds returned to baseline after suctioning of the contrast agent from the lungs and the SpO_2 remained above 85%. At this point, thoracoscopic fistula resection was attempted. The initial pneumothorax parameters were: CO_2 inflation pressure 3 mmHg with flow rate adjusted to 1 to 2 L/min under pressure controlled ventilation with PIP 20 to 23, PEEP 4 to 5 mmHg, frequency 30 to 32 breaths/min, and I:E 1.5 to 1.8. In spite of the normal bronchial breath sounds after suctioning, there was persistent hypoxemia and increased airway resistance during thoracoscopy. Intermittent manual assist ventilation was adopted to maintain oxygenation to the greatest extent possible to ensure that cerebral oxygen saturation did not fall below 20% of baseline. But finally, considering the safety of the patient and difficult exposure the procedure was converted to an open access. Arterial blood gas analysis before, during, end operation, during thoracoscopy、thoracotomy and at the time of entering NICU are summarized in the Table 1.

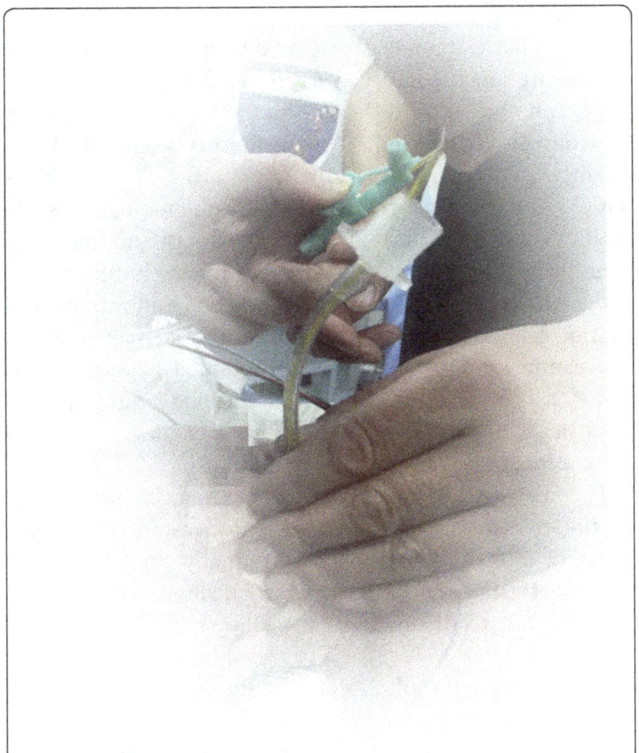

Fig. 3 Large amounts of bilious aspirate were cleared via endotracheal suction

Ventilator management during thoracotomy remained problematic, with high airway pressure, low tidal volume, and intermittent hypoxemia during thoracotomy. Breathing parameters include pressure-controlled ventilation combined with intermittent manual inflation management to maximize tidal volume and inhalation time to ensure oxygen supply. And the peak inspiratory pressure was limited to less than 28 mmHg. The patient developed a metabolic acidosis with base excess = − 11 and lactate = 4.5, which was corrected by intravenous sodium bicarbonate infusion. In view of the long operation time, about 8 ~ 10 ml/kg of intravenous isotonic saline including glucose (1 ~ 2% isotonic solution with sugar) supplementation and equal volume of RBC transfusions according to blood loss were given to maintain effective perfusion of the microcirculation and adequate blood pressure and urine output. Phenylephrine was prepared

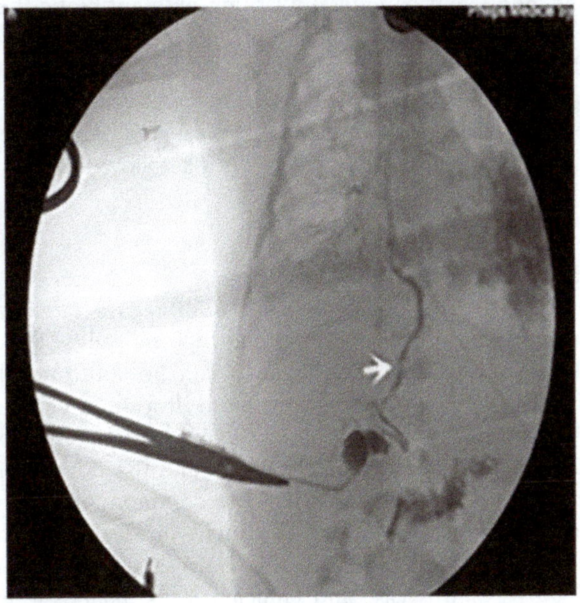

Fig. 4 Intraoperative cholangiography shows the connection between the biliary tract and the right main bronchus. The distal bile duct is patent. The white arrow indicates the biliary tract

to maintain the blood pressure within 20% of the baseline value if needed. The ScO_2% fluctuated in response to fluctuations in the SpO_2, and at one point, the ScO_2 fell to 38% (basal value 58%). Although this was a fairly short-term episode, it is nonetheless worthy of attention. When the SpO_2 improved, the ScO_2% returned to approximately 50%.

A retrograde methylene blue injection was performed for precise positioning of the fistula, and once again, both lungs were infiltrated and immediate suctioning was required. The total operative time was approximately 5.5 h, and the infant remained intubated postoperatively and was transferred to the neonatal intensive care unit (NICU) after surgery. Postoperative histopathological examination confirmed that the resected fistula originated from the bile duct. Biliary epithelial cells were found at the margin of the bronchial fistula and there was interstitial cholestasis.

Postoperative course

Normal oxygenation and arterial blood gases were maintained by CPAP ventilation with PEEP of 5 cm H_2O and FiO_2 of 0.4 (see Table 1 for blood gas values). Prolonged postoperative ventilator support was necessary because of persistent pneumonia, and the initial attempt to remove the thoracic tube failed because of acute pneumothorax and subcutaneous emphysema. The patient also had cholestasis and developed a chylothorax during the recovery stage. Drainage of chylous fluid from the thoracostomy tube gradually diminished as gastrointestinal decompression and use of intravenous methylprednisolone, NPO, and parenteral nutrition with antibiotic therapy were continued, and oral feeding was resumed without adverse reactions once the thoracic drainage was minimized. After 43 days in hospital, the infant recovered well and was stable for discharge. There were no neurological complications during follow-up after 4 months.

Discussion and conclusion

Congenital bronchobiliary fistula (CBBF) is a rare malformation with low morbidity and high mortality. When CBBF is suspected, the diagnosis can be confirmed by MRI, 3D-CT, or bronchoscopy, and ultrasound can also provide valuable clues. Bronchoscopy, which can show the bronchial opening of the fistula and the flow of bile through that opening, is the most common method of diagnosis [6–8]. Definitive treatment of CBBF requires surgical resection [1]. From the relatively long period of diagnosis of this case and clinician lacks diagnostic experience, it fully illustrates the rarity of the disease. Relatively long diagnosis time exacerbates lung inflammation and changes in lung consolidation.

Although there have now been dozens of repairs reported, so far only one, in a 3-year old girl (weight 10 kg), has focused on anesthesia management [3], and perioperative anesthesia management in a low birth-weight neonate with impaired respiratory physiology would be different [9]. Low birth weight and incomplete lung development are only two of the many challenges in anesthesia management during resection of CBBF in neonates. CBBF presents with nonspecific symptoms, and recurrent chest infection, fever, dyspnea, and pulmonary consolidation may all be signs of the anomaly, which may also be accompanied by congenital heart defects. All of these factors will affect the anesthesiologist's decision-making during the perioperative management of cardiovascular and respiratory function [10–13]. In our case, the patient's already compromised lung function was further compromised after both lungs were infiltrated by the contrast agents that were necessary to locate and identify the fistula, and this caused further difficulty in providing effective ventilation and resulted in obstinate hypoxemia. Fortunately, there was some improvement after suctioning and manual-assist ventilation. In addition, surgery times may be prolonged during resection of CBBF, particularly when there are other congenital biliary defects to be repaired. Anesthesia management is also particularly challenging when surgery is performed in neonates less than 1 month after birth and in the presence of congenital heart disease and bilateral lung consolidations [14].

Given that the main problems during the perioperative period are inadequate ventilation and hypoxia, 116 papers can be retrieved according to search strategy ((((Anesthe*[Title] AND (Chemical pneumonia OR Hypoxemia OR Hypercapnia OR dyspnea))) OR (Anesthe*[-Title] AND thoracoscop*)) OR (bronchobiliary fistula AND Anesthe*[Title]) Filters: English; Infant: birth-23 months in on pubmed database. After excluding literatures which are not related to newborns and infants and or not related to perioperative anesthesia management, 25 related literatures are finally obtained (Table 2). But there is only one article describing directly the anesthesia of neonatal tracheobiliary fistula, which is a short report of a three-year-old child [3].

The reasons for intractable hypoxemia during surgery in the present case, which presented as intraoperative hypoxia, metabolic acidosis, and finally an inability to tolerate thoracoscopic surgery, requiring conversion to open thoracotomy, included the following:

1) Although auscultation of the lungs indicated normal air movement with only slightly coarsened breath sounds during thoracoscopy, elevated airway pressures and low tidal volume with hypercapnia were noted. Ventilation was acceptable after

Table 2 Literature search results related to anesthesitic management of tracheobiliary fistula operation in children

Year	Author	Research type	Operation type	Age	Weight	Number of patients	focus point
2018	Mohtar S [4]	Retrospectively	Thoracoscopy	< 3 months	1–21 kg	60	Extraluminal bronchial blocker
2018	Vika Fatafehi [9]	Retrospectively	Surgery lasting < 45 min	Pediatric	–	1090	Desaturation
2019	McCann ME [10]	Review	All	Infant	–	–	Brain injury, CBF
1998	Semin Perinatol [15]	Review	All	Micropremie	–	–	Anesthetic considerations
2016	King MR [11]	Retrospective analysis	All	1–20 Y	1–120 kg	446	Desaturation
2015	Wei K [16]	Case report	Emergent inguinal herniorrhaphy	21 Ds	3.8 kg	1	Hypercapnia
2011	Broemling N [17]	Review	Thoracic/thoracotomy	Neonate	–	–	anesthetic management
2005	Choudhry DK [5]	Review	Thoracic surgery	Infants and Children	–	–	Single lung ventilation devices
2005	Krosnar S [18]	Retrospective	Thoracoscopic surgery	Children	–	8	Anesthetic management of TEF/EA
2016	Razlevice I▯26	Prospective study	Thoracic or urologic surgery	< 3 months	–	44	Cerebral oxygen desaturation
1972	Smith AL [19]	Review	All	–	–	–	Cerebral blood flow and metabolism
2008	Sola A [20]	Review	All	Neonate	–	–	Oxygen toxicity
1994	Keenan RL [21]	Retrospective analysis	Noncardiac surgery	0–1 Y	–	4645	Bradycardia during anesthesia in Infants
2004	Means LJ [22]	Review	Laparoscopic/thoracoscopic surgery	–	–	–	Anesthetic management
2010	De Armendi AJ [23]	Case report	Proximal hypospadias repair	8 M	8.4 kg	1	Hypercapnia
2015	Ehlers M [12]	Case series	Thoracic surgery	0–3 M	2.1–4.0 kg	3	Hypercapnea and low cardiac output
1999	Petrat G [24]	Review	Minimally-invasive surgery	–	–	–	Anesthetic considerations
2016	Chiluveru SA [16]	Case report	Right lobectomy for CPAM	6 M	4 kg	1	Pulmonary hypertension
1993	Tobias JD [25]		Laparoscopic and Thoracoscopic procedures	Children	–	–	Air embolism
1999	Gunawardana RH [26]	Prospective study	Cleft lip and palate surgery	3 M-5Y	–	200	Low HB and brydicardia
1999	Chen KB [27]	Case report	Thoracotomy	Preterm infant	500 g	1	Preterm infant anesthesia of PDA
2008	McHoney M [13]	Prospective study	Thoracoscopy	1D-15Y	–	–	CO2 excretion, thermoregulation
1992	Kinouchi K [14]	Prospective study	All	1 M-12Y	–	61	Respiratory infection
1980	Welle P [28]	Prospective study	No abstract	Neonate	–	–	Transcutaneous oxygen monitoring
1994	Rowe R [29]	Case series report	Thoracoscopy	Pediatric	–	9	Anesthetic management

M months; *D* days *Y* years; *CPAM* congenital pulmonary airway malformation; *CBF* cerebral blood flow; *TEF/EA* tracheoesophageal fistula; *HB* hemoglobin; *PDA* patent ductus arteriosus

conversion to thoracotomy, but the bilateral chemical pneumonitis combined with acid reflux pneumonia and partial lung consolidations, which are characterized by inflammatory cell infiltration, alveolar epithelial cell destruction, degeneration, increased capillary wall permeability, interstitial pulmonary edema, and thickened, edematous alveolar membranes, ultimately caused insufficient ventilation leading to hypoxemia that severely compromised the PaO_2 [30].

2) The establishment of an iatrogenic pneumothorax followed by surgical compression of the lungs during thoracotomy led to atelectasis, reduced respiratory area, and hypoxia. Compression of the mediastinum during thoracotomy caused the heart rate and blood pressure to plummet twice, but the heart rate and blood pressure recovered spontaneously as soon as the compression was relieved.
Intraoperative problems that are commonly reported during thoracoscopic surgery include desaturation, transient hypotension requiring vascular expansion, hypercapnia (> 45 mmHg), hypothermia (< 34.9 °C), and metabolic acidosis [22]. Some of these require conversion to an open approach, while some are corrected without interruption of surgery. Significant risk factors for complications during thoracoscopic resection of CBBF also include young age of the patient, low body temperature, thoracic insufflation, high insufflation pressure and flow, and length of surgery [16, 18, 24, 27, 31]
3) The presence of a bronchobiliary fistula causes direct air leak from the fistula into the biliary system during mechanical ventilation, which further contributes to decreased effective ventilation and low PaO_2.
4) V/Q mismatch occurs during pneumothorax or open thoracotomy in a lateral position because of reduced perfusion at the lung bases, and this can also contribute to insufficient ventilation in neonates, with a decrease in total tidal volume causing deficient minute ventilation and hypoxemia [32, 33].
5) Tracers that are used to locate the bronchial opening and trace the fistula may infiltrate the lungs, causing transient increase in airway pressures and reduced oxygenation. In our case, these adverse effects on respiratory gas exchange were partially ameliorated by immediate suctioning and by the use of the lowest effective doses contrast agent and methylene blue.
6) Congenital heart diseases, such as atrial septal defect, can cause pulmonary hypertension. Right-to-left shunt occurs during hypoxia and CO_2 accumulation causes refractory hypoxemia. In this case, the reasons for the difficulty in keeping the SaO_2 above 85% were complex, and whether there was a right-to-left shunt remains unknown. Perioperative echocardiography or TEE may assist in diagnosis, but these were not performed in this case [17, 34–36].

Finally, intraoperative monitoring of cerebral oxygen saturation provided strong evidence of perioperative balance of cerebral oxygen supply and demand. Noninvasive real-time monitoring is an advantage in the neonate [37]. A baseline cerebral perfusion value of 25%, or > 250 min of the area under the AUC curve, is thought to be of clinical value as a predictor of an increased risk of postoperative neurological complications. Cerebral oxygen saturation is related to Hb, NIBP, PaO_2, $PaCO_2$, and other factors. Elevated $PaCO_2$ during cerebral hypoxia stimulates cerebral vasodilation and increases cerebral perfusion. However, cerebrovascular autoregulation is limited in neonates, and additional care must be taken during the perioperative period to monitor and maintain the balance of cerebral oxygen supply and demand in this especially vulnerable group [20, 38, 39]. Fortunately, in the present case, after 4 months of follow-up, the patient showed no sign of any adverse CNS effects.

In summary, for newborns with CBBF, a rare anomaly with a high mortality rate, for which surgery is the only definitive treatment, the most prominent anesthesia challenges are hypoxemia, increased airway resistance, impaired ventilation, and the risk of metabolic acidosis, particularly during prolonged surgeries. Careful perioperative anesthesia management and close cooperation among the entire neonatal medical team are the key factors in successful management of this rare condition. Traditional thoracotomy may be safer and more appropriate for neonate combined with extremely risk factors.

Abbreviations

CBBF: Congenital bronchialbiliary fistula; ScO2%: Cerebral tissue oxygen saturation; SpO2: PULSE oximetry saturation; PIP: Peak airway pressure; PEEP: Positive end expiratory lung pressure; CPAP: Consistent positive airway pressure

Acknowledgements

We thank the General Surgery Team for having respected our management conducts in this case and our wish to publish this case for educational purposes.

Authors' contributions

H.Y. and P.Z. were involved in the care of the patient and did the writing of the paper. Y.D. was involved in the care of the patient and collaborated on paper writing. G.Z. collaborated on paper writing and review of the paper. All authors read and approved the final manuscript.

References

1. Günlemez A, Tugay M, Elemen L, Türker G, Gürcan NI, Demir H, Gürbüz Y, Hosten T. Surgical experience in a baby with congenital broncho-biliary fistula. Ann Thorac Surg. 2009;87(1):318–20.
2. Li TY, Zhang ZB. Neonatal congenital bronchobiliary fistula:a case report and literature review. World J Clin Cases. 2019;7(7):881–90.
3. Chandran R, Batra RK, Agarwala S, Mishra R. Selective bronchial blockade with Fogarty catheter in a child with acquired bronchobiliary fistula. Paediatr Anaesth. 2013;23(4):373–5.

4. Mohtar S, Hui TWC, Irwin MG. Anesthetic management of thoracoscopic resection of lung lesions in small children. Paediatr Anaesth. 2018;28(11): 1035–42.
5. Choudhry DK. Single-lung ventilation in pediatric anesthesia. Anesthesiol Clin North Am. 2005;23(4):693–708.
6. Tommasoni N, Gamba PG, Midrio P, Guglielmi M. Congenital tracheobiliary fistula. Pediatr Pulmonol. 2000;30(2):149–52.
7. Bringas Bollada M, Cabezas Martín MH, Martínez Sagasti F, Ortuño AF. Congenital bronchobiliary fistula diagnosed in adult age. Med Int. 2006; 30(9):475–6.
8. Chawla SC, Jha P, Breiman R, Farmer D, Gooding C. Congenital tracheobiliary fistula diagnosed with contrast-enhanced CT and 3-D reformation. Pediatr Radiol. 200838(9):999–1002.
9. Lemoto VF H'u, Sugimoto K, Kanazawa T, Matsusaki T, Morimatsu H. The incidence of desaturation during anesthesia in adult and pediatric patients: a retrospective study. Acta Med Okayama. 2018;72(5):467–78.
10. McCann ME, Lee JK, Inder T. Beyond anesthesia toxicity: anesthetic considerations to lessen the risk of neonatal neurological injury. Anesth Analg. 2019;129(5):1354–64.
11. King MR, Anderson TA, Sui J, He G, Poon KY, Coté CJ. Age-related incidence of desaturation events and the cardiac responses on stroke index, cardiac index, and heart rate measured by continuous bioimpedance noninvasive cardiac output monitoring in infants and children undergoing general anesthesia. J Clin Anesth. 2016;32:181–8.
12. Ehlers M, Pezzano C, Leduc L, Brooks J, Silva P, Oechsner H, Crnkovic A, Galay I, Afroze F. Use of jet ventilation in thoracoscopic tracheo-esophageal fistula repair-can both surgeons and anesthesiologists be happy? Paediatr Anaesth. 2015;25(8):860–2.
13. McHoney M, Mackinlay G, Munro F, Capek A, Aldridge L. Effect of patient weight and anesthetic technique on CO2 excretion during thoracoscopy in children assessed by end-tidal CO2. J Laparoendosc Adv Surg Tech A. 2008; 18(1):147–51.
14. Datta PK, Pawar DK, Baidya DK, Maitra S. Dextrose-containing intraoperative fluid in neonates: a randomized controlled trial. Paediatr Anaesth. 2016; 26(6):599–607.
15. Spaeth JP, O'Hara IB, Kurth CD. Anesthesia for the micropremie. Semin Perinatol. 1998;22(5):390–401.
16. Wei K, Xu H, Liao W, Zhang C, Yao W. A newborn tolerated severe hypercapnia during general anesthesia: a case report. J Med Case Rep. 2015; 9:196.
17. Chiluveru SA, Dave NM, Dias RJ, Garasia MB. Congenital pulmonary airway malformation with atrial septal defect and pulmonary hypertension for lobectomy-anesthetic considerations. Ann Card Anaesth. 2016;19(2):372–4.
18. Kalfa N, Allal H, Raux O, Lardy H, Varlet F, Reinberg O, Podevin G, Héloury Y, Becmeur F, Talon I, Harper L, Vergnes P, Forgues D, Lopez M, Guibal MP, Galifer RB. Multicentric assessment of the safety of neonatal videosurgery. Surg Endosc. 2007;21(2):303–8.
19. Smith AL, Wollman H. Cerebral blood flow and metabolism: effects of anesthetic drugs and techniques. Anesthesiology. 1972;36(4):378–400.
20. Sola A. Oxygen in neonatal anesthesia: friend or foe? Curr Opin Anaesthesiol. 2008;21(3):332–9.
21. Keenan RL, Shapiro JH, Kane FR, Simpson PM. Bradycardia during anesthesia in infants. An epidemiologic study. Anesthesiology. 1994;80(5):976–82.
22. Means LJ, Green MC, Bilal R. Anesthesia for minimally invasive surgery. Semin Pediatr Surg. 2004;13(3):181–7.
23. De Armendi AJ, Mayhew JF, Cure JA. Another cause of hypercapnia during induction of anesthesia. Paediatr Anaesth. 2010;20(11):1055.
24. Krosnar S, Baxter A. Thoracoscopic repair of esophageal atresia with tracheoesophageal fistula: anesthetic and intensive care management of a series of eight neonates. Paediatr Anaesth. 2005;15(7):541–6.
25. Tobias JD. Anesthetic considerations for endoscopic procedures in children. Semin Pediatr Surg. 1993;2(3):190–4.
26. Gunawardana RH, Gunasekara SW, Weerasinghe JU. Anesthesia and surgery in pediatric patients with low hemoglobin values. Indian J Pediatr. 1999; 66(4):523–6.
27. Chen KB, Tu KT, Cheng HC, Wu YL, Chang JS. The anesthetic management of a preterm infant weighing 500 grams undergoing ligation of patent ductus arteriosus--a case report. Acta Anaesthesiol Sin. 1999;37(2):89–92.
28. Welle P, Hayden W, Miller T. Continuous measurement of transcutaneous oxygen tension of neonates under general anesthesia. J Pediatr Surg. 1980; 15(3):257–60.
29. Rowe R, Andropoulos D, Heard M, Johnson K, DeCampli W, Idowu O. Anesthetic management of pediatric patients undergoing thoracoscopy. J Cardiothorac Vasc Anesth. 1994;8(5):563–6.
30. Kinouchi K, Tanigami H, Tashiro C, Nishimura M, Fukumitsu K, Takauchi Y. Duration of apnea in anesthetized infants and children required for desaturation of hemoglobin to 95%. The influence of upper respiratory infection. Anesthesiology. 1992;77(6):1105–7.
31. Petrat G, Weyandt D, Klein U. Anesthetic considerations in pediatric laparoscopic and thoracoscopic surgery. Eur J Pediatr Surg. 1999;9(5):282–5.
32. Edwards AD, Wyatt JS, Richardson C, Delpy DT, Cope M, Reynolds EO. Cotside measurement of cerebral blood flow in infants by near infrared spectroscopy. Lancet. 1988;2(8614):770–1.
33. Smith HL, Jones JG. Non-invasive assessment of shunt and ventilation/ perfusion ratio in neonates with pulmonary failure. Arch Dis Child Fetal Neonatal Ed. 2001;85(2):F127–32.
34. Hoon SK, Kang SW, Kwak SH, Kim J. Hypoxia due to positive pressure ventilation in Edwards' syndrome: a case report. J Int Med Res. 2018;46(2): 895–900.
35. Lichtenstein DA, Mauriat P. Lung ultrasound in the critically ill neonate. Curr Pediatr Rev. 2012;8(3):217–23.
36. Broemling N, Campbell F. Anesthetic management of congenital tracheoesophageal fistula. Paediatr Anaesth. 2011;21(11):1092–9.
37. Razlevice I, Rugyte DC, Strumylaite L. Assessment of risk factors for cerebral oxygen desaturation during neonatal and infant general anesthesia: an observational, prospective study. BMC Anesthesiol. 2016;16(1):107.
38. Kussman BD, Wypij D, DiNardo JA, Newburger JW, Mayer JE Jr, del Nido PJ, Bacha EA, Pigula F, McGrath E, Laussen PC. Cerebral oximetry during infant cardiac surgery: evaluation and relationship to early postoperative outcome. Anesth Analg. 2009;108(4):1122–31.
39. Durduran T, Zhou C, Buckley EM, Kim MN, Yu G, Choe R, Gaynor JW, Spray TL, Durning SM, Mason SE, Montenegro LM, Nicolson SC, Zimmerman RA, Putt ME, Wang J, Greenberg JH, Detre JA, Yodh AG, Licht DJ. Optical measurement of cerebral hemodynamics and oxygen metabolism in neonates with congenital heart defects. J Biomed Opt. 2010;15(3):037004.

16

A prospective study on elective surgical inpatient satisfaction with perioperative anaesthesia service at ayder comprehensive specialized hospital, mekelle, ethiopia

Kore Menjie Benwu* and Hagos Gebregziabher Gebremedhin

Abstract

Background: Patient satisfaction is a subjective and challenging perception, linking physical, expressive, psychological, societal, and cultural factors. Dissatisfaction arises if the patient feels an inconsistency between expected and delivered care. Usually health care satisfactions are very high and according to many studies levels of satisfaction are above 85% and patient's satisfaction in terms of anesthesia is not very different. The aim of this study was to assess patient's satisfaction with perioperative anesthesia service and associated factors.

Methods: Institution-based cross-sectional study was conducted from December to January, 2017/8 at the Ayder Comprehensive Specialize Hospital. The data were collected using structured interviewer-administered questionnaire prepared to collect data on demographic character of the patients, determinant factors which could affect the patient satisfaction level on anesthesia service. Epi Info version 6 was used to record the data and SPSS version 20 was used for the analysis. Descriptive statistics were used to explore the socio-demographic characteristics of patients; factors possibly related to satisfaction level and overall satisfaction were summarized as frequencies and percentages.

Results: One hundred twenty consecutive patients were originally enrolled in the study that took over 1 Month. The overall proportion of patients who satisfied with anaesthesia services was 88.33%. Nausea and vomiting, pain, shortness of breath and cold were factors which affected patient satisfaction negatively.

Conclusion and recommendation: Compared with the other studies done at home and abroad; the overall proportion of patients, in Ayder comprehensive specialized hospital, who responded for satisfaction with perioperative anesthesia service is low. Patient satisfaction level should be determined regularly and all bodies should work to decrease the factors which decrease the satisfaction level.

Keywords: Patient satisfaction, Perioperative anaesthesia service, Associated factors, Operation

* Correspondence: lulakm2020@gmail.com
Mekelle University College of Health Science Department of Anesthesia, Po-box 1871, Mekelle, Ethiopia

Background

Patient satisfaction is a subjective and challenging perception, linking physical, expressive, psychological, societal, and cultural factors. Dissatisfaction happens if the patient feels an inconsistency between expected and delivered care. Because of the complexity and duration of the surgery, the pathophysiology of the disease is difficult to measure patient satisfaction with perioperative anesthesia care. Usually health care satisfactions is very high and according to many studies levels of satisfaction is above 85% and patient's satisfaction in terms of anesthesia is not very different [1, 2].

Anesthetists now a days are considered to have greater participation in preoperative evaluation and postoperative care this should allow prior identification and treatment of postoperative adverse effects. They are expected to describe professional obligation of patient care which relate to direct anesthetist and patient interactions, he/she must earn respect and trust from the patients through detailed discussion on anesthetic plan and responding for any kind of concerns about the anesthesia [3–7]. Visiting the patient and discussing the perioperative issues of the anesthesia and patient concerns significantly enhance patient satisfaction, regardless of the type of anesthesia performed [7–12].

Of patients who have got general anesthesia and local anesthesia for different kinds of surgery, 87% of patient was satisfied, 0.5% dissatisfied and 12.5% had no opinion [13]. Whereas another study discovered that 21.54% of patients succeeded an overall satisfaction less than 85%, and female, and educated patients were less satisfied [14].

In Ethiopia, health coverage is inadequate and of poor quality, and the country has exceptionally poor health status compare to other low-income countries [15]. And dissatisfaction with anesthesia has been reported to be associated with a 12-fold risk of global dissatisfaction with day case surgery and, to the investigator's knowledge, researches on elective inpatient satisfaction has rarely been reported in the literature [16–20]. Therefore we conducted this research to identify the satisfaction level of patients who have got surgery in Ayder Comprehensive Specialized Hospital and the result of this study will also use as baseline assessment for any further researchers and policy makers since there is not adequate studies on the subject area.

Methods

Study area, period and study design

Institution-based cross sectional-study design was used among patients who were scheduled for different kinds of surgery from surgical, orthopedics, medical, and gynecologic ward. The study was conducted from December 1/2017 to January 1/2018 at Mekelle University Ayder Comprehensive Specialized Hospital. Mekelle University Ayder Comprehensive Specialized Hospital is found in the Tigray regional state which is 780km far from the capital city of Ethiopia.

Sample size and sampling procedure

Using consecutive sampling procedure all elective patients (120) from surgical, orthopedics, medical, and gynecologic ward that were operated upon under general or regional anesthesia during study were included.

Data collection

Pre-tested structured questionnaire was prepared by reviewing previously done studies on the topic of a prospective study on elective surgical inpatient satisfaction with perioperative anaesthesia service [13, 14, 20]. The questionnaire was first prepared in English language by English language expert and then translated into Amharic by Amharic language expert, then to Tigrigna which is the local language of the patient in the study area by Tigrigna language expert. After the data has been collected the information acquired from the study participants changed to Amharic then to English by respective language experts.

Two data collectors who had experience on clinical data collection used after debriefing on the data collection methods by the principal investigators. Pretest on 10 patients was done before the actual data collection date and some of the terms were rephrased which were not clear for the participants. Data comprehensiveness and uniformity was checked by the investigators.

Data collection was done on socio-demographic characteristics and factors associated with perioperative anesthesia management of patients, satisfaction level and general satisfaction on perioperative anesthesia management after 24 h of operation using face to face interview. Before getting to the operation theater participants were educated about the standard care should provide for any patients on the context of anesthesia like detail information about the type of anesthesia the expected postoperative complications, having parts on the selection of anesthesia and others. After 24 h of their operation participants were asked to respond for whether they were involved on the decision of the type of anesthesia they could have, adequate information about the type of anesthesia they will have, had they any unnecessary disturbing events, whether they got relief for their any kind of discomfort on the postoperative time and level of their satisfaction and overall satisfaction.

Data analysis

Epi Info version 6 was used to record the data and SPSS version 20 was used for the analysis. Descriptive statistics were used to explore the socio-demographic characteristics of patients; factors possibly related to satisfaction level and overall satisfaction were summarized as frequencies and percentages. Chi-square tests were employed. Variables associated with satisfaction of participants on perioperative anesthesia management in chi-square tests analysis were included and *P*-values less than 0.05 were considered to be statistically significant in all cases.

Exclusion criteria

Patients were excluded if they have current history of mental illness, if he/she was operated previously in our hospital, critically ill (ASA 3–6) patient and patients who unable to communicate, patients who admitted to intensive care unit for further management, and pregnant patients were also excluded.

Definition of terms

- **ASA 1**: A normal healthy patient.
- **ASA 2**: A patient with a mild systemic disease
- **ASA 3**: A patient with a severe systemic disease that is not life-threatening.
- **ASA 4**: A patient with a severe systemic disease that is a constant threat to life.
- **ASA 5**: A moribund patient who is not expected to survive without the operation. The patient is not expected to survive beyond the next 24 h without surgery.
- **ASA 6**: A brain-dead patient whose organs are being removed with the intention of transplanting them into another patient [21]

Table 1 Socio demographic characteristics of surgical inpatients who has gone through surgery in Ayder comprehensive specialized Hospital, Mekelle, Ethiopia 2017/18

Characteristics	Category	Number	Percentage
Sex	Male	59	49.1%
	Female	61	50.9%
Payment status	Paying	107	89.16%
	Free	13	10.84%
Marital status	Single	32	26.7%
	Married	72	58.3%
	Divorced	8	7.00%
	Widowed	8	7.00%
Educational level	Primary school	89	74.17%
	Secondary school	25	20.83
	Higher education	6	5.00%

Result

Socio demographic characteristics of the participants

One hundred twenty consecutive patients were originally enrolled in the study that took over 1 month. None of them refused to fill out the questionnaire. As shown in Table 1 the baseline characteristics of the final 120 participants were active and 49.1% of them were male (Table 1).

As described in Table 1, from these 120 patients, 100 of them received general anesthesia and 20 of them received regional anesthesia. Of the respondents 89 (94.17%) completed primary school and 6 (5%) had certificate for diploma or above. The Paying status of participants was asked in the preoperative time and 89.16% of the participants responded that they are categorized under paying patients for every service they got (Table 1).

Association between satisfaction level and determinant factors

Chi-square test analysis was done to test the satisfaction level of participants with different parameters. General question that indicates the satisfaction rate of the patient on the anesthesia service was provided for the participants. From these participants106 (88.33%) of theme responded that they are satisfied on the anesthesia service. Furthermore, from the total patients who responded their satisfaction on perioperative anesthesia service only 56 (91.80%) of them were female. Then again, the male participants were 2 times more dissatisfy than the female participants though it is not statically significant (chi-square = 1.45, $P = 0.2285$). Participants were categorized in four group of age to test the association between the satisfaction level and age. As a result, the younger and the oldest participants were less satisfied on the perioperative anesthesia service than the middle age group which is statically significant (chi-square = 12.689, $P = 0.0054$).

Some Complication and specific tasks which are directly related to the type of anesthesia might decrease the satisfaction rate of the patient. The association indicates the type of the anesthesia and the satisfaction level. It was cheeked that patients who were operated under general anesthesia were 2 times more dissatisfied than who underwent their operation under regional anesthesia. However, the difference on the satisfaction level is not statically significant (chi-square = 2.733, $P = 0.0983$). Moreover, chi-square test analysis was also done to test the satisfaction level between participants who were visited and not visited by the anesthesia provider a day before the day of the operation. As a result, participants who were visited

Table 2 Association between different parameters versus satisfaction rate of surgical inpatients that had undergone surgery at Ayder comprehensive Specialized Hospital, Mekelle, Ethiopia 2017/18

Variable		Satisfied	Not satisfied	Chi square	*p*-value
Sex	Male	50	9	1.45	0.2285
	Female	56	5		
Age (Year)	15–24	11	7	12.689[a]	0.0054
	25-44	44	4		
	45–64	46	2		
	65+	5	1		
Education status	Primary	89	0	40.151 [a]	< 0.0001
	Secondary	15	10		
	Higher	2	4		
Types of anaesthesia	General	91	9	2.733 [a]	0.0983
	Regional	15	5		
Preoperative evaluation	Visited	104	8	27.102 [a]	< 0.0001
	Not-visited	2	6		

[a]Yates corrected chi-square

by the anesthesia provider were 4 times more satisfied than those who were visited by the anesthesia provider (chi-square = 27.102, $P < 0.0001$) which is statically significant. Education level is also one important factor for patient satisfaction and participants were classified in three groups to cheek the satisfaction level. Accordingly, the analysis shows that participants who has higher education were more dissatisfied than the other group which is statically significant (chi-square = 40.151, $P < 0.0001$) (Table 2).

Different perioperative complications, which might affect the satisfaction level, were put in to the chi-square analysis to test the value of clinical factors of patient satisfaction. The incidence rate of patients who had pain in perioperative time in general anesthesia were 2 times more than the participants who were operated in regional anesthesia group. Besides, the relationship between pain and satisfaction among the group in the chi-square test analysis is not strong (chi-square = 0.6047, $P = 0.4374$).

Dyspnea was also one of the concerns that was raised by the patient for the decrement of the satisfaction level. Subsequently, 18.75% of the patients who went through their operation under general anesthesia are dissatisfied; whereas all patients who were operated under regional anesthesia and who has dyspnea were satisfied. Nevertheless, chi-square test analysis shows that the difference between the group is not statically significant

Table 3 Association between different perioperative complications versus satisfaction of surgical inpatients that had undergone surgery at Ayder comprehensive Specialized Hospital, Mekelle, Ethiopia 2017/18

Variable		Satisfied	Not satisfied	Chi-square	*P*- Value
Pain	Regional anesthesia	1	0	0.6047 [a]	0.4374
	General anesthesia	11	3		
Dyspnoea	Regional anesthesia	2	0	0.112 [a]	0.7379
	General anesthesia	13	3		
Shivering	Regional anesthesia	2	1	0.375 [a]	0.5403
	General anesthesia	0	0		
Cold	Regional anesthesia	3	2	0.16 [a]	0.6892
	General anesthesia	4	2		
Nausea and vomiting	Regional anesthesia	2	2	6.331[a]	0.0119
	General anesthesia	38	1		

[a]Yates corrected chi-square

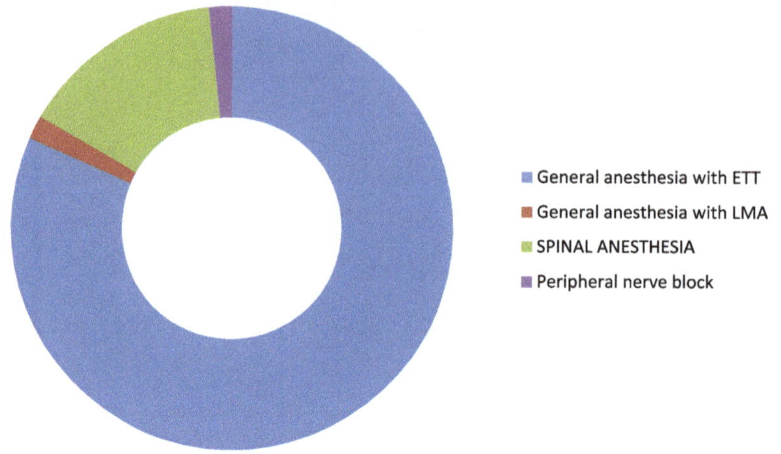

Fig. 1 Types of anesthesia used for different kinds of surgery at Ayder comprehensive Specialized Hospital, Mekelle, Ethiopia 2017/18

(chi-square = 0.0112, $P = 0.7379$). Nausea and vomiting was also another concern raised by the patients and these affect their satisfaction level. Thus, 50% of the patients who went through their operation under regional anesthesia were dissatisfied and 2.26% of the patients were from general anesthesia group. Then, chi-square test analysis shows strong relationship between nausea and vomiting and dissatisfaction among the group (chi-square = 6.331, $P = 0.0119$) (Table 3).

The types of anesthesia was also analyzed where the majority which is 100 (83.33%) of the patients had got general anesthesia. Moreover, 98 (98%) was operated under general anesthesia with endotracheal tube (ETT). Conversely, the remaining 2 (2%) was operated under general anesthesia with laryngeal mask airway (LMA) (Fig. 1). Types of surgery was also recorded and from 120 patients 43 (35.83%) were general surgery cases, 25 (20.83%) orthopedic cases, 8 (6.67%) cardiothoracic cases, 13 (10.83%) ENT cases, 21 (17.50%) gynecology cases and 10 (8.33%) urology cases (Fig. 2). Among the 120 patients who undergone surgery, 27 (22.5%) were associated to co-morbidities and of which 7 (5.83%) were asthmatic, 13 (10.83%) were hypertensive, and 7(5.83%) were diabetic patients shown in figure 3 and figure 4 respectively) (Figs. 3 and 4). Using the America Society of Anesthesiologist (ASA) standard, the overall health status of the patients was determined. Thus, of the total 78 (65%) were ASA 1 patients and 42 (35%) were ASA 2 patients (Fig. 5). Using Likert scale all patients were asked for the degree of satisfaction they had at recovery room when they are ready for transfer to their ward; 25 (21%) and 4 (20%) of the participants responded they are very satisfied, 56 (49%) and 7 (35%) responded satisfied, 32 (26%) and 6 (30%) responded neutral, 7 (4%) and 3 (15%) participants responded that they are dissatisfied on anesthesia service they have got from general and spinal anesthesia respectively. From both groups no participant response for very dissatisfied (Fig. 6). The professional approach to the patient which is getting consent of the patient for any kind of procedure is done. And this includes the decision of the anesthesia management in which it significantly affects the anesthetic satisfaction rate; participants

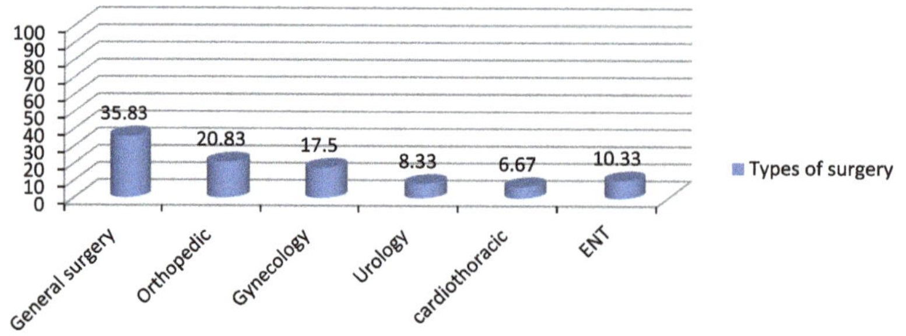

Fig. 2 Shows the Types of procedure done at Ayder comprehensive specialized Hospital, Mekelle, Ethiopia 2017/18

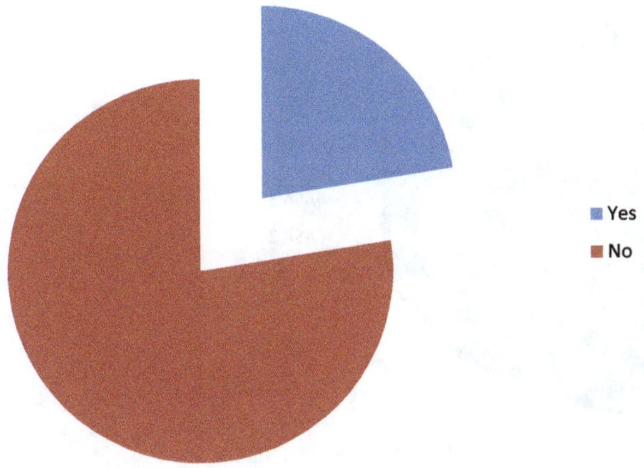

Fig. 3 Presence of associated morbidity on patients those who got surgery at Ayder comprehensive specialized Hospital, Mekelle, Ethiopia 2017/18

were asked whether they think that they get best help from their anesthesia provider. Hence, 67 (67%) of them are from the general anesthesia group and 14 (70%) of them are from the regional anesthesia group who felt that the anesthesia provider did best for them. And similarly, they were asked whether the anesthesia provider got consent for any procedure done to the participant and did they get the opportunity to ask questions and give opinion on the anesthetic management. Accordingly, 20 (20%) from general anesthesia group and 5 (25%) from regional anesthesia group responded that they had discussion and gave their opinion on the type of anesthesia they have got (Fig. 7). Specific question was provided which address the desire of the participant on having the same kind of anesthesia management by the same anesthetist if they have the same kind of operation. Thus 55 (47%) participants from the general anesthesia group and 14 (70%) participants from the spinal anesthesia group want to have the same kind of anesthesia intervention and management (Fig. 8).

Discussion

Our study showed that the overall proportion of participants who said we were satisfied with perioperative anesthesia services in Mekelle University Ayder Comprehensive Specialized Hospital was 88.33%. This finding was low compared with other studies done abroad and home [4, 18, 19, 22]. This can be secondary to poor preoperative assessment because the patient was not included on the selection of anesthesia type, and there was poor perioperative patient handling. On the other hand, some reference studies show that the technique of anesthesia was general anesthesia with patient controlled analgesia. And that minimizes the postoperative pain incidence and maximizes the satisfaction rate. And another reason for the low satisfaction level in our study is nausea and vomiting (39 and 20%), difficulty to breath in the immediate postoperative time (16 and 10%) and pain (14 and 5%) were the factors which had high percentage form factors which can decrease the satisfaction level in general and regional anesthesia respectively.

In this study the extreme age group (15–24 yrs. and 65 + yrs.) were less satisfied than the middle age groups ($P = 0.0054$), the result of this study matches with study done in Gonder University Hospital [20]. Patient dissatisfaction rate was high at the age of 20–39 years old. But the result of our study did not match with study done in Japan. This difference might be due to small number of patients were included in mentioned age group in Japan's study [23].

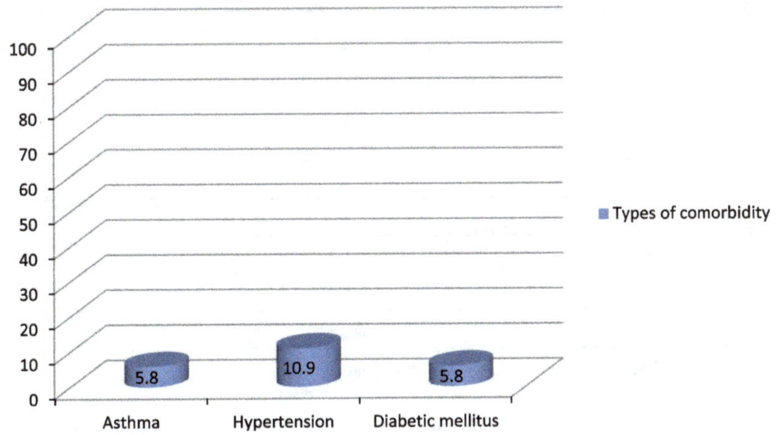

Fig. 4 Types of associated morbidity on patients those who got surgery at Ayder comprehensive specialized hospital, Mekelle, Ethiopia 2017/18

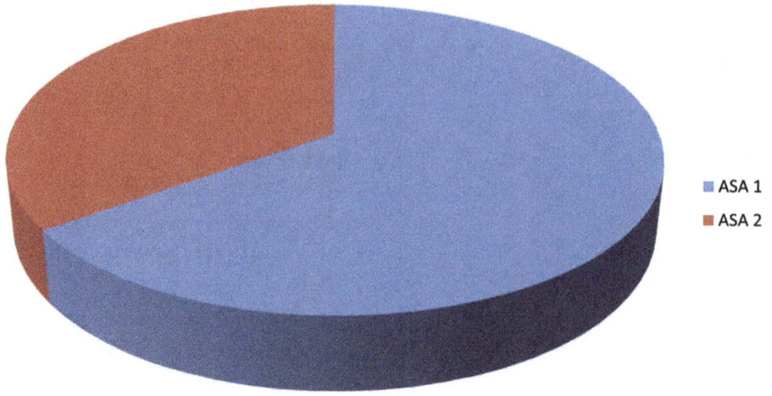

Fig. 5 Shows physical status of patients who were operated at Ayder comprehensive Specialized Hospital Mekelle, Ethiopia 2017/18

According to some studies, satisfaction rate is affected by the sex of the participants where female participants are less satisfied than male [1, 20]. But in this study female participant are more satisfied than male which was 91.80 and 84.75% respectively ($P = 0.2285$). This difference could be explained by the duration of stay in the reference study [1, 20] which was very short. Moreover, the type of surgery in our study was not life threating and preoperative hospital stay was not long for female patients. And this is because the waiting list for surgery from female side is not that much.

In our study, those who were more educated had low level of satisfaction. 100 and 33.33% of participants had a maximum of primary school and went for higher education respectively ($P < 0.0001$). The result of our study matches with study done in Saudi Arabia which showed that the educated participants had low satisfaction level [14].

In this study, less participants who were operated under regional anesthesia (75%) were satisfied than participants operated upon general anesthesia (general vs regional, $P = 0.0983$). But the study conducted at University of Gonder Hospital [20] indicate that participants who were operated under regional anesthesia was satisfied than those who were operated under general anesthesia. This discrepancy might be explained as some of patients in our study had peripheral block which usually cause pain on multiple attempts.

In our study participants who were evaluated by the anesthesia provider in the preoperative time had high satisfaction level (92.86%) than those who didn't get the anesthetist visit a day before the surgery ($P < 0.0001$). This result is in line with a study done in Australia [24]; this could be because of reassurance of patients and knows more about types of anesthesia that they will have.

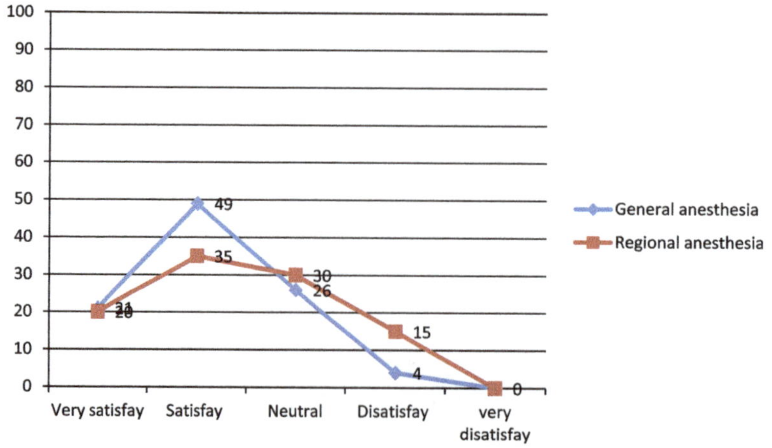

Fig. 6 Shows level of satisfaction of patients those who undergo their operation by regional and general anesthesia at Ayder comprehensive specialized Hospital mekelle Ethiopia 2017/18

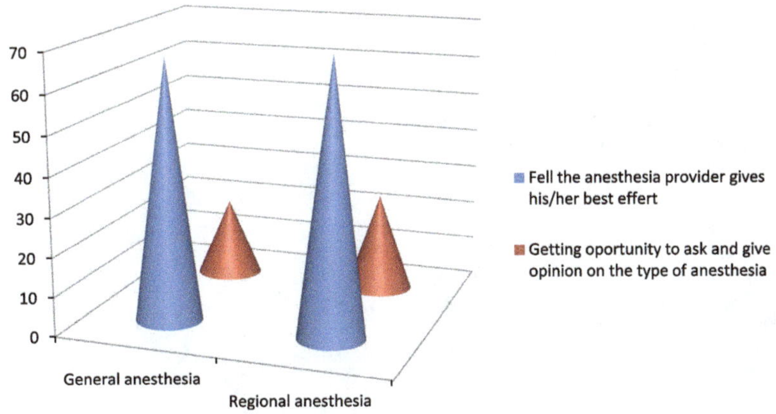

Fig. 7 Shows the attitude of the patients towards the anesthesia provider and the whole stay when they undergo their operation by general and spinal anesthesia at Ayder comprehensive specialized Hospital Mekelle Ethiopia 2017/18

Limitation of the study

Due to time constraint, small sample size was the limitation of the study. And this is because of the short time devoted between anesthesia and assessment of satisfaction.

Conclusion

Compared with the other studies done at home and abroad; the overall proportion of patients, in Ayder comprehensive specialized hospital, who responded for satisfaction with perioperative anesthesia service is low.

Recommendations

Patient satisfaction level should be done regularly at least once in a year. The official bodies of the hospitals, the anesthesia providers, nurses who work at ward and post anesthesia care unit have great responsibility to solve the precipitating factors for the low satisfaction level. In addition, the anesthesia provider should minimize the dissatisfying factors and increase factors exploiting satisfaction to reach at the final endpoint of patient satisfaction and quality of health service delivery. Training should also be given to anesthetists in the areas of the communication skills.

Abbreviations

ASA: America society of anesthesiology; BMI: Body mass index; ENT: Ear, nose and throat; ETT: Endotracheal tube; LMA: Laryngeal mask airway; LMP: Last menstrual period; MDGs: Millennium Development Goals; PONV: Post operative nausea and vomiting; SPSS: Statistical package for social sciences

Acknowledgments

Not applicable.

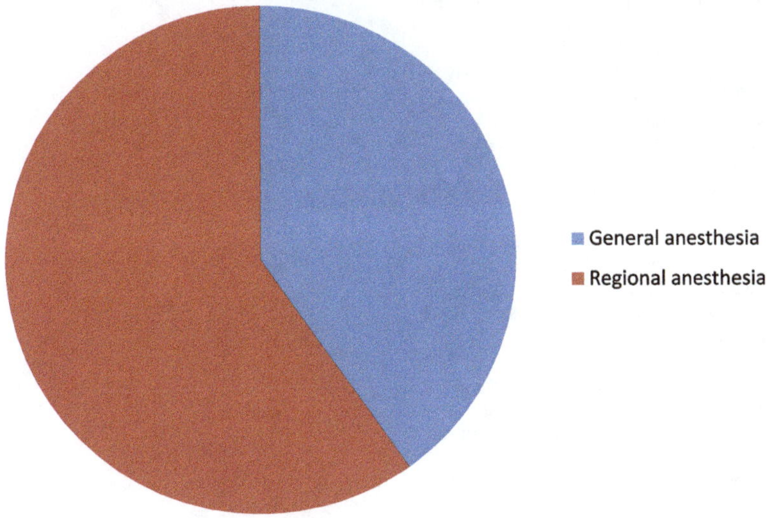

Fig. 8 Shows desire of the participants on having the same kinds of anesthesia if they have the same kinds of surgery at Ayder comprehensive specialized hospital Mekelle Ethiopia 2017/18

Authors' contributions

KMB Has presented ideas, statement of the problem, study materials, methodology, set the objectives, develop questionnaires. Has also participated in data analysis and writing results, discussion and conclusion. HGG Has participated in writing the literature, supervised the quality of data collection, analysis and developed tables and figures for results sections. He has also participated in editing the proposal and the result/research. All authors read and approved the final manuscript.

References

1. Auquier P, Pernoud N, Bruder N, et al. Development and validation of a perioperative satisfaction questionnaire. Anesthesioloy. 2005;102:1116–23.
2. Fung D, Cohen M. Measuring patient satisfaction with anaesthesia care: a review of current methodology. Anesth Analg. 1998;87:1089–98.
3. Heppner DL, Badner AM, Hurwitz S, Gustatson M, Tsen LC. Patient satisfaction with preoperative assessment in a preoperative assessment testing clinic. Anesthesia Analg. 2004;98:1099–105.
4. Evaluation of Patient Satisfaction and Recovery Time Following Different Anesthetic techniques at the San Ignacio University Hospital. Rev Col Anesthesia. 2010;38(2):178–202.
5. Gill TM, Feinstein AR. A critical appraisal of the quality-of-life measurements. JAMA. 1994;272:619–26.
6. Abbey A, Andrews FM. Modelling the psychosocial determinants of life quality. Soc Indic Res. 1985;16:1–34.
7. Klock PA, Roizen MF. More or better—educating the patient about the anesthesiologist's role as perioperative physician. Anesth Analg. 1996;83: 671–2.
8. Lee A, Lum ME. Measuring anaesthetic outcomes. Anaesth Intensive Care. 1996;24:685–93.
9. Vyhunthan G, Aeshana de Silva NG. Audit to evaluate preoperative visit to patient by anaesthetist. Sri Lankan Journal of Anaesthesiology. 2012;20(2): 88–91.
10. Kouki et al, Greek surgical patients satisfactiondevopress. Patient Prefer Adherence. 2012:6:569–578.
11. Yucelt U. An investigation of causes of patient satisfaction/dissatisfaction with physician services. Health Mark Q. 1994;12:11–28.
12. Tielsch JM, Steinberg EP, Cassard SD, et al. Preoperative functional expectations and postoperative outcomes among patients undergoing first eye cataract surgery. Arch Ophthalmol. 1995;113(10):1312–8.
13. Wołowicka L, et al. Patient satisfaction with anesthesia as a measure of quality of anesthesia care. Folia Med Cracov. 2001;42(4):219–26 https://www.ncbi.nlm.nih.gov/pubmed/12815782/.
14. Baroud ND, Nofal HW, Ahmad AN. Patient satisfaction in anesthesia. A modified Iowa satisfaction in anesthesia scale. Anesth Essays Res. 2010;4: 85–90 https://www.ncbi.nlm.nih.gov/pubmed/25885236.
15. Girma S, et al. Human resource development for health in Ethiopia: challenges of achieving the millennium development goals. Ethiop J Health Dev. 2007;21:3.
16. Myles PS, William DL, Handratam M, Anderson H, Weeks AM. Patient satisfaction after anesthesia and surgery; result of a prospective surgery of 10811 patients. Br J Anesthesia. 2000;84(1):6–10.
17. Kouki P, Matsota P, Christodoulaki K, et al. Greek surgical patients' satisfaction related to preoperative anesthetic services in an academic institute. Patient Prefer Adherence. 2012;569(78):6.
18. Lehman M, et al. Postoperative patient compliant prospective interviews study of 12276 patients. J Ansth Clin. 2010;22(1):13–21.
19. Belihun A, Alemu M, Mengistu B. A Prospective Study on Surgical Inpatient Satisfaction with Perioperative Anesthetic Service 2015 6; 3 8.
20. Gebremedhn E, et al. Patient satisfaction with anesthesia with anaesthesia services and associated factors at the University of Gondar Hospital. 2013;8: 377. https://www.ncbi.nlm.nih.gov/pmc/articles/PMC4549915/
21. DJ Doyle; Emily American Society of Anesthesiologists Classification (ASA Class) October 6, 2017. https://www.ncbi.nlm.nih.gov/books/NBK441940.
22. Fernandez MB, et al. Assessing patient satisfaction with cataract surgery under topical anesthesia supplemented by intracameral lidocain combined with sedation. Arq Bras Oftalmol. 2013;76(6):345–9.
23. Nakahashi K, Motozu Y, Sasaoka N, Hirai K, Kitaguchi K, Furuya H. Patient satisfaction with anesthesia care. Masui. 2004;53(10):1136–42.
24. Pollard JR, Coyle PJ, Gilbert LR, Beck EJ. Intraoperative awareness in a regional medical system. A review of 3 years' data. Anesthesiology. 2007; 106(2):269–74.

17

Photoacoustic gas monitoring for anesthetic gas pollution measurements and its cross-sensitivity to alcoholic disinfectants

Jennifer Herzog-Niescery[1*], Thomas Steffens[2], Martin Bellgardt[1], Andreas Breuer-Kaiser[1], Philipp Gude[1], Heike Vogelsang[1], Thomas Peter Weber[1] and Hans-Martin Seipp[2]

Abstract

Background: Real-time photoacoustic gas monitoring is used for personnel exposure and environmental monitoring, but its accuracy varies when organic solvents such as alcohol contaminate measurements. This is problematic for anesthetic gas measurements in hospitals, because most disinfectants contain alcohol, which could lead to false-high gas concentrations. We investigated the cross-sensitivities of the photoacoustic gas monitor Innova 1412 (AirTech Instruments, LumaSense, Denmark) against alcohols and alcoholic disinfectants while measuring sevoflurane, desflurane and isoflurane in a laboratory and in hospital during surgery.

Methods: 25 mL ethyl alcohol was distributed on a hotplate. An optical filter for isoflurane was used and the gas monitor measured the 'isoflurane' concentration for five minutes with the measuring probe fixed 30 cm above the hotplate. Then, 5 mL isoflurane was added vaporized via an Anesthetic Conserving Device (Sedana Medical, Uppsala, Sweden). After one-hour measurement, 25 mL isopropyl alcohol, N-propanol, and two alcoholic disinfectants were subsequently added, each in combination with 5 mL isoflurane. The same experiment was in turn performed for sevoflurane and desflurane. The practical impact of the cross-sensitivity was investigated on abdominal surgeons who were exposed intraoperatively to sevoflurane. A new approach to overcome the gas monitor's cross-sensitivity is presented.

Results: Cross-sensitivity was observed for all alcohols and its strength characteristic for the tested agent. Simultaneous uses of anesthetic gases and alcohols increased the concentrations and the recovery times significantly, especially while sevoflurane was utilized. Intraoperative measurements revealed mean and maximum sevoflurane concentrations of 0.61 ± 0.26 ppm and 15.27 ± 14.62 ppm. We replaced the cross-sensitivity peaks with the 10th percentile baseline of the anesthetic gas concentration. This reduced mean and maximum concentrations significantly by 37% ($p < 0.001$) and 86% ($p < 0.001$), respectively.

Conclusion: Photoacoustic gas monitoring is useful to detect lowest anesthetic gases concentrations, but cross-sensitivity caused one third falsely high measured mean gas concentration. One possibility to eliminate these peaks is the recovery time-based baseline approach. Caution should be taken while measuring sevoflurane, since marked cross-sensitivity peaks are to be expected.

Keywords: Gas pollution, Occupational gas exposure, Photoacoustic gas monitoring, Cross-sensitivity, Isoflurane, Sevoflurane, Desflurane, Recovery time

* Correspondence: j.herzog-niescery@klinikum-bochum.de
[1]Department of Anesthesiology, Katholisches Klinikum Bochum, Ruhr-University Bochum, St. Josef Hospital, Gudrunstraße 56, 44791 Bochum, Germany

Background

Occupational anesthetic gas exposure is attracting growing interest, since studies have shown that low-dose exposure to volatile anesthetics (VA) increases the number of DNA strand breaks and the micronuclei frequencies in lymphocytes and epithelial cells [1, 2]. Although exposure levels of healthcare professionals have been minimized, it still is good clinical practice to reduce gas pollution 'as low as reasonably achievable' [3]. The Occupational Safety and Health Administration of the United States recommends the control of VA exposure by engineering controls, good work practices, use of personal protective equipment, administrative controls, and personnel exposure and environmental monitoring. The latter is especially significant, because it demonstrates the effectiveness of the gas control program and should be performed every six months [4].

Different approaches are available to evaluate the personnel's exposure, but measurements in the individual breathing zones are commonly performed, either by time-integrated or real-time air-sampling. A dosimeter is an example for time-integrated sampling. It measures the mean pollution level, but the minimum sampling duration is > 15 min and it is not possible to get an instant feedback [4]. Hence, real-time measurements performed by gas analyzers are preferred, because they present mean and maximum concentrations continuously and enable an immediate feedback of the current VA exposure. Their low analytical detection limits allow to detect trace concentrations of 0.005 ppm. However, it is known that their accuracy may vary when they are used together with organic solvents such as alcohols [5, 6]. This is problematic for VA measurements in hospitals, because many commonly used substances contain alcohol, which may lead to a misjudgment of the actual pollution (Table 1).

We investigated the cross-sensitivities of a photoacoustic gas monitor against alcohols and alcoholic disinfectants (AD) while measuring isoflurane (ISO), sevoflurane (SEVO), and desflurane (DES) in the air. Characteristic curves and an approach to deal with these interferences are presented.

We hypothesized that there is a cross-sensitivity for all three VA and that the elimination of the cross-sensitivity would reduce the average false-high VA concentration significantly by 30%. This practical impact of the cross-sensitivity was investigated on abdominal surgeons who were exposed intraoperatively to sevoflurane.

Methods

Laboratory experiments were performed at the University of Applied Sciences, Giessen, Germany, in 2018. VA pollution measurements were conducted in a German University hospital (Katholisches Klinikum Bochum, St. Josef Hospital). The study was approved by the local ethics committee in December 2015 (No. 5184–14; Ethikkommission der Ruhr-Universität Bochum, Germany). Written informed consent was obtained from all participants included in this study. Measurements were performed according to the Declaration of Helsinki.

Photoacoustic gas monitoring

All measurements were conducted with the photoacoustic gas monitor Innova 1412 (AirTech Instruments, LumaSense, Denmark). This analyzer identifies any gas that absorbs infrared light by using the photoacoustic infrared detection method with specific optical filters. The operating principle is as follows: A pump sucks in a sample of air into a sealed measurement cell, where pulsed infrared laser light is transferred through an optical filter. The monitored gas selectively absorbs the transmitted light, which leads to volume variations caused by increasing and decreasing temperature. This results in an acoustic signal in the measurement cell, which is proportional to the investigated gas concentration.

The gas monitor was calibrated by the manufacturer with optical filters for VA measurements (UA 0970: SEVO and DES, wavelength 8.2 μm; UA 0971: ISO, wavelength 8.5 μm) and for water vapor (SB0527, lower detection limit 50 ppm). Filters for VA measurements had a bandwidth of 6% and analytical detection limits of 0.006 ppm for SEVO, 0.005 ppm for DES and 0.005 ppm for ISO at 20 °C, 1 atm pressure and for a sample integration time of 5 s. Filters for alcohols were not used in this study to demonstrate any cross-sensitivity. A measurement interval lasted 35 s and depended on the size of the measurement cell, the length of the sampling probe, time to flush both with fresh air (30 s), and on the sample integration time (5 s). An autocalibration was performed by the gas monitor prior to each change of the VA filter. According to the manufacturer, the reproducibility of the measured anesthetic gas concentration by the photoacoustic gas monitor is ±1% of the measured value.

Experimental setup

The tests were conducted in a laboratory sized 36.5 m^3. The door and the windows were kept closed. A hotplate was placed on a table and heated to 37 °C. The measuring probe of the photoacoustic gas monitor was fixed on a stand at a distance of 30 cm above the hotplate. A fan was used for a uniform distribution of air (Fig. 1).

Baseline values

First, baseline values for ISO, SEVO and DES were determined to detect any contamination in the air. The gas monitor was calibrated to measure ISO, SEVO or DES, but neither VAs, nor interfering agents were used. A measurement interval lasted 10 min each.

Table 1 Commonly used disinfectants and alcoholic components which may be interfering substances while using the gas monitor. n (right column) = number of alcoholic components

Alcohol / Disinfectant	Ethyl alcohol	Isopropyl alcohol	N-propanol	Benzyl alcohol	1-tetra-decanol	Biphenyl-2-ol	Glycerol	
Hand disinfection (hygienic or preoperative)								*n*
Ethyl alcohol 80 vol.%	X							1
Isopropyl alcohol 70 vol.%		X						1
N-propanol 60 Vol.%			X					1
AHD 2000®	X							1
Aktivin® DHH		X						1
Aseptoman®		X						1
Aseptoman® viral	X		X					2
Aseptopur®		X						1
Descoderm®		X						1
Desderman® pure	X	X				X		3
Hospisept®	X		X					2
Poly-Alcohol Hands Antiseptic		X						1
Promanum pure®	X	X						2
Skinman® clear			X				X	2
Skinman® complete	X							1
Skinman® complete pure	X							1
Skinman® soft		X			X			2
Skinsept® F		X						1
Softa-Man®	X		X					2
Softa-Man® acute	X		X					2
Spitacid®	X	X		X				3
Sterillium®		X	X		X			3
Sterillium® classic pure			X		X			2
Sterillium® med	X		X		X			3
Sterillium® virugard	X				X			2
Skin antiseptics								n
Cutasept®-F, –G		X						1
Kodan® tincture forte		X	X	X		X		4
Octeniderm®		X	X					2
Poly Alcohol colourless		X						1
Surface disinfection								n
Amocid Lysoform®						X		1
Bacillol® AF	X	X	X					3
Mikrozid® AF liquid	X		X					2
Total [n]	15	17	13	2	5	3	1	

Volatile anesthetics

An Anesthetic Conserving Device (ACD; Sedana Medical, Uppsala, Sweden) was used to vaporize the VAs. Therefore, a compressed air bottle with a flow rate of 480 L/h was combined with the ACD, which was flushed with liquid VA (6 in Fig. 1). The gas monitor was equipped with the optical filter for the VA of interest. As soon as the VA concentration in the air had reached the baseline value, a bolus of 5 mL liquid VA was injected into the ACD and the gas pollution measured for one hour. Regression lines, which appear as linear curves when using a semi logarithmic diagram, were calculated after the maximum concentration was reached by the formula $c = a \cdot \exp.(-b \cdot t)$ with c: VA concentration [ppm]; a: factor to calculate the regression; b: gradient; t: time.

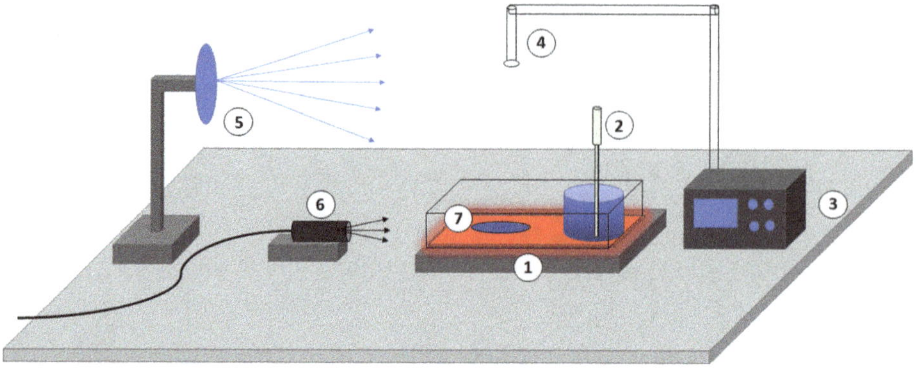

Fig. 1 Experimental setup. A hotplate (1) was heated to 37 °C and its temperature controlled by a thermometer (2). The gas monitor's (3) measuring probe was fixed on a stand (4). A fan was used for a uniform distribution of air (5). An Anesthetic Conserving Device was used for vaporization of the volatile anesthetic (6). The interfering agents were distributed on the hotplate (7)

Volatile anesthetics and interfering agents

An optical filter for ISO was used and 25 mL ethyl alcohol was distributed on the hotplate. After ten minutes of measurement, 5 ml ISO was injected into the ACD as described above, followed by a one-hour measurement. Subsequently, 25 mL isopropyl alcohol, N-propanol, AD I (isopropyl alcohol 45 vol%, N-propanol 30 vol%), and AD II (isopropyl alcohol 72 vol%) were added, each agent in combination with 5 mL ISO. Regression lines were calculated as described above.

The same tests were in turn performed with SEVO and DES.

Approach to eliminate cross-sensitivity peaks

The approach is based on the recovery time, which is the time needed to reduce the gas concentration in the room by two log steps (corresponds to a reduction of 99%). The recovery time was calculated according to DIN EN ISO 14644 [7] and depended primarily on the type of air-conditioning, the supply air volume, the volume of the operating room, and on the position of the exhaust air slots.

To demonstrate practical significance of this approach, the gas monitor was calibrated for SEVO and the VA exposure measured during abdominal surgery in the surgeons' individual breathing zones (25 cm around nose and mouth). The use of interfering agents was documented in time. VA concentrations and cross-sensitivity peaks were analyzed and the 'actual' SEVO pollution estimated.

Statistical analysis

IBM SPSS version 20 (IBM Corp., Armonk, NY) was used for statistical analysis. After testing variables for normality using the Kolmogorov-Smirnov test and Lilliefors correction, statistical significance was determined using Students t-test and Mann–Whitney U test. Linear regression analysis was performed. Continuous variables are shown as mean (standard deviation (SD)) or median (interquartile range (IQR)). A p-value < 0.05 (two-sited test, error probability $< 5\%$) was considered statistically significant.

The sample size required for measurements in hospital is based on a pilot study of 10 surgeons, who were exposed to a mean SEVO concentration of 0.58 ± 0.27 ppm including cross-sensitivity. For an α-risk of 0.05 with a power of 80% at least 16 measurements are needed to demonstrate a 30% reduction of the average SEVO concentration by elimination of the cross-sensitivity.

Results

Baseline values

Mean ± SD baseline values were 0.05 ± 0.01 (median: 0.05, IQR: 0.001) ppm for ISO, 0.01 ± 0.01 (median: 0.01, IQR: 0.001) ppm for SEVO, and 0.04 ± 0.01 (median: 0.05, IQR: 0.001) ppm for DES ($n = 5$ per VA).

Volatile anesthetics

The concentrations of all three VAs increased within approximately five minutes to a maximum of 21.01–23.99 ppm. The decay curves corresponded to recovery times of 52 min and exponential functions with $R^2 = 0.999$ for ISO, $R^2 = 0.995$ for SEVO, and $R^2 = 0.999$ for DES) (n = 5 per VA) (Fig. 2).

Volatile anesthetics and interfering agents

The gas monitor detected VA concentrations, although only alcohols and AD were used (n = 5 per interfering agent and for each VA) (Fig. 3 a-c). Consistently, highest cross-sensitivity peaks were caused by isopropyl alcohol, followed by AD, ethyl alcohol and N-propanol.

The simultaneous use of VA and interfering agent led to a false-high 'VA concentration' and extended the recovery time (Fig. 3d). Further, the strength of the cross-sensitivity reaction was influenced by the measured VA (SEVO > DES, ISO) (Table 2).

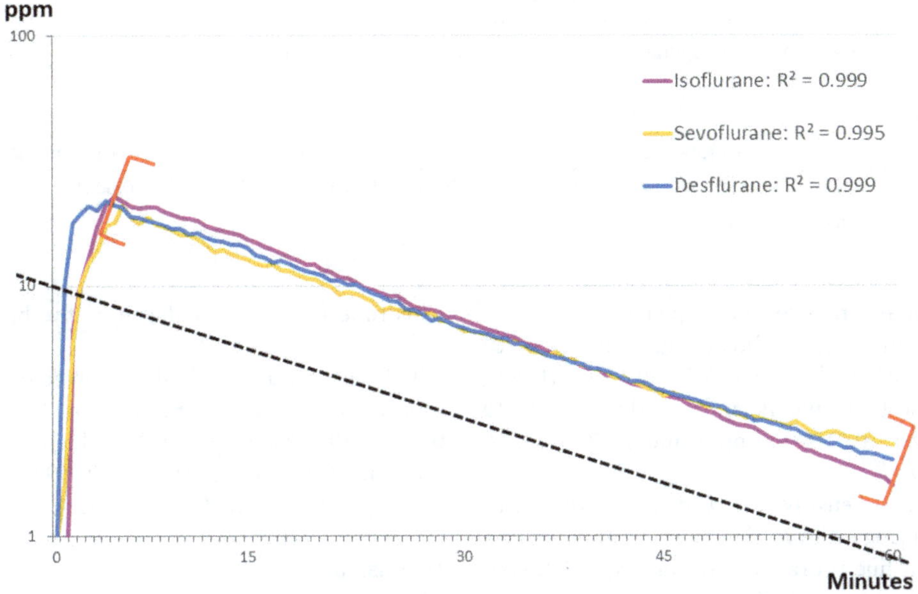

Fig. 2 Decay curves were similar for all gases (isoflurane: y = 29.691e-0.028x; sevoflurane: y = 22.508e-0.024x; desflurane: y = 24.956e-0.025x). R^2: exponential function with linear regression; calculations started after the maximum concentration was reached (red brackets). The recovery time was 52 min (dotted black line). $N = 5$ per anesthetic gas

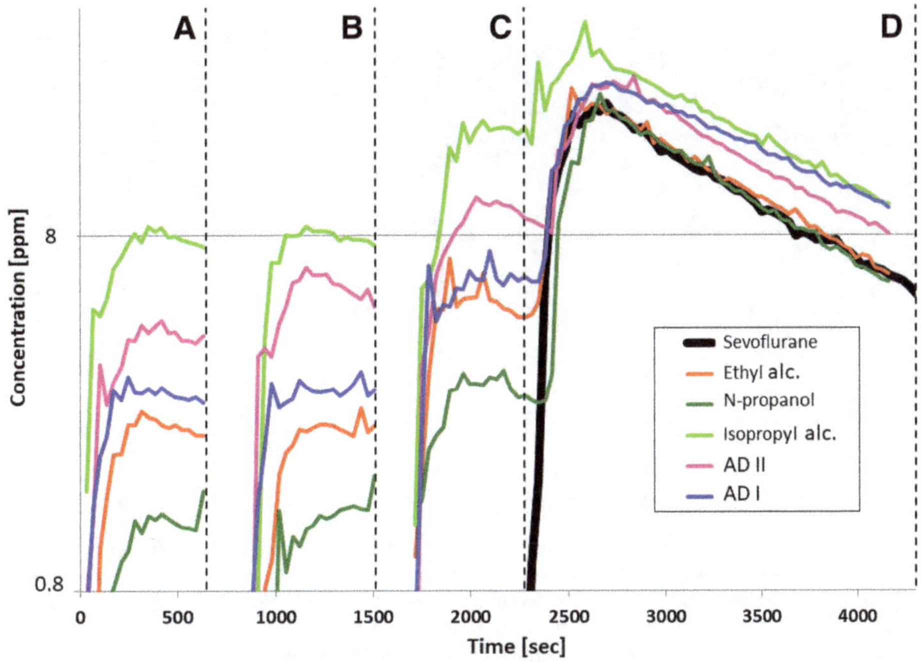

Fig. 3 The gas monitor with filters for isoflurane (**a**), desflurane (**b**), or sevoflurane (**c**) mistakenly detects anesthetic gases, although alcohols and alcoholic disinfectants (**ad**) were used ($n = 5$ per interfering agent). The strength of the cross-sensitivity was highest for isopropyl alcohol (alc.). **d** shows the increase of the actual sevoflurane concentration (black line) by interfering agents

Table 2 Impact of the volatile anesthetic on the strength of the cross-sensitivity reaction for different interfering substances. Boldface entries refer to a significant value (level of significance: $p < 0.05$). * = sevoflurane caused higher false-high 'VA' pollution levels than desflurane or isoflurane; # = desflurane caused higher false-high 'VA' pollution levels than isoflurane. $N = 5$ per interfering agent and for each VA

Anesthetic gas	Desflurane					Sevoflurane				
	Ethyl alcohol	N-propanol	Isopropyl alcohol	AD I	AD II	Ethyl alcohol	N-propanol	Isopropyl alcohol	AD I	AD II
Isoflurane	**0.042#**	0.329	0.383	0.457	**< 0.001#**	**< 0.001***	**< 0.001***	**< 0.001***	**< 0.001***	**< 0.001***
Sevoflurane	**< 0.001***	**< 0.001***	**< 0.001***	**< 0.001***	**< 0.001***	–	–	–	–	–

Approach to eliminate cross-sensitivity peaks

SEVO exposure in surgeon breathing zone ($n = 20$) was not distinguished between VA and interfering agents. The false-high mean and maximum SEVO concentrations were 0.61 ± 0.26 ppm and 15.27 ± 14.62 ppm, respectively.

To overcome cross-sensitivity, a 10th percentile baseline is drawn for logarithmic data with recovery time marked. A straight line is drawn from the upper left corner (0/log 10; intersection X-Y-axis) to the X-axis and moved to the peak's maximum. The intersection with the curve marks the end of the cross-sensitivity peak. This time interval is replaced by the baseline concentration (Fig. 4).

This technique resulted in corrected mean and maximum SEVO concentrations of 0.38 ± 0.09 ppm and 0.91 ± 0.49 ppm, respectively, which is a significant reduction of 38% for mean ($p < 0.001$) and 86% for maximum ($p < 0.001$) SEVO concentrations.

Discussion

This study investigated a photoacoustic gas monitor's cross-sensitivities against alcohols and AD while measuring VA pollution.

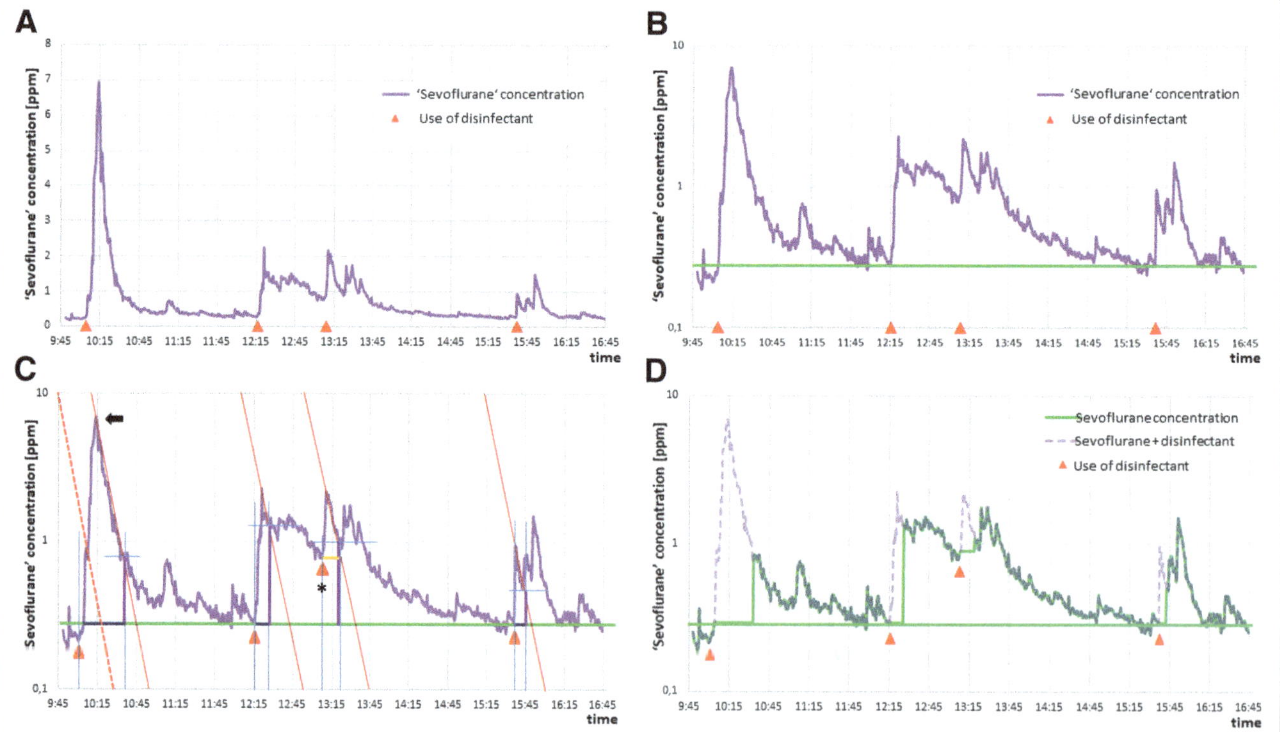

Fig. 4 Approach to eliminate cross-sensitivity peaks. **a** shows the false-high 'sevoflurane exposure' of a surgeon (purple line; [ppm] mean: 0.73 ± 0.70, maximum: 6.93; red triangle: use of disinfectant). After logarithmic presentation of the data (purple line in **b**), the 10th percentile baseline is drawn (green line; here 0.29 ppm), and the recovery time is marked (red dotted line in **c**; here 39 min). This line is moved to the peak's maximum (black arrow in **c**). The intersection with the curve marks the end of the cross-sensitivity peak (blue cross in **c**). This time interval is replaced by the baseline concentration (dark blue line in **c**). If interfering agents are used before the decay curve has reached the baseline concentration (back star in **c**) the cross-sensitivity interval should not be replaced by the 10th percentile, but by the measured concentration at the beginning of the cross-sensitivity peak (orange in **c**). In this example the 'corrected' mean and maximum sevoflurane concentrations were 0.53 ± 0.33 ppm and 1.76 ppm, which is a reduction by 28% (**d**)

In principle, photoacoustic gas monitoring is an excellent method to detect waste anesthetic gases in the air. The low detection limits allow for identification of the smallest concentrations of VAs and the immediate feedback of the VA exposure makes the gas monitor valuable in practice, because it may attract attention and help reduce the occupational gas burden. However, its cross-sensitivity to alcohols is problematic, because interfering agents are regularly used in the perioperative setting (e.g. for skin disinfection or surgical hand disinfection). This study aimed to investigate this phenomenon, since it is not considered in most clinical studies and the false-high 'VA' concentrations may stir unjustified fears [8–11].

The photoacoustic gas monitor's manufacturer advises that cross-sensitivities may occur, but no information is given about the impact of the interfering agent on the measured value, the decay curve, or its significance in the clinical environment [12]. Instead, the use of additional optical filters is recommended, but this assumes that all interfering agents are known. Although it is a possible approach in an experimental setting, this is difficult in hospitals. The gas monitor can simultaneously be used with filters for the VA, water vapor, and up to four alcohols. However, this still may be insufficient as other substances interferer as well (e.g. permanent marker: ethyl alcohol and 4-chloro-3-methylphenol). Another restriction is the high costs of the optical filters. Therefore, an alternative method should be known to eliminate cross-sensitivity peaks. The presented approach can be quickly performed without technical equipment; even the recovery time can be verified in the appropriate documents for every operating room (according to ISO 14644-3 for turbulent ventilation systems) [7].

Our experiences suggest that this approach is suitable for high, as well as low cross-sensitivity peaks. Its particular value is that it considers the cross-sensitivity's maximum, which falsely increase the mean VA concentration mostly. Each peak is replaced by the 10th percentile baseline and not just waived, which takes the actual VA concentration into account. However, it should be noted that the VA pollution during cross-sensitivity peaks is not measured but estimated. Thus, it is possible that the actual VA concentration is higher than the baseline value during a cross-sensitivity peak, which is a limitation (corrections lead to false-low VA concentrations).

In this study the elimination of the cross-sensitivity reduced the false-high mean and maximum 'VA' concentration by 37 and 86%, respectively. These percentages could be higher, if larger amounts of disinfectants are used [5]. This demonstrates the great impact of the cross-sensitivity on VA measurements.

Another finding was that the strength of the cross-sensitivity reaction was influenced by the measured anesthetic gas (SEVO > DES, ISO). This can be explained by the VA's different infrared spectra, which range between 3.2 and 3.6 μm, but the absorption is highest for SEVO [12]. Consequently, it is most important to consider the gas monitor's cross-sensitivity while measuring SEVO.

This study has a few limitations. First, we demonstrated the gas monitor's cross-sensitivity for selected alcohols and disinfectants only, which are regularly used in hospitals. Isopropyl alcohol caused strongest peaks, however, other alcohols might show different cross-sensitivity characteristics. Further, we used 25 mL in the experimental setting only, although larger amounts are usually used in clinical routine. Much larger amounts would have increased the time to eliminate the alcohol out of the room, which correlates with increased false-high VA measurements. Nevertheless, this would not affect the approach to eliminate the cross-sensitivity peaks. Thirdly, for accuracy of the presented method, the use of every interfering agent must be documented. This might be difficult for substances, which contain 'veiled' interfering agents (e.g. permanent markers). Furthermore, measurements of the baseline values demonstrated that trace concentrations of interfering agents are always detectable, even in an experimental setting. Lastly, the ACD is not registered for DES, because it can boil in the agent line due to its low boiling point, which may result in an unintended emission of gas boluses [3]. However, we did not observe an uneven discharge of the anesthetic.

Conclusions

Photoacoustic gas monitoring is an excellent method to detect trace concentrations of anesthetic gases, but clinicians are often unaware of its cross-sensitivity and overestimate VA pollution levels. This can be avoided by measurements with different optical filters or by post-hoc corrections using the described recovery time-based approach, which had reduced the false-high mean VA concentration by one third and the maximum concentration by 86% on average in this study. Caution should be taken while measuring SEVO concentrations, since marked cross-sensitivity peaks are to be expected.

Abbreviations

ACD: Anesthetic Conserving Device; AD: Alcoholic disinfectants; DES: Desflurane; IQR: Interquartile range; ISO: Isoflurane; SD: Standard deviation; SEVO: Sevoflurane; VA: Volatile anesthetic

Acknowledgements

Not applicable.

Authors' contributions

JHN planned the experiments and the study in hospital, is responsible for ethical approval, collected, analyzed and interpreted the data, and wrote the manuscript. TS planned the experimental part of the study and interpreted the data regarding the cross-sensitivity. MB collected the data during surgery in hospital and helped with the statistical analysis. ABK is responsible for data collection and analysis in hospital. PG prepared the figures and was a major contributor in writing the manuscript. HV prepared the tables, collected data in hospital and revised the manuscript critically. TPW interpreted the data and revised the manuscript. HMS conducted the experiments in the laboratory, analyzed and interpreted the data, developed the recovery-time based approach and helped writing the manuscript. All authors read and approved the final manuscript.

Authors' information

Not applicable.

Author details

[1]Department of Anesthesiology, Katholisches Klinikum Bochum, Ruhr-University Bochum, St. Josef Hospital, Gudrunstraße 56, 44791 Bochum, Germany. [2]Department of Life Science Engineering, University of Applied Sciences, Giessen, Germany.

References

1. Çakmak G, Eraydın D, Berkkan A, Yağar S, Burgaz S. Genetic damage of operating and recovery room personnel occupationally exposed to waste anaesthetic gases. Hum Exp Toxicol. 2018. https://doi.org/10.1177/0960327118783532.
2. Wiesner G, Schiewe-Langgartner F, Lindner R, Gruber M. Increased formation of sister chromatid exchanges, but not of micronuclei, in anaesthetists exposed to low levels of sevoflurane. Anaesthesia. 2008;63:861–4.
3. Herzog-Niescery J, Seipp HM, Weber TP, Bellgardt M. Inhaled anesthetic agent sedation in the ICU and trace gas concentrations: a review. J Clin Monit Comput. 2018;32:667–75.
4. Occupational Safety and Health Administration (OSHA). Anesthetic gases: guidelines for workplace exposures. 2000. http://www.osha.gov/dts/osta/anestheticgases/index.html Accessed: 30th November 2018.
5. Herzog-Niescery J, Botteck NM, Vogelsang H, Gude P, Bartz H, Weber TP, et al. Occupational chronic sevoflurane exposure in the everyday reality of the anesthesia workplace. Anesth Analg. 2015;121:1519–28.
6. Walder B, Lauber R, Zbinden AM. Accuracy and cross-sensitivity of 10 different anesthetic gas monitors. J Clin Monit. 1993;9:364–73.
7. Deutsches Institut für Normung, European Standard. International Organization for Standardization (DIN EN ISO): cleanrooms and associated controlled environments - part 3: test methods (ISO 14644). Berlin, Germany: Beuth Verlag GmbH; 2017.
8. Hoerauf K, Funk W, Harth M, Hobbhahn J. Occupational exposure to sevoflurane, halothane and nitrous oxide during paediatric anaesthesia. Waste gas exposure during paediatric anaesthesia. Anaesthesia. 1997;52:215–9.
9. Byhahn C, Heller K, Lischke V, Westphal K. Surgeon's occupational exposure to nitrous oxide and sevoflurane during pediatric surgery. World J Surg. 2001;25:1109–12.
10. Blokker-Veldhuis MJ, Rutten PM, De Hert SG. Occupational exposure to sevoflurane during cardiopulmonary bypass. Perfusion. 2011;26:383–9.
11. Schebesta K, Lorenz V, Schebesta EM, Hörauf K, Gruber M, Kimberger O, et al. Exposure to anaesthetic trace gases during general anaesthesia: CobraPLA vs. LMA classic. Acta Anaesthesiol Scand. 2010;54:848–54.
12. Luma Sense® Technologies. Innova 1412i multi-gas monitoring instruments. Manual. https://innova.lumasenseinc.com/manuals/1412i/. Accessed 30th November 2018.

18

Anaesthetic management of a large paraganglioma resection in a woman with isolated L-looped transposition of the great arteries

Ling Lan, Penghao Liu, Yuan Tian, Bo Zhu, Le Shen* and Yuguang Huang

Abstract

Background: Reports of anaesthetic management of paraganglioma resection in patients with isolated L-transposition of the great arteries (L-TGA) are rare. We focus on the preoperative evaluation, intraoperative management, and postoperative care of a frail patient with "physiologically corrected" L-TGA for paraganglioma resection.

Case presentation: We performed general anaesthesia for a 46-year-old patient with "physiologically corrected" L-TGA undergoing open large retroperitoneal paraganglioma resection. Although the preoperative medical therapy had attained its goals, the patient went through three periods of severe episodic hypertension and tachycardia as tumour manipulation released catecholamines. Goal-directed fluid therapy based on pulse pressure variation (PPV) and point-of-care transesophageal echocardiography (TEE) imaging enabled anaesthesiologists to make rapid judgments and to regulate blood pressure in a timely manner, thereby reducing the risk of heart failure caused by massive rapid fluid bolus therapy. The patient was transferred to the intensive care unit because of intraoperative hemodynamic changes and significant blood loss. Despite transient myocardial injury (elevated troponin I), no lethal arrhythmia or complications occurred perioperatively, and the patient recovered well and was discharged 1 week later.

Conclusions: Goal-directed fluid therapy combined with the adoption of TEE could effectively guide fluid administration, which is helpful for anaesthesia management during operation. We recommend the routine use of TEE in such cases.

Keywords: Paraganglioma, L-transposition of the great arteries, Goal-directed fluid therapy, Transesophageal echocardiography, Case report

* Correspondence: pumchshenle@163.com
Department of Anaesthesiology, Peking Union Medical College Hospital, Peking Union Medical College and Chinese Academy of Medical Sciences, 100730 Beijing, P.R. China

Background

Pheochromocytoma or paraganglioma (PPGL) is a rare neuroendocrine tumour, with an incidence of 0.6 cases per 100,000 person years [1]. L-transposition of the great arteries (L-TGA) is another rare form of congenital heart disease (CHD) characterized by atrioventricular and ventriculoarterial discordance, with a published incidence ranging from 0.02 to 0.07 per 1000 live births, comprising less than 1% of all CHDs [2]. Resecting a PPGL is a high-risk surgical procedure, especially for patients with heart issues. Additionally, a multidisciplinary team is required to reduce peri-anaesthetic risks and result in good perioperative outcomes [3]. Cardiovascular and hemodynamic variables must be monitored closely. However, there have been no standard guidelines for fluid administration during PPGL surgery. After preoperative vasodilation and adequate volume expansion, intraoperative goal-directed fluid therapy may be recommended for guiding fluid administration. We report a case of the anaesthetic management of a successful resection of a large paraganglioma in a woman with isolated L-TGA. Goal-directed fluid therapy and the application of intraoperative transoesophageal echocardiography (TEE) could effectively assess the patient's cardiac structure and function and guide fluid administration, which are helpful for anaesthesia management during operation.

Case presentation

We obtained written informed patient consent for this case report. A 46-year-old woman presented to the hospital with paroxysmal dizziness accompanied by visual blurring. Her vital signs, bilateral carotid ultrasound and cranial CT were normal. Admission electrocardiogram (ECG) showed that Q waves and ST segment elevated greater than 0.1 mv and T wave inversion in the right-sided precordial leads,which indicated an inferior myocardial infarction, whereas the level of troponin I was normal. Fast echocardiography revealed congenital heart disease with "physiologically corrected" L-TGA. The echo showed left atrial and anatomic right ventricular enlargement, moderate tricuspid insufficiency and a small amount of pericardial effusion. The preoperative value of NT-proBNP was 148 pg/ml. Because of "physiologically corrected" L-TGA, she did not have any symptoms of discomfort until she was middle-aged. The paroxysmal dizziness and visual blurring could be caused by orthostatic hypotension, which may reflect a low plasma volume or systemic ventricular dysfunction and systemic atrioventricular valve regurgitation. Fast ultrasound also showed a big solid and cystic tumor in the abdomen. Abdominal CT prescribed by the consultant urologist confirmed an 8.5-cm solid and cystic tumor of the left retroperitoneum with haemorrhagic changes inside, closely related to the left adrenal gland. After contrast enhancement, the tumour was significantly enhanced, and a clearance delay was observed. The plasma fractionated metanephrine test showed that normetanephrine was 7.76 nmol/L and metanephrine was 0.66 nmol/L. Iobenguane I-131 scintigraphy showed high uptake of the tumour. Biochemical and radiological evaluation indicated the diagnosis of benign paraganglioma [4], and the surgery was scheduled 2 weeks later. She had not been treated at other hospitals before and she denied there had been a similar situation in her family. The patient was unmarried, and her parents were both died at their early age because of the so called "heart disease".

For preoperative treatment [5], doxazosin was given 2~4 mg PO qd for 2 weeks. The preoperative treatment was prolonged because of the patient's poor compliance. She did not take the medicine and monitor BP on time at home. At the time of surgery, she had been in the hospital for another 1 week and was on phenoxybenzamine 10 mg PO bid. Adrenergic blockade was accompanied by a high-sodium diet (5000 mg per day) and generous fluid intake (2.5 l per day). During preoperative preparation in the hospital, the patient had no symptoms of discomfort, and the hemodynamic variables were stable with a BP of 100~110/70~80 mmHg and an HR of 60~80 bpm.

When the patient arrived in the operating room, standard American Society of Anaesthesiologists monitors (e.g., blood pressure, electrocardiography, oxygen saturation) were applied. Her blood pressure (BP) was 108/73 mmHg, her heart rate (HR) was 70 bpm, and her pulse oximeter saturation was 100% while breathing room air. The bispectral index monitor (BIS) was used, and the baseline data were 97. The BIS declined to 86 when midazolam 1 mg iv was administered to allay patient's anxiety. After a large-bore venous access was placed, the arterial catheter was placed under local anaesthesia prior to induction. Anaesthesia was then induced smoothly with propofol 2 mg/kg iv, lidocaine 1 mg/kg iv, fentanyl 2 μg/kg iv and rocuronium 1 mg/kg iv. Her trachea was intubated, and 8~10 ml/kg tidal volume-controlled ventilation without positive end-expiratory pressure (PEEP) was applied for the patient to an $EtCO_2$ of 35~45 mmHg. Anaesthesia was maintained with remifentanil 0.1~0.3 μg/kg/min and 1~1.5% sevoflurane in nitrous oxide/oxygen to keep the BIS between 40 and 60. After the insertion of a right internal jugular central venous line, a TEE probe was placed, and the examination showed that the left atrium was associated with the morphologic right ventricle through the tricuspid valve (Fig. 1a), and the aorta was connected to the morphologic right ventricle (Fig. 1b). An additional movie file shows this in more detail [see Additional file 1].

The operation was performed through an arc incision along the left rib margin. The whole process were

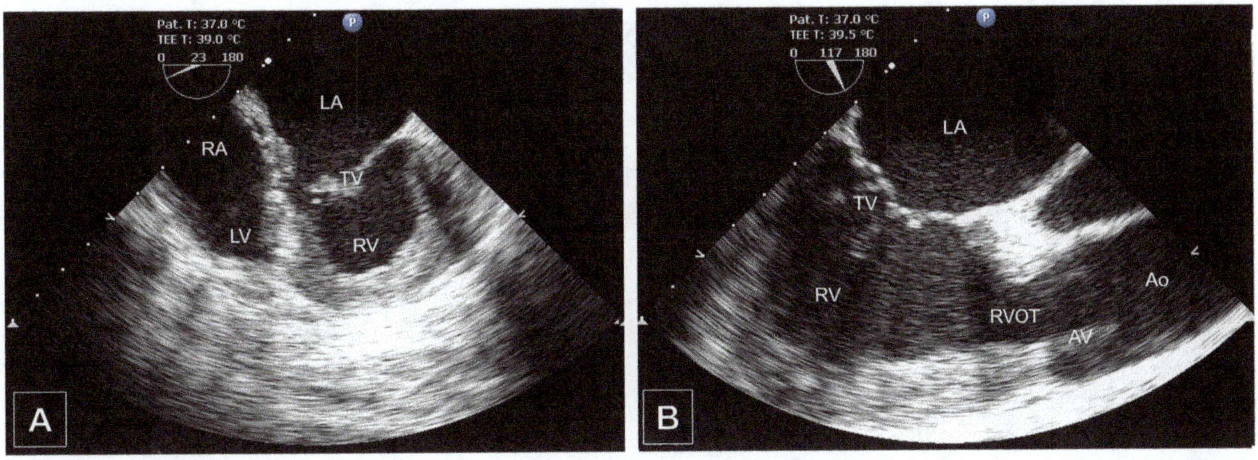

Fig. 1 a Intraoperative transoesophageal ultrasound of the middle esophageal four-chamber view. The left atrium (LA) was associated with the morphologic right ventricle (RV) through the tricuspid valve (TV), and the right atrium (RA) was associated with the morphologic left ventricle (LV) through the mitral valve. **b** Intraoperative transoesophageal ultrasound of the middle oesophageal aortic valve long-axis view. The aorta (Ao) was connected to the morphologic right ventricle through the aortic valve (AV)

divided into two phases based on the ligation of the blood supply to the tumour. Phase I included the portion of surgery during which the tumour was dissected and the vascular supply was isolated before the clamping of the effluent vein. Phase II was the portion of surgery after the effluent vein was clamped. During the induction and initial dissection, the hemodynamic variables were relatively stable, with a mean arterial BP of 65~85 mmHg, HR of 50~80 bpm and PPV of 5%~ 7%. However, BP and HR increased during tumour manipulation because of the release of catecolamine (Fig. 2 simulated the release process of catecholamine). There were mainly three episodes of systolic BP increases to 170~200/100~110 mmHg and HR increases to 110~130 bpm, all lasting approximately 5 mins (Fig. 3). These elevations were treated with continuous infusion of sodium nitroprusside 0.5~3 μg/kg/min and repeated intravenous bolus injections of phentolamine 1 mg and esmolol

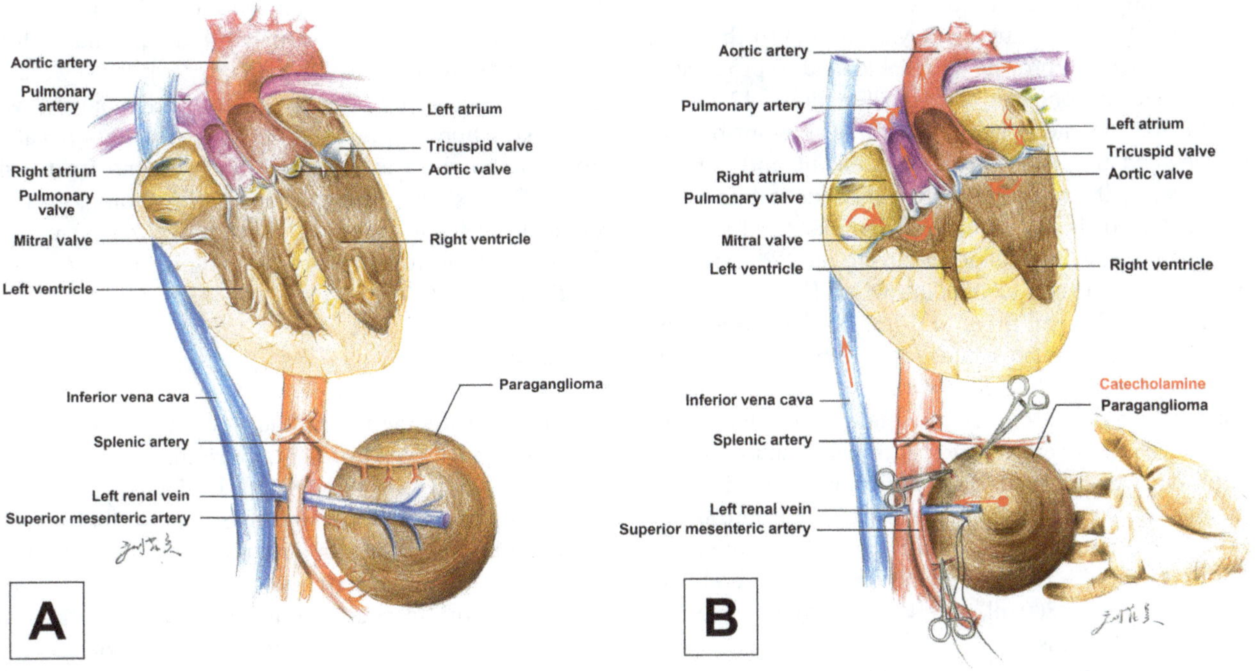

Fig. 2 a Normal status of the patient without catecholamine release. **b** Status of hemodynamic fluctuation with catecholamine release. Red arrow showing the pattern of blood flow during surgery in this patient

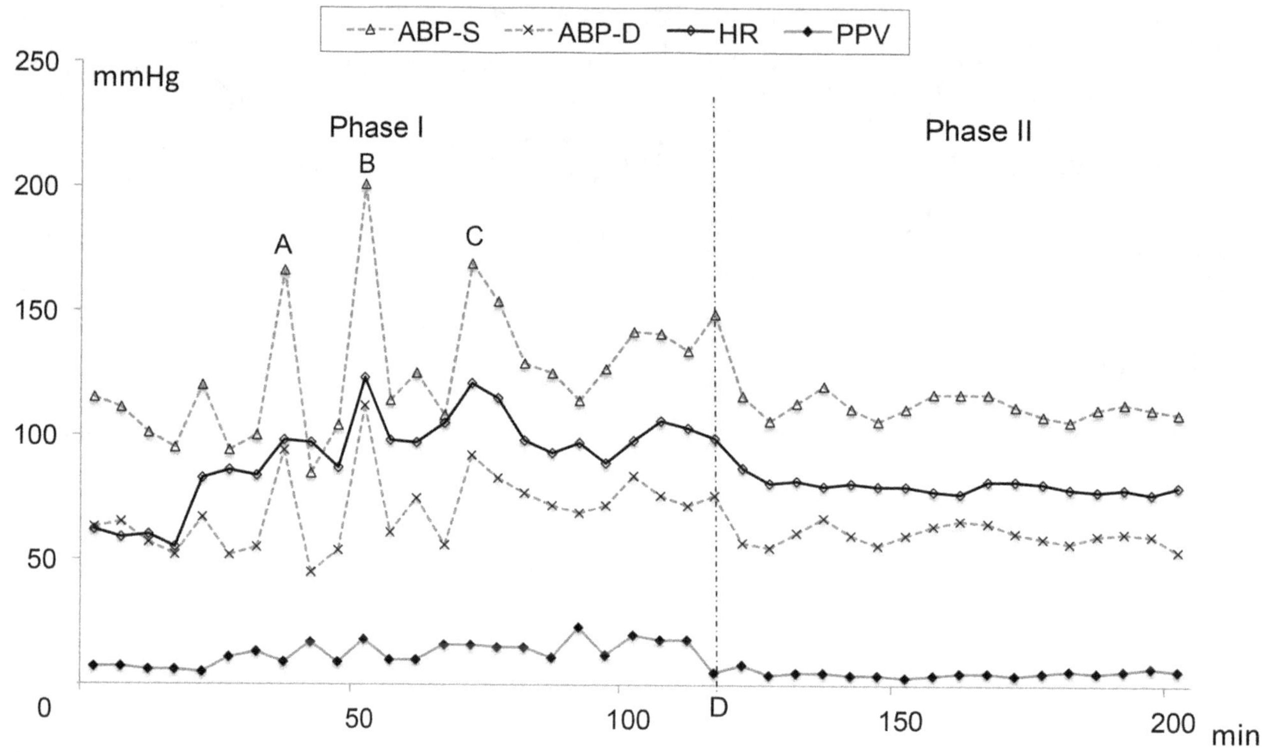

Fig. 3 Intraoperative hemodynamic changes in two phases based on the ligation of the blood supply to the tumour. Point **a**, point **b** and point **c** were the three main episodic hypertension instances in Phase I, which occurred before the clamping of the effluent vein. Point **d** was the time when the effluent vein was clamped. Arterial blood pressure-systolic (ABP-S); arterial blood pressure-diastolic (ABP-D); heart rate (HR); pulse pressure variation (PPV)

10~20 mg. The PPV varied above 15% during the episodic hemodynamic fluctuations. The hypotension was first treated by fluid bolus therapy according to the PPV. TEE was used to provide a reliable and reproducible index of the morphologic RV (the functional LV) end-diastolic volume and ejection fraction. The point-of-care image helped us assess cardiac movement and volume status, especially when hemodynamic fluctuations violently occurred. In addition, TEE demonstrated moderate tricuspid valve regurgitation during the BP increases, but function returned to baseline when BP normalized. According to the real-time TEE image, the intraoperative fluid administration strategy was to mainly maintain reasonable the morphologic RV (the functional LV) filling pressure but to try to limit crystalloid administration to avoid volume overload and acute heart failure. Once the tumour was removed, the sodium nitroprusside infusion was discontinued, and a norepinephrine infusion of 0.05~0.15 μg/kg/min was started to prevent hypotension because the PPV was 3%~ 8%. Intraoperative blood loss was approximately 800 ml, and 4 units of allogeneic red blood cells were infused.

The patient was transferred to the intensive care unit (ICU) because of intraoperative hemodynamic changes and significant blood loss. She was extubated and discharged from the ICU on the first postoperative day. Although the levels of troponin I and NT-proBNP after surgery were both slightly higher than normal, which met the diagnosis of myocardial injury [6], there were no lethal complications. One week later, the patient was discharged home smoothly. During a follow-up call 1 month later, she was very satisfied with the treatment, except for a slight incision pain. Her pathologic testing revealed "cellular changes consistent with paraganglioma" with positive immunostaining for chromogranin A, SDHB and S100.

Discussion

PPGLs are catecholamine-secreting tumours of chromaffin cells with frequent germline, somatic, or postzygotic mutations in genes. At present, more than 17 pathogenic genes are known to be related to PPGL. Hereditary PPGL accounts for 35%~ 40%, showing familial inheritance, and is one of the manifestations of some hereditary syndromes. Among germline genetic mutations, the highest mutant frequency was in SDHB (10.3%). The PGL4 gene, also known as SDHB, was first identified in 2001 and is also linked to the development of PPGL [7]. Patients with germline SDHB gene mutations less commonly develop multiple tumours. However, the tumours can be distributed in all locations, most commonly in the abdomen. The pathological immunohistochemical staining of SDHB was positive in this patient, which further confirmed the preoperative diagnosis.

According to the different signal transduction pathways involved in the gene mutation of PPGLs, the genes can be mainly divided into two categories. Cluster 1 is related to the hypoxia-related pathway. Cluster 2 promotes tumour growth by activating MAPK and/or mTOR signalling pathways [8]. A common feature of cluster 1 tumours is the activation of hypoxia-inducible factors (HIFs). Patients who had chronic hypoxemia due to cyanotic congenital heart disease were at increased risk for developing PPGL. A population-based retrospective analysis provided direct evidence that patients with CHD had a higher risk of developing PPGL than those with noncyanotic CHD and patients without CHD [9]. PPGL in patients with cyanotic CHD has led to a growing recognition that their cooccurrence is more than coincidence. Vaidya and her colleagues reported that the high frequency (80%) of mutations in EPAS1 in patients with cyanotic CHDs contrasts with rates of only 5 to 6% in cohorts of unselected patients with PPGLs [10]. In addition to chronic hypoxemia, transcription factors are physiologically induced in response to low cellular oxygen levels (hypoxia). Pseudohypoxia occurs when HIF pathways are constitutively activated, regardless of oxygen levels. The patient we reported had isolated L-TGA without any cardiac defects, which was "physiologically corrected" and had no hypoxia because systemic deoxygenated venous blood returns to the pulmonary circulation and oxygenated pulmonary venous blood returns to the systemic circulation [2, 11]. Although the patient did not develop true hypoxemia, cluster 1 genetic mutations could result in the aberrant and constitutive activation of HIFs even under normal levels of oxygen.

The perioperative management of patients with PPGLs has been reviewed in the literature [3, 12–14]. Although no large-scale study has been performed to report perioperative anaesthesia management in patients with PPGLs and CHD, many single-episode cases have been reported about the perioperative management experience in patients with PPGLs and CHD. In particular, cases of cyanotic CHD, including Tetralogy of Fallot and univentricular and Fontan heart disease, have been reported [15, 16]. However, reports of anaesthetic management in patients with isolated L-TGA and paraganglioma are rare.

For preoperative assessment, her BP was normal, and her symptoms were less common for patients with the classic triad of PPGLs, which consists of episodic headache, sweating, and tachycardia [5]. Arrhythmias were another concern because of L-TGA and potential intraoperative catecholamine release. Her preoperative ECG was misinterpreted as an inferior myocardial infarction. These are the characteristic ECG findings of L-TGA because the interventricular septum is depolarized in the opposite direction of normal [17]. In addition, patients with L-TGA are at increased risk for AV heart block and heart failure as adults due to a progressive decline in morphologic right ventricular function. The risk of complete heart block rises over time, with a 2% per year increase in incidence because of progressive fibrosis with advancing age. By 45 years of age, > 30% of patients with isolated L-TGA develop clinical congestive heart failure [18], although there were no signs of catecholamine-induced cardiomyopathy in this patient.

Regarding intraoperative management, many patients who undergo paraganglioma resection exhibit labile BP, arrhythmias, and tachycardia during surgery, though most can be managed without lasting morbidity or mortality [19]. However, our patient was at particular risk from hemodynamic changes and acute morphologic right heart failure. Because of the large tumour size, open adrenalectomy was chosen as recommended by the endocrine society clinical practice guidelines to ensure complete tumour resection and prevent tumour rupture [5]. Open resection could avoid the effects of CO_2-peritoneum on hemodynamic (catecholamine release, decreased preload, increased afterload, tachycardia, and hypertension). Although adequate filling pressures were necessary in this patient for her tumour resection, intravascular fluid overload was a concern considering her history of subclinical right ventricular dysfunction. A systematic review has demonstrated that a PPV of at least 13 to 15% is strongly associated with volume responsiveness [20]. In this case, goal-directed fluid therapy was adopted, and PPV was used as an indicator of fluid responsiveness. Besides,the point-of-care TEE could be helpful for anaesthesia management during operation. But it requires experienced operators for TEE monitoring.

Postoperative concerns for patients after PPGL resection include recovery of normal adrenergic function with stable BP, potential for rebound hypoglycaemia, and possible adrenal insufficiency. Fortunately, the patient recovered very well despite a brief period of hypotension and myocardial injury. She did not suffer from hypoglycaemia or persistent adrenal dysfunction.

Conclusions

Goal-directed fluid therapy combined with the adoption of TEE could effectively guide fluid administration, which is helpful for anaesthesia management of paraganglioma resection in patients with isolated L-TGA. We recommend the routine use of TEE in such cases.

Additional file 1. Loops 1: Middle esophagus four-chamber view. The normal right atrium (RA) is connected to the triangular-shaped ventricle (the morphologic left ventricle) by means of mitral valve with two leaflets at a higher attachment point. The ventricle has small muscle trabeculae. The left atrioventricular valve has the lowest attachment point, suggesting tricuspid valve. The enlarged left atrium (LA) is connected to the round ventricle (the morphologic right ventricle) by the tricuspid valve, which has a thick muscular trabecula. Loops 2: Middle esophagus aortic valve long axis view. The Aorta is closer to the front of the body, and part of the normal riight ventricular structure is missing. The left atrium is enlarged and connected to the morphologic Right Ventricle (the functional left ventricle) by the tricuspid valve.

Abbreviations

L-TGA: L-transposition of the great arteries; PPGL: Pheochromocytoma or paraganglioma; CHD: Congenital heart disease; TEE: Transesophageal echocardiography; PPV: Pulse pressure variation; BP: Blood pressure; HR: Heart rate; ECG: Electrocardiogram; BIS: Bispectrality index; $EtCO_2$: Capnography; ICU: Intensive care unit; HIFs: Hypoxia-inducible factors; LA: Left atrium; LV: Left ventricle; RA: Right atrium; RV: Right ventricle; RVOT: Right ventricle outflow tract; AV: Aortic valve; TV: Tricuspid valve; Ao: Aorta; ABP-S: Arterial blood pressure-systolic; ABP-D: Arterial blood pressure-diastolic

Acknowledgements

Not applicable.

Authors' contributions

LL contributed to the clinical conduct of the case, data collection, and writing of the manuscript. BZ and YT contributed to the intraoperative TEE assessment. PHL contributed to the preparation of the accompanying figures and materials. LS contributed to the analysis and interpretation of the collected data and revision of the manuscript. YGH first came up with the idea of collecting the rare case and substantively revised the manuscript. All authors have read and approved the manuscript.

References

1. Berends AMA, Buitenwerf E, de Krijger RR, Veeger N, van der Horst-Schrivers ANA, Links TP, et al. Incidence of pheochromocytoma and sympathetic paraganglioma in the Netherlands: a nationwide study and systematic review. Eur J Intern Med. 2018;51:68–73.
2. Ravishankar C. L-transposition of the great arteries. Pediatr Crit Care Med. 2016;17:S344–6.
3. Kinney MA, Warner ME, vanHeerden JA, Horlocker TT, Young WF Jr, Schroeder DR, et al. Perianesthetic risks and outcomes of pheochromocytoma and paraganglioma resection. Anesth Analg. 2000;91: 1118–23.
4. Neumann HPH, Young WF Jr, Eng C. Pheochromocytoma and Paraganglioma. N Engl J Med. 2019;381:552–65.
5. Lenders JW, Duh QY, Eisenhofer G, Gimenez-Roqueplo AP, Grebe SK, Murad MH, et al. Pheochromocytoma and paraganglioma: an endocrine society clinical practice guideline. J Clin Endocrinol Metab. 2014;99:1915–42.
6. Vascular Events In Noncardiac Surgery Patients Cohort Evaluation Study I, Devereaux PJ, Chan MT, Alonso-Coello P, Walsh M, Berwanger O, et al. Association between postoperative troponin levels and 30-day mortality among patients undergoing noncardiac surgery. JAMA. 2012;307:2295–304.
7. Astuti D, Latif F, Dallol A, Dahia PL, Douglas F, George E, et al. Gene mutations in the succinate dehydrogenase subunit SDHB cause susceptibility to familial pheochromocytoma and to familial paraganglioma. Am J Hum Genet. 2001;69:49–54.
8. Dahia PL. Pheochromocytoma and paraganglioma pathogenesis: learning from genetic heterogeneity. Nat Rev Cancer. 2014;14:108–19.
9. Opotowsky AR, Moko LE, Ginns J, Rosenbaum M, Greutmann M, Aboulhosn J, et al. Pheochromocytoma and paraganglioma in cyanotic congenital heart disease. J Clin Endocrinol Metab. 2015;100:1325–34.
10. Vaidya A, Flores SK, Cheng ZM, Nicolas M, Deng Y, Opotowsky AR, et al. EPAS1 mutations and Paragangliomas in cyanotic congenital heart disease. N Engl J Med. 2018;378:1259–61.
11. Wallis GA, Debich-Spicer D, Anderson RH. Congenitally corrected transposition. Orphanet J Rare Dis. 2011;6:22.
12. Sesay M, Tauzin-Fin P, Gosse P, Ballanger P, Maurette P. Real-time heart rate variability and its correlation with plasma catecholamines during laparoscopic adrenal pheochromocytoma surgery. Anesth Analg. 2008;106: 164–70 table of contents.
13. Kiernan CM, Du L, Chen X, Broome JT, Shi C, Peters MF, et al. Predictors of hemodynamic instability during surgery for pheochromocytoma. Ann Surg Oncol. 2014;21:3865–71.
14. Wang W, Li P, Wang Y, Wang Y, Ma Z, Wang G, et al. Effectiveness and safety of laparoscopic adrenalectomy of large pheochromocytoma: a prospective, nonrandomized, controlled study. Am J Surg. 2015;210:230–5.
15. Kasaliwal R, Sarathi V, Pandit R, Budyal SR, Bukan A, Kakade H, et al. Pheochromocytoma and tetralogy of Fallot: a rare but potentially dangerous combination. Endocr Pract. 2014;20:e80–5.
16. Song MK, Kim GB, Bae EJ, Lee YA, Kim HY, Min SK, et al. Pheochromocytoma and paraganglioma in Fontan patients: common more than expected. Congenit Heart Dis. 2018;13:608–16.
17. Warnes CA. Transposition of the great arteries. Circulation. 2006;114:2699–709.
18. Filippov AA, Del Nido PJ, Vasilyev NV. Management of Systemic Right Ventricular Failure in patients with congenitally corrected transposition of the great arteries. Circulation. 2016;134:1293–302.
19. Livingstone M, Duttchen K, Thompson J, Sunderani Z, Hawboldt G, Sarah Rose M, et al. Hemodynamic stability during Pheochromocytoma resection: lessons learned over the last two decades. Ann Surg Oncol. 2015;22:4175–80.
20. Marik PE, Cavallazzi R, Vasu T, Hirani A. Dynamic changes in arterial waveform derived variables and fluid responsiveness in mechanically ventilated patients: a systematic review of the literature. Crit Care Med. 2009;37:2642–7.

19

Distant survival for patients undergoing surgery using volatile versus IV anesthesia for hepatocellular carcinoma with portal vein tumor thrombus

Xiao-Yan Meng[1,2†], Xiu-Ping Zhang[3†], Zhe Sun[3†], Hong-Qian Wang[1] and Wei-Feng Yu[1,2*]

Abstract

Background: Whether anesthesia type is associated with the surgical outcome of Hepatocellular carcinoma (HCC) patients with portal vein tumor thrombus (PVTT) remains to be determined. This study aims to investigate the impact of volatile inhalational anesthesia (INHA) versus total IV anesthesia (TIVA) on the survival outcomes in HCC patients with PVTT.

Methods: A cohort of in-patients whom were diagnosed of HCC with PVTT in Eastern Hepatobiliary Surgery Hospital, Shanghai, China, from January 1, 2008 to December 24, 2012 were identified. Surgical patients receiving the INHA and TIVA were screened out. The overall survival (OS), recurrence-free survival (RFS) and several postoperative adverse events were compared according to anesthesia types.

Results: A total of 1513 patients were included in this study. After exclusions are applied, 263 patients remain in the INHA group and 208 in the TIVA group. Patients receiving INHA have a lower 5-year overall survival rate than that of patients receiving TIVA [12.6% (95% CI, 9.0 to 17.3) vs. 17.7% (95% CI, 11.3 to 20.8), $P = 0.024$]. Results of multivariable Cox-regression analysis also identify that INHA anesthesia is significantly associated with mortality and cancer recurrence after surgery compare to TIVA, with HR (95%CI) of 1.303 (1.065, 1.595) and 1.265 (1.040, 1.539), respectively. Subgroup analysis suggested that in more severe cancer patients, the worse outcome related to INHA might be more significant.

Conclusion: This retrospective analysis identifies that TIVA is associated with better outcomes compared with INHA. Future prospective studies clinical and translational studies are required to verify this difference and investigate underlying pathophysiology.

Keywords: Hepatocellular carcinoma, Portal vein tumor Thrombus, Volatile inhalational anesthesia, Total IV anesthesia

* Correspondence: ywf808@sohu.com
†Xiao-Yan Meng, Xiu-Ping Zhang and Zhe Sun contributed equally to this work.
[1]Department of Anesthesiology, Eastern Hepatobiliary Surgery Hospital, the Second Military Medical University, 225 Changhai Road, Shanghai, China
[2]Department of Anesthesiology, Ren Ji Hospital, School of Medicine, Shanghai Jiao Tong University, 160 Pudian Road, Shanghai, China

Background

Volatile inhalational (INHA) and IV anesthesia (TIVA) are two methods commonly used in general anesthesia maintenance. Currently, several researches reported that INHA was associated with worse postoperative outcomes compare to INHA in certain types of cancers. Dr. Wigmore et al. [1] did a retrospective analysis which firstly compared long-term survival in more than 7000 patients undergoing elective cancer surgeries, and reported that mortality of patients accepted INHA is approximately 50% greater than those accepted TIVA. Since then, more studies reported similar results in different cancers [2]. Besides from these clinical evidences, animal researches also reported that administration of volatile inhalational agents was associated with upregulation of tumorigenic growth factors including hypoxia-inducible factors (HIFs) and insulin-like growth factor (IGF) [3, 4], which are highly associated with progression angiogenesis and cell proliferation in tumor.

Although the underlying mechanism remains unclear, these results have drawn due attention that anesthesia technique might be an independent risk factor for postoperative outcomes of most cancers, including liver cancer. Of note, previous studies also reported that the MAC of sevoflurane is lower in patients with end-stage liver cancer [5]. Thus, we hypothesize that INHA might be associated with lower 5-year overall survival (OS) compared with TIVA in hepatocellular carcinoma (HCC) patients with portal vein tumor thrombus (PVTT), an end-stage liver cancer with a high recurrence rate and reduced median survival time (MST) [6–9], in considering that in these end stage cancer patients, even subtle differences in medication might lead to significant effects on long-term outcome.

Methods

Study design

We retrospectively identified all patients who underwent aggressive surgical liver resection for selected HCC patients with PVTT at Eastern Hepatobiliary Surgery Hospital from January 1, 2008 to December 24, 2012. Exclusion criteria including: (1) no surgical treatment performed; (2) received mixed inhalational and intravenous anesthesia; (3) received additional procedures with different anesthesia or for other diseases afterwards; (4) received extra sedation in ICU or in general ward after surgery; (5) less than 18 years old; (6) had an urgent or emergence surgery and (7) incomplete follow-up data. The research was approved by the Ethics Committee of the Eastern Hepatobiliary Surgical Hospital of China. Written informed consents to record clinical follow up data were obtained from participants or their surrogates during hospitalization.

Baseline data retrospectively extracted including anesthetic technique, year of surgery, age at the time of surgery, sex, American Society of anesthesiologists' (ASA) physical status classification, pre-existing diagnosis of diabetes or hypertension, HBV surface antigen (HBsAg) and HCV anti-body (HCV-ab). Data related to patients' preoperative liver function, cytonecrosis and cancer statue were also documented, including Child-Pugh score, alpha-fetoprotein (AFP), type of PVTT, tumor diameter as well as alanine aminotransferase (ALT) and aspartate aminotransferase (AST) levels.

Outcomes

The primary outcome was 5-year OS. Secondary outcomes were (1) recurrence-free survival (RFS); (2) 30-day mortality; (3) a set of major adverse cardiac events (MACE) that included myocardial infarction (MI), cardiac arrest, or newly diagnosed malignant arrhythmia; (4) multiple organ dysfunction (MOD) primarily induced of acute hepatic failure postoperatively; (5) blood loss and blood transfusion; (6) hospital length of stay (7) postoperative ALT and AST were also recorded.

Anesthesia techniques

Patients were divided based on INHA or TIVA they received for maintenance of anesthesia. Patients in the TIVA group received continuous infusions of propofol, and those in the INHA group received sevoflurane. Supplementary opioid for maintaining were used at the discretion of the anesthetist in all patients, including sufentanil and/or remifentanil, with the highest dose no more than 50 mg and 2 mg, respectively. No other sedative-hypnotic drugs were used during maintenance.

Type of anesthesia was according to the anesthetist's decision, mainly depending on their preference and proficiency of the anesthesia technique. Details of the surgical process as previously described [10].

Statistical analyses

The Kaplan–Meier method was used to calculate the overall survival and recurrence-free survival of patients from the date of surgery to the date of events. A univariable Cox regression analysis was applied, and for variables with P less than 0.1 were then included into the multivariable model to identify risk factors.

Secondary outcomes were compared using chi-square or Mann-Whitney-Wilcoxon tests as appropriate. Missing values (all less than 5%) were filled by the average value of the variable. Significant difference defined as $P < 0.05$ in all analysis (SPSS version 22.0; IBM Inc., USA).

Results

Baseline characters and survival for all patients

A total of 1523 patients whom are diagnosed of HCC with PVTT are delivered in the study period. After exclusions applied, 471 patients are included in the analysis, with 263 patients in the INHA group and 208 in the TIVA (Fig. 1). The mean age is 48.6 years old; The majority of patients are male (90.6%), had a grade of ASA II (88.3%) and Child-Pugh A (88.4%); 410 (87.0%) of patients have large hepatocellular carcinoma (> 10 cm).; 408 (86.6%) are identified with HBsAg−+, including 4 with both HBsAg− + and HCV-ab+. Only 4 patients are identified with HCV-ab− + alone, which is not enough for effective analysis. Five-year survival rate for all patients is 14.8% (95% CI, 11.3 to 17.6), with median survival time of 9.0 month (95% CI, 7.9 to 10.0). The patient characteristics in two groups are described in Table 1.

Five-year OS and RFS

Results of Kaplan–Meier survival analysis show that, compare with TIVA, INHA is associated with a worse 5-year OS rate [17.7% (95% CI, 11.3 to 20.8 VS. 12.6% (95% CI, 9.0 to 17.3)); $P = 0.024$, Fig. 2a], as well as a worse 5-year RFS rate[15.4% (95% CI, 12.6 to 18.1) VS. 11.7% (95% CI, 9.7 to 13.8); $P = 0.032$, Fig. 2b]. On univariable analysis, 6 potential risk factors have $P < 0.1$ are included in multivariable model (Supplementary table 1). Results of multivariable analysis also suggest that INHA is an independent risk factor for mortality [HR (95%CI), 1.303 (1.065, 1.595)] and cancer recurrence [HR (95% CI), 1.265 (1.040, 1.539); Table 2] in 5 years after surgery.

Other secondary outcomes

Other outcomes including 30-day mortality rate, postoperative MACE and MOF rate, as well as blood loss, blood transfusion and length of stay in hospital are similar in both groups (Table 3). Postoperative serum biomarker of ALT and AST are compared (with incomplete data), the results suggest a minor liver cytonecrosis of TIVA after surgery (Supplementary Figure 1).

Subgroup analysis

In multivariable model, four more variables are screened out as independent risk factors for 5-year OS and RFS: Child-Pugh, AFP level, diameter of hepatocellular carcinoma and PVTT type. We then did a subgroup

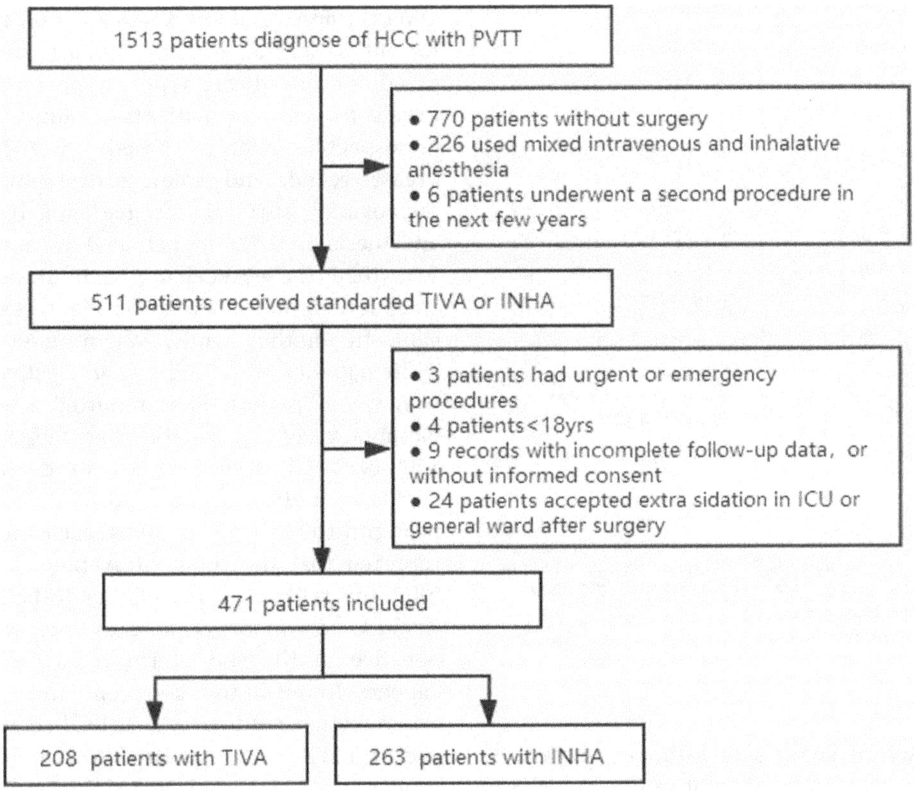

Fig. 1 Flow diagram detailing the selection of patients included in the retrospective analysis. INHA = volatile inhalational; TIVA = total IV anesthesia

Table 1 Patient baseline characters

Variables	TIVA ($N = 208$)	INHA ($N = 263$)	P value
	N (%)	N (%)	
Sex (male)	188 (90.4)	239 (90.9)	0.856
HBsAg − +[a]	182 (87.5)	226 (85.9)	0.619
ASA			
II	186 (89.4)	229 (87.1)	0.191
III	22 (10.6)	30 (11.4)	
IV	0 (0)	4 (1.5)	
Child-Pugh			
A	184 (88.5)	233 (88.6)	0.662
B	22 (10.6)	25 (9.5)	
C	2 (0.4)	5 (1.1)	
AFP (ug/L)			
< 25	30 (14.4)	54 (20.5)	0.109
25–399	39 (18.8)	45 (17.1)	
400–999	12 (5.8)	25 (9.5)	
≥ 1000	127 (61.1)	139 (52.9)	
Tumor Diameter (cm)			
< 5	1 (0.4)	2 (0.8)	0.546
5–9.9	22 (10.6)	36 (13.7)	
≥ 10	185 (88.9)	225 (85.6)	
PVTT			
1	30 (14.4)	40 (15.3)	0.716
2	131 (63.0)	163 (62.0)	
3	47 (22.1)	60 (22.8)	
Year of surgery			
2008	70 (33.7)	79 (30.0)	0.882
2009	33 (15.9)	42 (16.0)	
2010	31 (14.9)	46 (17.5)	
2011	31 (14.9)	37 (14.1)	
2012	43 (20.7)	59 (22.4)	
	Mean (SD)	Mean (SD)	
Age (yr)	48.0 (10.94)	49.0 (9.73)	0.078
	Median (IQR)	Median (IQR)	
WBC (10^9/L)	5.5 (4.2, 7.3)	5.4 (4.3, 7.1)	0.06
ALT (U/L)	47.8 (31.0, 66.0)	45.0 (29.1, 67.3)	0.903
AST (U/L)	49.0 (37.0, 69.0)	52.0 (35.0, 71.0)	0.820

ASA American Society of Anesthesiologists, *PVTT* Portal vein tumor thrombus, *INHA* Volatile inhalational anesthesia, *TIVA* Total IV anesthesia, *WBC* White blood cells, *NLR* Neutrophil–lymphocytes ratio

[a] Including 4 patients with HBsAg− + and anti-HCV − +

Kaplan–Meier survival analysis to estimate the association of anesthesia type on postoperative OS and RFS in different sub-variable groups, there were Child-Pugh A; Child-Pugh B&C; tumor diameter < 10 cm; tumor diameter ≥ 10 cm; AFP < 400μg/L; AFP ≥ 400μg/L; PVTT typeI; PVTT typeII; PVTT typeIII (Figs. 3, 4, 5, and 6). The results suggest that INHA was associated with significant lower OS and RFS rate compare with TIVA in several sub-variable groups indicating more severe liver cancer status, including tumor diameter ≥ 10 cm (Fig. 4b, d); AFP ≥ 400μg/L (Fig. 5b, d); PVTT typeIIand PVTT typeIII (Fig. 6c, e, f).

Discussion

This retrospective analysis evaluates long-term OS, RFS and several short-term postoperative adverse events in 1513 HCC patients with PVTT receiving INHA and TIVA. We identify that patients receiving INHA using sevoflurane had a lower 5-year OS and RFS rate than that of patients receiving TIVA using propofol. On multivariable Cox regression analysis, we identify that INHA is an independent risk factor for mortality and cancer recurrence in 5-year after surgery. In subgroup analysis, our results suggest that patients accepted INHA, compare with those who accepted TIVA, have worse survival rates when there are in severe liver cancer status. No significant differences in postoperative adverse events and 30-day mortality are found between the two groups in this study.

Clinical evidence of anesthesia type on surgical outcomes

Recently, several clinical studies have been investigated for anesthesia type on postoperative outcomes in elective cancer patients. Enlund et al. [6] did a retrospective analysis based on 2838 patients with breast, rectal, and colon cancer, they reported that the overall survival for patients receiving propofol anesthesia is 4.7% higher at 1-yr and 5.6% higher at 5-yr than those receiving sevoflurane. But after balance for confounders, this differences are not significant. In another study, Wigmore et al. [1] analyzed 7030 patients who underwent elective cancer surgery over a 3-yr period, They reported a worse outcome in patients receiving volatile anesthesia, with a HR of 1.46 (95% CI, 1.29 to 1.66) for death, compare with TIVA. In addition, Yan et al. [7]. designed a randomized controlled trail in 80 breast cancer patients, they reported that the total intravenous anesthesia can inhibit the release of vascular endothelial growth factor C (VEGF-C) in breast surgery, yet with no significant benefice in the short-term recurrence rate of breast cancer. Importantly, a recent meta-analysis with 9 retrospective studies and 1 RCT concluded that, the use of TIVA was associated with improved RFS in all cancer types and improved OS in several certain types of cancers [2]. These studies have achieved consistent results that TIVA anesthesia has a better long-term

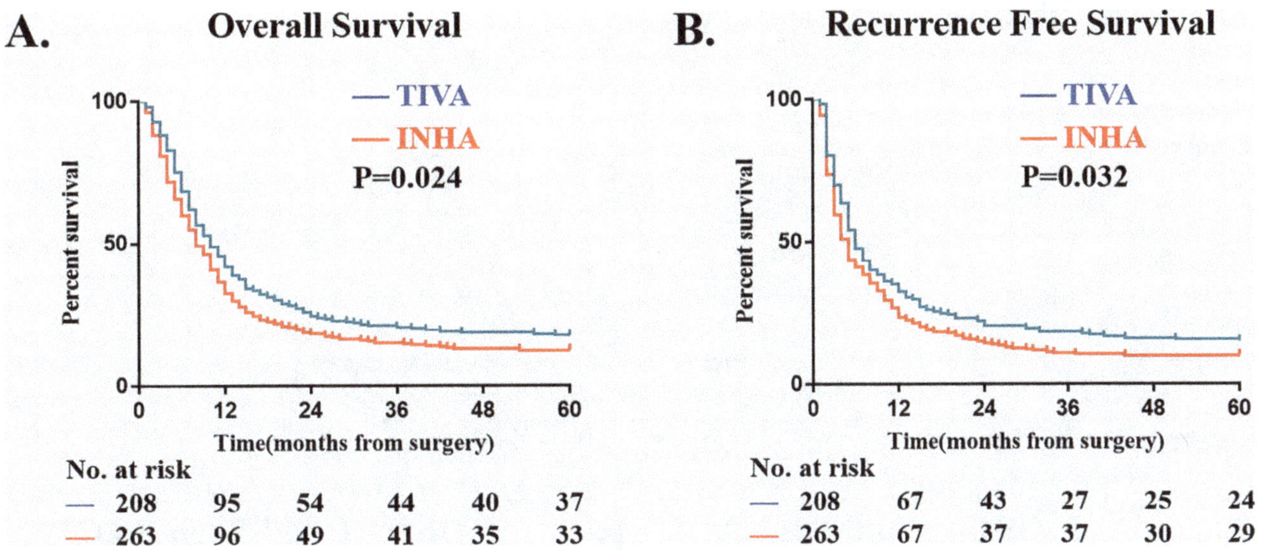

Fig. 2 Kaplan–Meier survival curves from the date of surgery by anesthesia type for (**a**) overall survival in patients before matching ($P = 0.007$), (**b**) overall survival in patients after matching ($P = 0.044$), (**c**) recurrence-free survival in patients before matching ($P = 0.020$), (**d**) recurrence-free survival in patients after matching ($P = 0.081$). INHA = volatile inhalational; TIVA = total IV anesthesia

prognosis for patients undergoing tumor resection compared with INHA. However, the population these studies enrolled varies a lot. Yet meaningful conclusions on whether TIVA is superior to INHA for all cancer patients or just for certain types of cancer are difficult to define. To this end, the current study sort to compare the long-term survival rate in TIVA and INHA in HCC patients with PVTT.

Laboratory evidence of anesthetics on tumors metastasis and recurrence

Over the years, numerous animal and laboratory studies have been investigated for the mechanism of anesthetic agents on primary tumors metastasis and recurrence. Cellular immune system and tumor proliferation-associated factors are considered to play a key role in it. For instance, propofol has been demonstrated to have a preservation effective on T lymphocyte activity and Th1 cytokine secretion, or even inhibits tumor growth in animal model [8, 9, 11]. Of note, T lymphocytes and NK cells are two major cytotoxic effector cells that participate in cell-mediated immune responses. Meanwhile, researches also proved that sevoflurane could inhibit primary leukocyte integrin lymphocyte function and could induced lymphocyte apoptosis through downregulation of Lymphocyte Function-associated Antigen 1 (LFA-1), thus promoting tumor recurrence and metastasis [12]. Moreover, studies both in vivo [13] and in patients undergoing breast cancer surgery [14] have reported an inhibitory effect of anesthetic agents on natural killer cell function, and further promotes tumor recurrence. This inhibitory effect is probably related to the dysfunction in CD16 cell and CD107α NK receptor after exposure to sevoflurane [15]. More recently, Bellanti et al. [16] demonstrated that

Table 2 Cox proportional hazard regression analyses: multivariable model for overall survival and recurrence-free survival

Variables	Overall Survival		Recurrence-Free Survival	
	HR (95% CI)	*P* Value	HR (95% CI)	*P* Value
Anesthesia type (INHA/TIVA)	1.303 (1.065, 1.595)	0.010	1.265 (1.040, 1.539)	0.019
Child-Pugh	1.897 (1.491, 2.414)	0.000	1.653(1.297, 2.105)	0.000
AFP (ug/L)	1.099 (1.010, 1.194)	0.027	1.071 (0.989, 1.160)	0.093
Tumor Diameter (cm)	1.606 (1.183, 2.181)	0.002	1.492(1.123, 1.983)	0.006
PVTT	1.160 (0.989, 1.360)	0.068	–	–

ASA American Society of Anesthesiologists, *PVTT* Portal vein tumor thrombus, *INHA* Volatile inhalational, *TIVA* Total IV anesthesia, *NLR* Neutrophil–lymphocytes ratio

Table 3 Adverse outcomes

	TIVA	INHA	*P* Value
	N (%)	N (%)	
Dichotomous Outcomes			
30-day Mortality	4 (2.1)	11 (4.7)	0.106
MACE	4 (2.1)	11 (4.7)	0.106
MOD	6 (3.3)	9 (3.9)	0.797
Blood Transfusion	80 (43.5)	78 (33.5)	0.189
	Median (IQR)	Median (IQR)	
Continuous Outcomes			
Blood Loss	400 (245,800)	400 (300,800)	0.301
Length of Stay (days)	15 (13,20)	16 (13,20)	0.920

IQR Interquartile range, *MACE* Major adverse cardiac events, *MOF* Multiple organ failure, *RR* Risk ratio

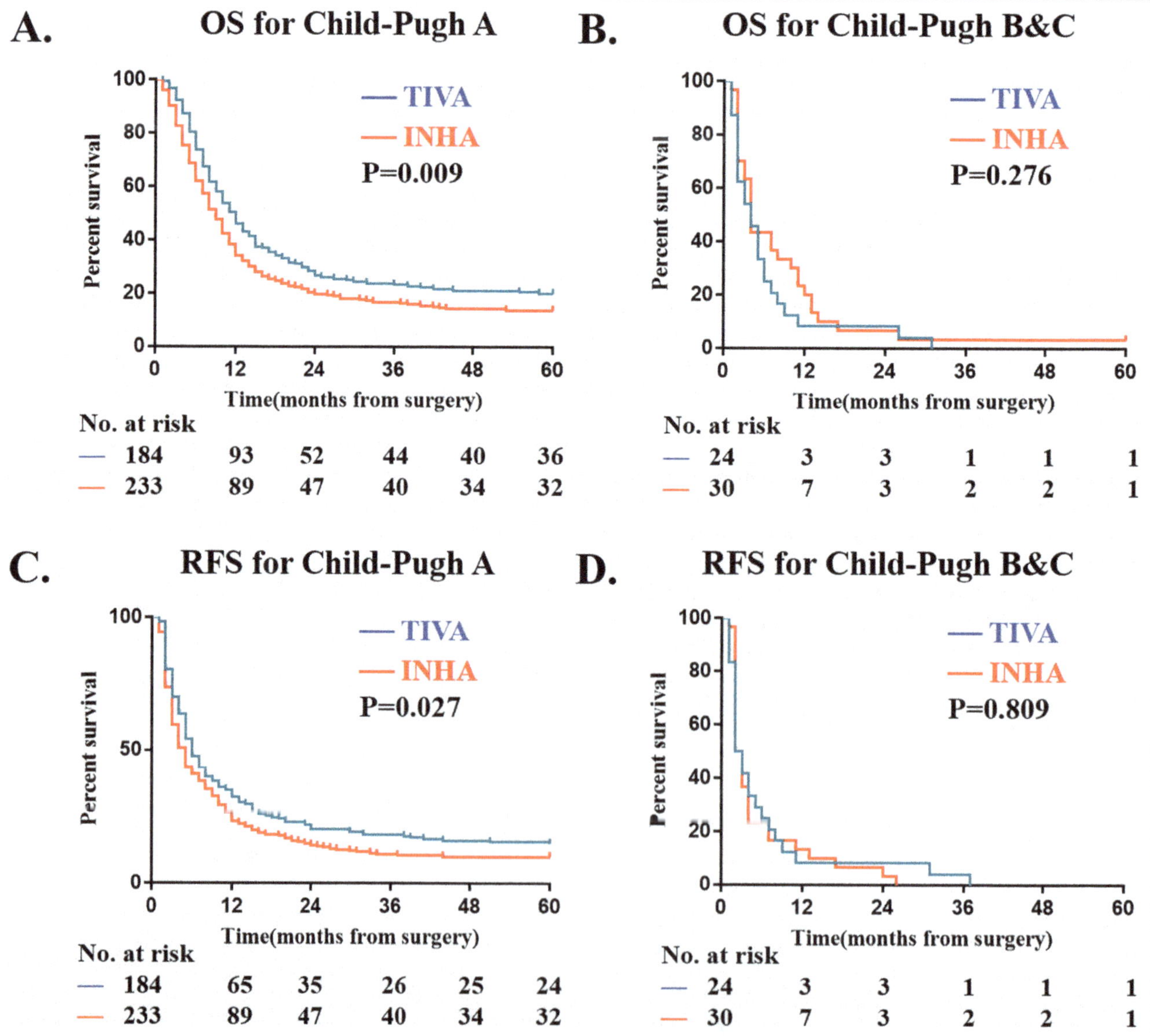

Fig. 3 Subgroup Kaplan–Meier survival analysis for anesthesia type on (**a**) OS in Child-Pugh A; (**b**) OS in Child-Pugh B&C; (**c**) RFS in Child-Pugh A; (**d**) RFS in Child-Pugh B&C

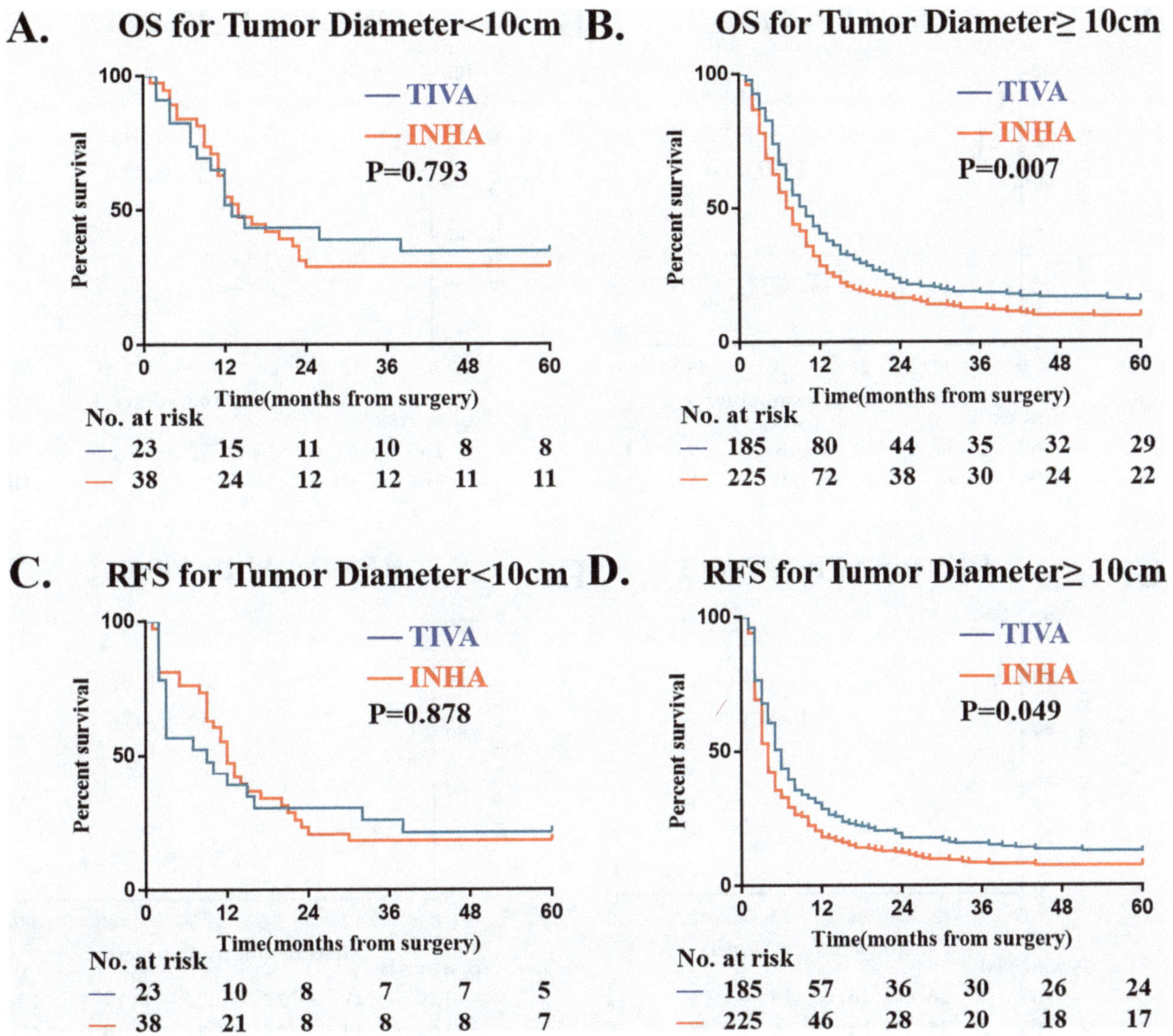

A. No. at risk	0	12	24	36	48	60
TIVA	23	15	11	10	8	8
INHA	38	24	12	12	11	11

B. No. at risk	0	12	24	36	48	60
TIVA	185	80	44	35	32	29
INHA	225	72	38	30	24	22

C. No. at risk	0	12	24	36	48	60
TIVA	23	10	8	7	7	5
INHA	38	21	8	8	8	7

D. No. at risk	0	12	24	36	48	60
TIVA	185	57	36	30	26	24
INHA	225	46	28	20	18	17

Fig. 4 Subgroup Kaplan–Meier survival analysis for anesthesia type on (**a**) OS in tumor diameter < 10 cm; (**b**) OS in tumor diameter ≥ 10 cm; (**c**) RFS in tumor diameter < 10 cm; (**d**) RFS in tumor diameter ≥ 10 cm

propofol, but not sevoflurane, prevents mitochondrial dysfunction and oxidative stress by limiting hypoxia-inducible factor 1 alpha (HIF-1α) activation in hepatic ischemia/reperfusion injury. According to their description, this change could be beneficial for liver function, as HIF-1α governs the transcription of genes controlling proliferation and metastasis of tumor cells [17, 18]. Additionally, previous researches already demonstrate that isoflurane administration could result in an up-regulation of HIF-1α in tumor [19]. However, there have no solid evidence to prove those theory in human body, while the molecular mechanisms of the different outcomes of the two anesthetic methods remains to be determined yet.

HCC with PVTT

HCC ranges as the fifth most common malignancy tumor [20]. Indeed, even worse prognosis is reported in HCC patients with PVTT, with a reported rate of 20% and a reduced median survival time (MST) of around 2–4 months compared to HCC patients without PVTT [21–24]. According to the Asia-Pacific guideline, surgery is recommended as one of the beneficial multidisciplinary treatments for PVTT.

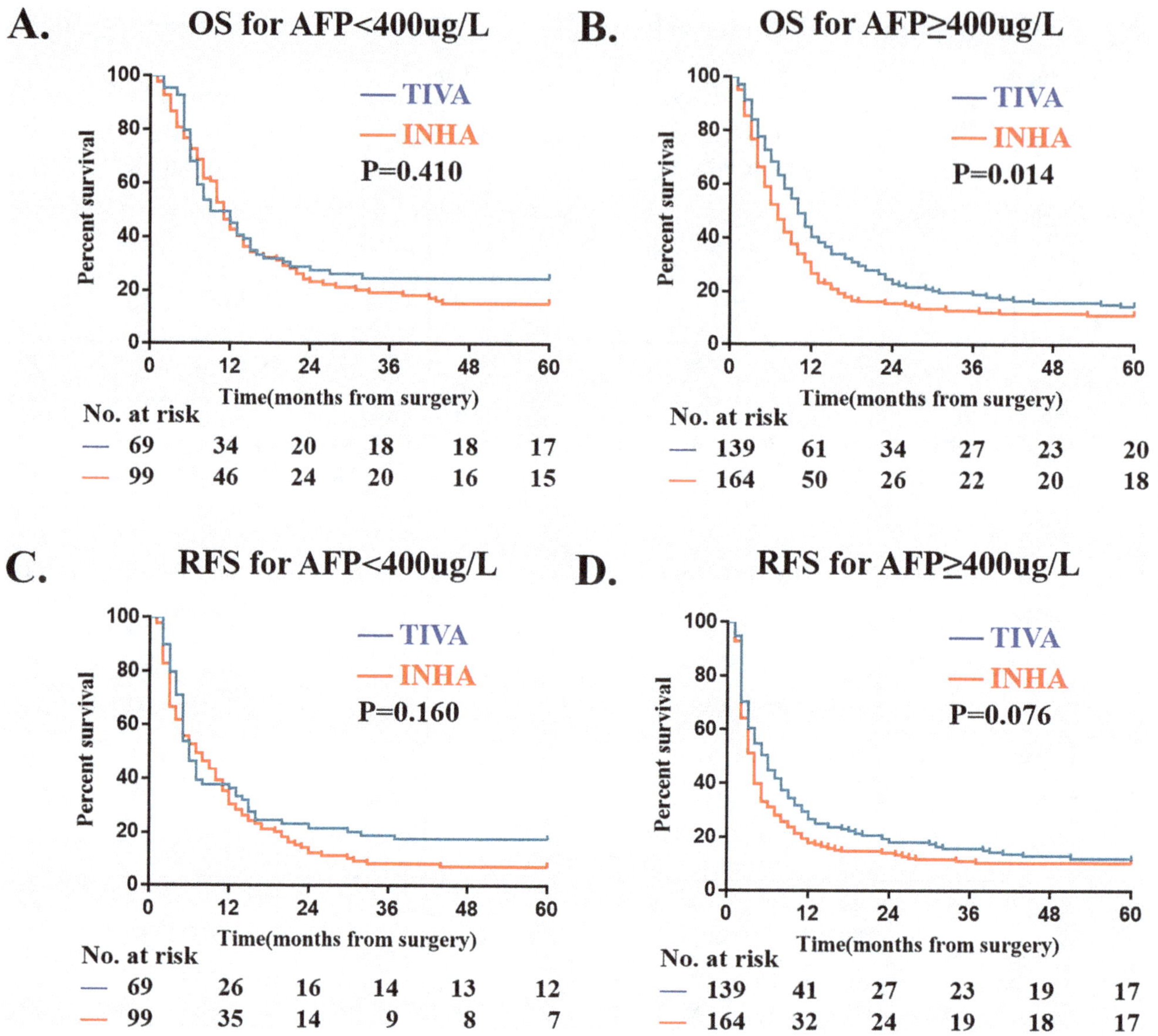

Fig. 5 Subgroup Kaplan–Meier survival analysis for anesthesia type on (**a**) OS in AFP < 400μg/L; (**b**) OS in AFP ≥ 400μg/L; (**c**) RFS in AFP < 400μg/L; (**d**) RFS in AFP ≥ 400μg/L

Moreover, aggressive surgical resection is associated with a longer survival outcome, and even provide chances for complete cure with type I and II PVTT [10, 25]. Meanwhile, recent studies reported that under advanced perioperative management and skilled surgical operation, the in-hospital mortality of HCC patients with PVTT arrives an acceptable rate ranging from 3.7 to 10% [26, 27]. However, the knowledge about risk factors for postoperative mortality, cancer recurrence and other side events of HCC patients with PVTT still remains insufficient. Our result provides with extra evidence that anesthesia type might be a risk factor for surgical outcomes of HCC patients with PVTT.

Limitations

Several methodological discrepancies and limitations of this study should be discussed. First, there might be inclusion bias exist in our cohort, as more than a thousand patients were excluded with only 471 enrolled. Meanwhile, the majority of included patients are male, with ASA score of II, Child-Pugh score of A, and tumor size over 10 cm. Second, certain clinical data of treatment are not collected, including perioperative chemoradiotherapy, detailed surgical techniques, and usage of opioids during surgery. Opioids have been reported to have an effect on tumor cell proliferation and angiogenesis, as well as on tumor recurrence and metastasis. However, it's hard to

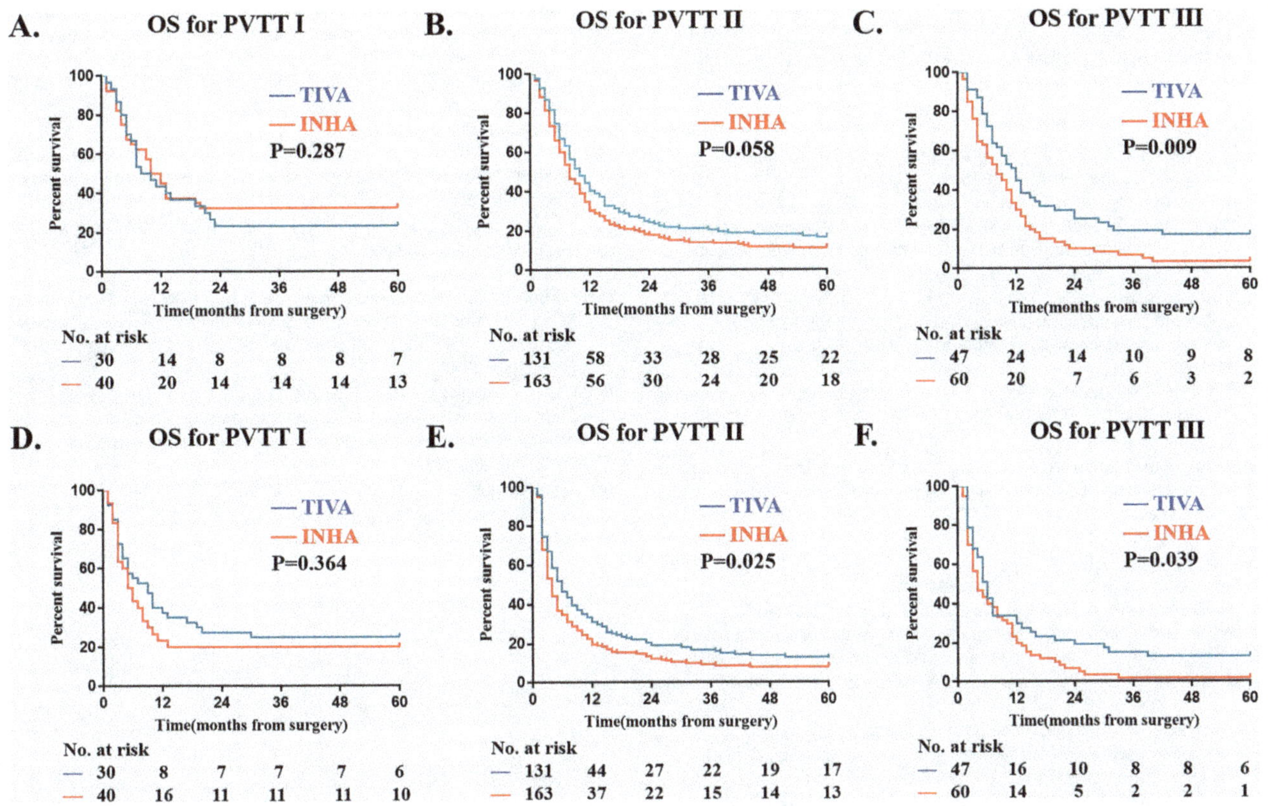

Fig. 6 Subgroup Kaplan–Meier survival analysis for anesthesia type on (**a**) OS in PVTT typeI; (**b**) OS in PVTT typeII; (**c**) OS in PVTT typeIII; (**d**) RFS in PVTT typeI; (**e**) RFS in PVTT typeII; (**f**) RFS in PVTT typeIII

accurately record and compare total amounts of opioid used in both groups during surgery, as they were administered both continuously or intermittently. In this study all patients accepted at least one of remifentanil or sufentanil treatment in standard dose. Besides, since this is a retrospective analysis based clinical records and follow up data, the reason for the choice of anesthesia type at that time point, as well as potential factors affecting this choice, are not recorded or balanced. Thus, prospective researches with rigorous study design and large sample size on this field are in urgent need.

In conclusion, this retrospective analysis of long-term outcomes identifies that INHA is associated with worse survival rate compare with TIVA, and the choice of anesthesia type might be an independent risk factor for survival of HCC patients with PVTT. For some sub-variable groups (including PVTT type I, Child-puge B&C, tumor diameter < 10 cm, AFP < 400μg/L) there was no difference in outcomes between TIVA and INHA. Future prospective researches are urgent to verify this difference and figure out underlying causes of it.

Abbreviations

HCC: Hepatocellular carcinoma; PVTT: Portal vein tumor thrombus; INHA: Volatile inhalational anesthesia; TIVA: Total IV anesthesia; OS: Overall survival; MST: Median survival time; HIFs: Hypoxia-inducible factors; IGF: Insulin-like growth factor; MACE: Major adverse cardiac events; MOD: Multiple organ dysfunction; ALT: Alanine aminotransferase; AST: Aspartate aminotransferase; NLR: Neutrophil-lymphocyte ratio; ASA: American Society of anesthesiologists' Assessment; AFP: Alpha-fetoprotein

Acknowledgements

The authors thank Han Wang, M.D. for his contributions to data analysis.

Authors' contributions

XYM helped conduct the study, analyze the data, and write the manuscript; XPZ helped conduct the study, analyze the data, ZS and HQW helped revise the manuscript; WFY helped design the study and revise the manuscript. The author(s) read and approved the final manuscript.

Author details

[1]Department of Anesthesiology, Eastern Hepatobiliary Surgery Hospital, the Second Military Medical University, 225 Changhai Road, Shanghai, China. [2]Department of Anesthesiology, Ren Ji Hospital, School of Medicine,

Shanghai Jiao Tong University, 160 Pudian Road, Shanghai, China. [3]Department of Hepatic Surgery, Eastern Hepatobiliary Surgery Hospital, the Second Military Medical University, 225 Changhai Road, Shanghai, China.

References

1. Wigmore TJ, Mohammed K, Jhanji S. Long-term survival for patients undergoing volatile versus IV anesthesia for cancer surgery: a retrospective analysis. Anesthesiology. 2015;60(6):240.
2. Yap A, Lopez-Olivo MA, Dubowitz J, Hiller J, Riedel B. Anesthetic technique and cancer outcomes: a meta-analysis of total intravenous versus volatile anesthesia. Can J Anaesth. 2019;66(5):546–61.
3. Huang H, Benzonana LL, Zhao H, Watts HR, Perry NJ, Bevan C, Brown R, Ma D. Prostate cancer cell malignancy via modulation of HIF-1α pathway with isoflurane and propofol alone and in combination. Br J Cancer. 2014;111(7): 1338–49.
4. Luo X, Zhao H, Hennah L, Ning J, Liu J, Tu H, Ma D. Impact of isoflurane on malignant capability of ovarian cancer in vitro ‡. Br J Anaesth. 2015;114(5): 831–9.
5. Fujita Y, Kimura K, Hamada H, Takaori M. Comparative effects of halothane, isoflurane, and sevoflurane on the liver with hepatic artery ligation in the beagle. Anesthesiology. 1991;75(2):313–8.
6. Enlund M, Berglund A, Andreasson K, Cicek C, Enlund A, Bergkvist L. The choice of anaestheticâ "sevoflurane or propofolâ" and outcome from cancer surgery: a retrospective analysis. Ups J Med Sci. 2014;119(3):251–61.
7. Yan T, Zhang GH, Wang BN, Sun L, Zheng H. Effects of propofol/ remifentanil-based total intravenous anesthesia versus sevoflurane-based inhalational anesthesia on the release of VEGF-C and TGF-β and prognosis after breast cancer surgery: a prospective, randomized and controlled study. BMC Anesthesiol. 2018;18(1):131.
8. He FY, Feng WZ, Zhong J, Xu W, Shao HY, Zhang YR. Effects of propofol and dexmedetomidine anesthesia on Th1/Th2 of rat spinal cord injury. Eur Rev Med Pharmacol Sci. 2017;21(6):1355–61.
9. Kushida A, Inada T, Shingu K. Enhancement of antitumor immunity after propofol treatment in mice. Immunopharmacol Immunotoxicol. 2007;29(3–4):477–86.
10. Shi J, Lai ECH, Li N, Guo WX, Xue J, Wan YL, Wu MC, Cheng SQ. Surgical treatment of hepatocellular carcinoma with portal vein tumor thrombus. Ann Surg Oncol. 2010;17(8):2073–80.
11. Liu J, Dong W, Wang T, Liu L, Zhan L, Shi Y, Han J. Effects of etomidate and propofol on immune function in patients with lung adenocarcinoma. Am J Transl Res. 2016;8(12):5748.
12. Yuki K, Astrof NS, Bracken C, Soriano SG, Shimaoka M. Sevoflurane binds and allosterically blocks integrin lymphocyte function-associated antigen-1. Anesthesiology. 2010;113(113):600–9.
13. Melamed R, Bar-Yosef S, Shakhar G, Shakhar K, Ben-Eliyahu S. Suppression of natural killer cell activity and promotion of tumor metastasis by ketamine, thiopental, and halothane, but not by propofol: mediating mechanisms and prophylactic measures. Anesth Analg. 2003;97(5):1331–9.
14. Buckley A, Quaid MS, Johnson P, Buggy D. Serum from women undergoing breast cancer surgery, randomized to propofol-paravertebral anaesthetic technique, maintain natural killer cell anti-tumour activity compared with sevoflurane-opioid technique. Eur J Anaesthesiol. 2014;31:2.
15. Buckley A, Mcquaid S, Johnson P, Buggy DJ, Hemmings HC. Effect of anaesthetic technique on the natural killer cell anti-tumour activity of serum from women undergoing breast cancer surgery: a pilot study. Br J Anaesth. 2014;113(suppl 1):i56–62.
16. Bellanti F, Mirabella L, Mitarotonda D, Blonda M, Tamborra R, Cinnella G, Fersini A, Ambrosi A, Dambrosio M, Vendemiale G. Propofol but not sevoflurane prevents mitochondrial dysfunction and oxidative stress by limiting HIF-1Î± activation in hepatic ischemia/reperfusion injury. Free Radic Biol Med. 2016;96:323–33.
17. Semenza GL. Hypoxia-inducible factors: mediators of cancer progression and targets for cancer therapy. Trends Pharmacol Sci. 2012;33(4):207–14.
18. Semenza GL. HIF-1 mediates metabolic responses to intratumoral hypoxia and oncogenic mutations. J Clin Investig. 2013;123(9):3664–71.
19. Li QF, Wang XR, Yang YW, Su DS. Up-regulation of hypoxia inducible factor 1alpha by isoflurane in Hep3B cells. Anesthesiology. 2006;105(6):1211–9.
20. Bruix J, Reig M, Sherman M. Evidence-based diagnosis, staging, and treatment of patients with hepatocellular carcinoma. Gastroenterology. 2016;150(4):835.
21. Bruix J, Sherman M. Management of hepatocellular carcinoma: an update. American association for the study of liver diseases (AASLD) practice guideline. Hepatology. 2011;53:1020–35.
22. Schöniger-Hekele M, Müller C, Kutilek M, Oesterreicher C, Ferenci P, Gangl A. Hepatocellular carcinoma in Central Europe: prognostic features and survival. Gut. 2001;48(1):103–9.
23. Balogh J, Victor D, Asham EH, Burroughs SG, Boktour M, Saharia A, Xian L, Ghobrial RM, Monsour HP. Hepatocellular carcinoma: a review. J Hepatocell Carcinoma. 2016;3:41–53.
24. Yeung YP, Lo CM, Liu CL, Wong BC, Fan ST, Wong J. Natural history of untreated nonsurgical hepatocellular carcinoma. Am J Gastroenterol. 2005; 100(9):1995–2004.
25. Kokudo T, Hasegawa K, Matsuyama Y, Takayama T, Izumi N, Kadoya M, Kudo M, Ku Y, Sakamoto M, Nakashima O. Survival benefit of liver resection for hepatocellular carcinoma associated with portal vein invasion. J Hepatol. 2016;65(5):938–43.
26. Chen JS, Wang Q, Chen XL, Huang XH, Liang LJ, Lei J, Huang JQ, Li DM, Cheng ZX. Clinicopathologic characteristics and surgical outcomes of hepatocellular carcinoma with portal vein tumor thrombosis. J Surg Res. 2012;175(2):243–50.
27. Chok KS, Cheung TT, Chan SC, Poon RT, Fan ST, Lo CM. Surgical outcomes in hepatocellular carcinoma patients with portal vein tumor thrombosis. World J Surg. 2014;38(2):490–6.

20

Anesthetic management of tracheal laceration from traumatic dislocation of the first rib

Penghui Wei[1†], Dong Yan[1†], Jiapeng Huang[2], Lili Dong[1], Ying Zhao[1], Fei Rong[1], Jing Li[1], Wenxi Tang[1*] and Jianjun Li[1*]

Abstract

Background: Tracheobronchial lacerations from trauma can be life-threatening and present significant challenges for safe anesthetic management. Early recognition of tracheal injuries and prompt airway control can be lifesaving.

Case presentation: A 56-year-old man with no significant medical history presented with difficulty breathing after a blunt trauma to his chest to the emergency room and was diagnosed with dislocation of the first rib and tracheal laceration after a chest tomography (CT) study. Subcutaneous emphysema in neck area quickly worsened indicating continuous air leak. Emergent surgical repair was scheduled. General anesthesia with maintaining spontaneous ventilation was performed and a 5.5 mm endotracheal tube was placed under the guidance of flexible bronchoscopy. Depth of anesthesia was maintained to achieve a Bispectral Index Score of 40–60. Once the offending first rib was removed, a 7.5 mm endotracheal tube was inserted distal to the laceration site with the guidance of flexible bronchoscopy. Once confirmed location of the endotracheal tube, cisatracurium was administered intravenously and the patient was managed on mechanical ventilation with interval positive pressure ventilation. The operation was successful and he was transferred to the ICU intubated. He then received elective surgical repairs for sternum fracture, multiple rib fractures and hemopneumothorax under general anesthesia on day 5 after the first surgery and was extubated on postoperative day 7. The subsequent course was uneventful. Comprehensive rehabilitation was done for 2 weeks and he was discharged home on postoperative day 41.

Conclusions: Early diagnosis and multidisciplinary collaborations are keys to the successful management of this patient. Flexible bronchoscopy is particularly useful in airway management for urgent trachea tracheal laceration repair.

Keywords: Tracheobronchial lacerations, First rib, Anesthetic management, Flexible bronchoscopy

Background

Traumatic tracheobronchial lacerations are relatively uncommon with incidence between 0.5 and 2% among patients with multiple injuries [1]. About 19% of tracheobronchial lacerations occur in the trachea only, 32% are in the left main stem bronchus only, and 47% are in the right main stem bronchus only [2]. Tracheobronchial lacerations are the second most common causes of death and more than 75% of patients die before they arrive to the emergency department [3, 4]. Tracheobronchial lacerations present unique challenges to the anesthesiologist, early recognition and prompt airway control are key for survival.

Tracheobronchial lacerations could be caused by blunt trauma, penetrating trauma or iatrogenic injuries from emergency intubations, multiple intubation attempts, and over-inflation of the tracheal cuff [1, 5].

* Correspondence: drsoup@163.com; Drsoup@163.com; ljj9573@163.com; Ljj9573@163.com
[†]Penghui Wei and Dong Yan contributed equally to this work.
[1]Department of Anesthesiology, Qilu Hospital of Shandong University (Qingdao), No.758 Hefei Road, Qingdao, People's Republic of China

Acute traumatic tracheal injury is rare to be seen by anesthesiologists because tracheobronchial lacerations usually result in acute airway obstruction and death at the scene of an accident or crime [6]. In recent years, more patients with tracheobronchial lacerations presented to the emergency department due to better pre-hospital evacuation procedures and heightened trainings [4]. Tracheobronchial lacerations from traumatic dislocation of the first rib is exceedingly rare.

The anatomical location of the first rib determines that significant dislocation could result in injuries of subclavian vessels, trunks of the brachial plexus, cervicothoracic ganglion, and trachea [7]. The first rib is not commonly dislocated in trauma because its articulations at the T1 vertebra and the manubrium are stabilized by strong ligaments [8]. In rare cases, traumatic first rib dislocations could injure subclavian artery, cervicothoracic ganglion, brachial plexus and trachea [7].

Case presentation

Written informed consent for the publication of this case was obtained from the patient. A 56-year-old man (height, 165 cm; weight, 70 kg) with no significant medical history presented to the emergency room complaining of right chest pain, chest congestion and shortness of breath after sustaining blunt trauma to the right chest. His vital signs were as follows: heart rate (HR), 91 beats/min; respiratory rate (RR), 34 breaths/min; blood pressure (BP), 108/71 mmHg; and initial pulse oximetry saturation (SpO_2) of 85%. Arterial blood gas: PH 7.35, $PaCO_2$ 47 mmHg, and PaO_2 49 mmHg. Flail chest and paradoxical breathing were evident. Significant subcutaneous emphysema in neck and anterior chest area was diagnosed with marked crepitus throughout. Computed Tomography (CT) scan showed massive subcutaneous emphysema, pneumomediastinum, multiple rib fractures, bilateral hemopneumothorax and compressive pneumothorax (Fig. 1 a and b). The sternocostal articulation displacement was seen and the sternal portion of the right first rib penetrated the posterior tracheal wall above the carina (Fig. 2). Chest tube was inserted to decompress pneumothoraxes and hemopneumothorax, and breathing difficulties were alleviated. Unfortunately, rapid worsening of subcutaneous emphysema indicated continuous air leak from laceration after 3 h. The patient developed respiratory distress and became hemodynamically unstable. Emergent CT demonstrated that the right first rib penetrated the posterior tracheal wall up to approximately 6 cm below the glottis and 6 cm above the carina (Fig. 3 a). The first rib divided the trachea into two parts, 5.3 mm in diameter on the left and 6.6 mm on the right (Fig. 3 b and c). The patient was quickly transferred to the operation room. He was agitated, in respiratory distress and his vital signs were: HR 108 beats/min; RR 30 breaths/min; BP 90/58 mmHg and SpO_2 80%. We maintained the hemodynamic stability with intravenous phenylephrine. A fiberoptic bronchoscope was immediately available with different sized endotracheal tubes. General anesthesia was induced with midazolam 2 mg, fentanyl 0.05 mg and 2%~ 5% sevoflurane while maintaining spontaneous ventilation. A sterile flexible fiberoptic bronchoscope loaded with a 5.5 mm endotracheal tube (outer diameter 7.3 mm) identified the laceration of the trachea and the endotracheal tube was advanced distally past the laceration site. He was spontaneously breathing with fraction of inspired oxygen 100%, tidal volume 330 ml, frequency 30, SpO_2 95% and end-tidal carbon dioxide partial pressure ($PetCO_2$) 40 mmHg. Depth of anesthesia was maintained to achieve a Bispectral Index Score of 40–60. The thoracic cavity was opened to expose the right first rib by the surgical team and the right first rib was removed approximately 30 min later (Fig. 4 a). A 7.5 mm endotracheal tube was then exchanged and positioned distally to the laceration with the guidance of flexible bronchoscopy. Once confirmed location of the endotracheal tube, cisatracurium 14 mg and fentanyl 0.15 mg were administered intravenously. The patient was managed on mechanical ventilation with

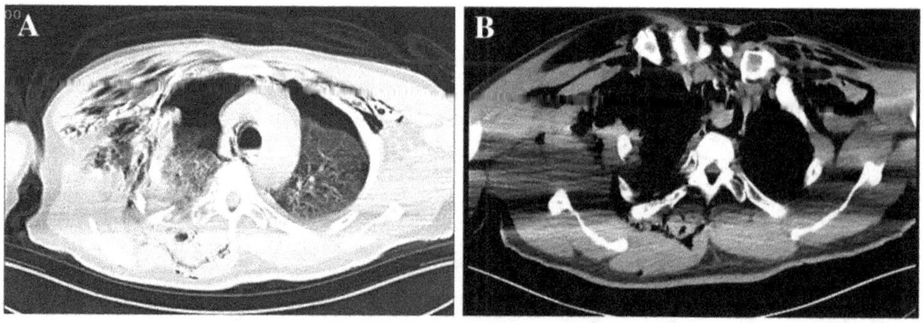

Fig. 1 Thoracic CT scan showing massive subcutaneous emphysema, pneumomediastinum, multiple rib fractures, bilateral hemopneumothorax and compressive pneumothorax on pulmonary (**a**) and mediastinal (**b**) window

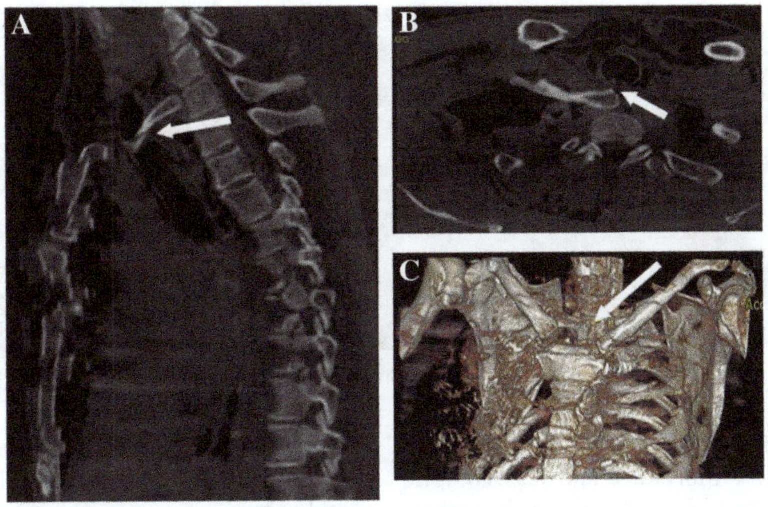

Fig. 2 CT scans of multi-slice technique showing the tracheal laceration secondary to the dislocation of right first rib. **a** Sagittal CT image of the chest. **b** Axial CT image of the chest. (C) Volume rendering of thorax

interval positive pressure ventilation. The respiratory parameters were: fraction of inspired oxygen 60%, tidal volume 550 ml, frequency12, airway peak pressure 22 cm H_2O, SpO_2 98% and $PetCO_2$ 38 mmHg. Direct surgical repair of the tracheal laceration was successful and he was transferred to the ICU intubated. In ICU, he was managed on the ventilator with synchronized intermittent mandatory ventilation and continuous positive airway pressure. In order to improve pulmonary function, elective surgical repairs of sternum fracture, multiple rib fractures and hemopneumothorax under general anesthesia were performed on day 5 after first surgery and the patient was extubated on postoperative day 7. Repeated CT demonstrated the integrity of tracheal wall (Fig. 4 b). Comprehensive rehabilitation was done for 2 weeks and he was discharged home on postoperative day 41.

Discussion and conclusions

In blunt trauma, approximately 80% of tracheobronchial lacerations occur near the carina at the distal trachea, typically in the posterior trachea wall due to lack of cartilaginous support [6]. Tracheal wall laceration from the first rib is a rare complication of

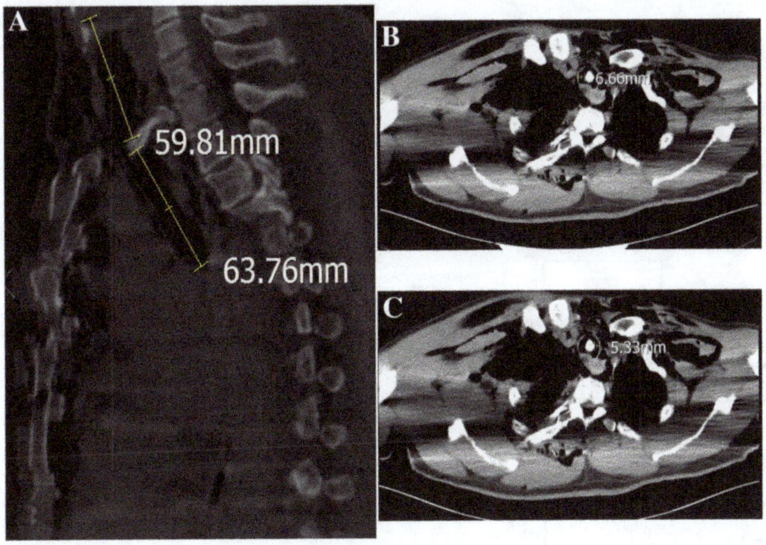

Fig. 3 Preoperative evaluation of Tracheobronchial lacerations by a high-resolution CT. **a** Sagittal CT image of the chest showing the posterior tracheal wall laceration up to 59.81 mm below the glottis and 63.76 mm above the carina. **b**, **c** Axial CT image of the chest showing the bone shadow in the trachea; the residual largest cavity of the trachea on the left was 5.33 mm in diameter and 6.66 mm on the right

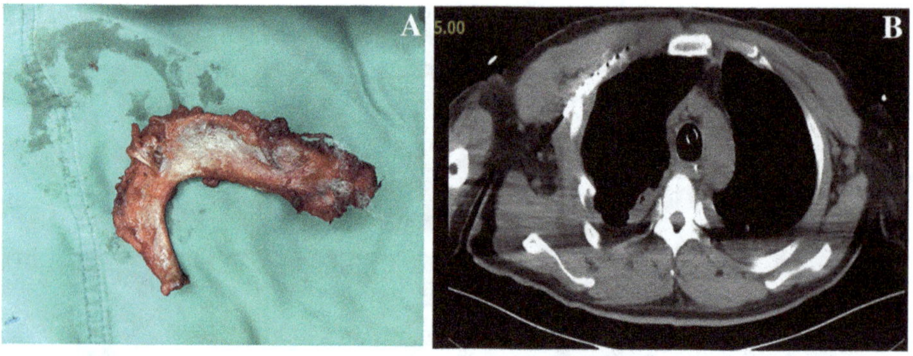

Fig. 4 **a** The right first rib was removed. **b** Postoperative chest CT-scan showing the integrity of posterior tracheal wall

blunt chest trauma. Early diagnosis and treatment are associated with fewer morbidity and less complications including infection and tracheobronchial stricture [9].

The diagnosis of tracheobronchial lacerations is based on high clinical suspicion and signs of subcutaneous emphysema, pneumothorax, or pneumomediastinum [10, 11]. CT scan of the chest should be the initial screening tool in hemodynamically stable patients suffering from multiple chest trauma [12]. A persistent pneumothorax with large air leak from a well-placed chest tube should raise the suspicion of potential airway injury. Other important radiographic findings that are associated with tracheobronchial tears include incorrect location or overdistention of the endotracheal tube cuff [13]. The gold standard for diagnosis is bronchoscopy, which can identify the details of the laceration and guide the accurate positioning of the endotracheal tube [11]. However, tracheobronchial tears may not be visible if the tracheal mucosa remains intact or is sealed by fibrin. In addition, expertise and availability of bronchoscopy can further delay the diagnosis [14]. On a supine CT examination, a classic "fallen-lung sign" is reported as being specific for a bronchial tear, which refers to the peripheral, rather than central, lung collapse occurring when the normal central bronchial anchoring attachments of the lung are disrupted. The collapsed lung falls toward the dependent portion of the hemithorax and is thus seen posteriorly when the patient is supine as during CT examination [13, 14]. No fallen-lung sign was observed in our case because the laceration site was located in the trachea not the mainstem bronchus.

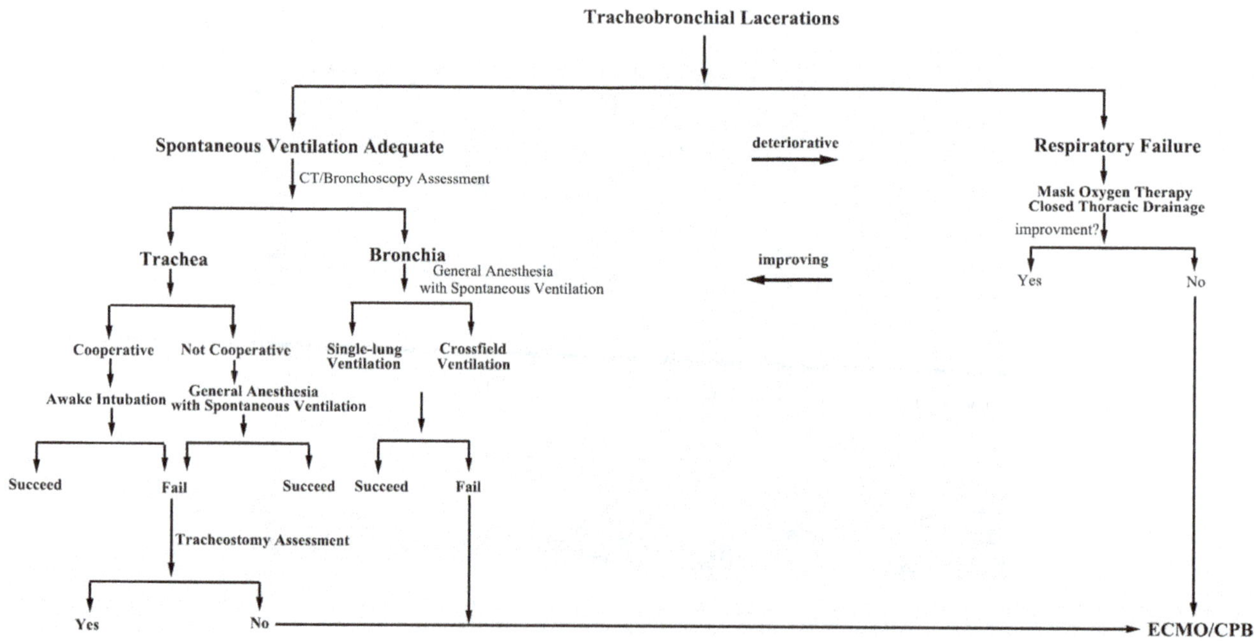

Fig. 5 The proposed difficult airway algorithm in patients with tracheobronchial lacerations

Management of small lacerations (lesions smaller than 1 cm) without surgical intervention may be possible if the endotracheal tube is able to stent the laceration and allow for wound healing [5, 15]. Lacerations larger than 1 or 2 cm or with extensive pneumomediastinum, progressive subcutaneous emphysema, and deteriorative ventilation should be addressed with primary repair [10]. In our case, we performed surgical removal of the first rib and repair of the trachea because the dislocated first rib could cause further tearing of the trachea and the chance of spontaneous healing was not likely. Patients with high suspicion of a tracheal laceration or clinically unstable with rapid drop in oxygenation, should be intubated immediately, under spontaneous ventilation with the guidance of a flexible bronchoscopy [1]. Other ventilatory management options include awake intubation with local anesthetic infiltration, cricothyrotomy, tracheostomy, extracorporeal membrane oxygenation (ECMO), cardiopulmonary bypass (CPB) and cross-field ventilation [4, 16]. In patients with tracheobronchial lacerations, we propose the following difficult airway algorithm (Fig. 5). Awake intubation with local anesthetic infiltration may be a safer option in many difficult airway management [4]. However, the patient was agitated and cannot cooperate when he was transferred to the operation room. In order to prevent larger tears caused by unintended movements during intubation, general anesthesia with spontaneous ventilation was performed. Our patient was not a candidate for either cricothyrotomy or tracheostomy due to the presence of the first rib and the position of the laceration. Crossfield ventilation and single-lung ventilation are generally preferred for patients with the carinal or bronchial injuries [14, 17]. Our patient was intubated with a small single-lumen tube initially with bronchoscopy guidance and ECMO was available in the operating room as backup.

Veno-venous ECMO has proven to be an effective therapy in patients with tracheobronchial lacerations and is difficult to intubate and ventilate [18]. ECMO allows surgical repair by providing adequate oxygenation while minimizing the risk of positive pressure ventilation on tracheobronchial leakage and mechanical dehiscence [19]. The use of ECMO instead of traditional cardiopulmonary bypass technique in tracheal surgery was supported by the lack of intracranial hemorrhage and unstoppable bleeding associated with high-dosed anticoagulants [16, 18].

Successful management of Tracheobronchial lacerations requires constant communications between the anesthesiologist and the surgeon. A multidisciplinary approach and effective communication led to successful outcome in the case.

In summary, we presented a rare case of tracheal laceration from a dislocated first rib. We highlighted the importance of multi-dimensional analysis of a high-resolution CT in diagnosing the tracheal laceration caused by the first rib. Flexible bronchoscopy is particularly useful for successful difficult airway management in urgent tracheobronchial laceration. The importance of effective communication between anesthesiologists and surgeons can't be over-emphasized in these challenging cases.

Abbreviations

BP: Blood pressure; CPB: Cardiopulmonary bypass; CT: Computed tomography; ECMO: Extracorporeal membrane oxygenation; HR: Heart rate; ICU: Intensive care unit; ID: Internal diameter; PetCO2: end-tidal carbon dioxide partial pressure; RR: respiratory rate; SpO_2: Pulse oximetry saturation

Acknowledgements

Not applicable

Authors' contributions

JJL and WXT conceived and designed the case report; and agreed to be accountable for all aspects of the work in ensuring that questions related to the accuracy or integrity of any part of the work were appropriately investigated and resolved. PHW, DY and JPH contributed to writing and revising the manuscript. LLD, YZ and FR performed the anesthesia. PHW, DY and JL contributed to collection of data. All authors read and approved the final manuscript.

Author details

[1]Department of Anesthesiology, Qilu Hospital of Shandong University (Qingdao), No.758 Hefei Road, Qingdao, People's Republic of China. [2]Department of Anesthesiology & Perioperative Medicine, University of Louisville, Louisville, KY, USA.

References

1. Karmy-Jones R, Wood DE. Traumatic injury to the trachea and bronchus. Thorac Surg Clin. 2007;17(1):35–46.
2. Kiser AC, O'Brien SM, Detterbeck FC. Blunt tracheobronchial injuries: treatment and outcomes. Ann Thorac Surg. 2001;71(6):2059–65.
3. Bertelsen S, Howitz P. Injuries of the trachea and bronchi. Thorax. 1972;27(2): 188–94.
4. Lee WT, Eliashar R, Eliachar I. Acute external laryngotracheal trauma: diagnosis and management. Ear Nose Throat J. 2006;85(3):179–84.
5. Singh P, Wojnar M, Malhotra A. Iatrogenic tracheal laceration in the setting of chronic steroids. J Clin Anesth. 2017;37:38–42.
6. Valerio P, Ivan M, Francisco R, Urena A, Ricard R, Ricardo M, Josep S, Ignacio E, Rosa V, Moya J. Survival after traumatic complete laryngotracheal transection. Am J Emerg Med. 2008;26(7):837 e833–4.
7. Stoddart S, Handy M, Cleland P, Wall D, Brown A. Traumatic dislocation of the first rib: a case report and review of the literature. Emerg Med Australas. 2017;29(6):746–8.
8. Christensen EE, Dietz GW. Injuries of the first costovertebral articulation. Radiology. 1980;134(1):41–3.
9. Wu MH, Tsai YF, Lin MY, Hsu IL, Fong Y. Complete laryngotracheal disruption caused by blunt injury. Ann Thorac Surg. 2004;77(4):1211–5.
10. da Silva Costa A Jr, Juliano Perfeito JA, Succi JE, Villaca Leao LE, Rymkiewicz E, da Matta CA, Sandrini MM. A video-assisted endotracheal suture technique for correction of distal tracheal laceration after intubation. Ann Thorac Surg. 2012; 93(6):2073–5.
11. Paik JH, Choi JS, Han SB, Jung HM, Kim JH. Complete cervical tracheal transection caused by blunt neck trauma: case report. Ulus Travma Acil Cerrahi Derg. 2014;20(6):459–62.
12. Le Guen M, Beigelman C, Bouhemad B, Wenjie Y, Marmion F, Rouby JJ. Chest computed tomography with multiplanar reformatted images for diagnosing traumatic bronchial rupture: a case report. Crit Care. 2007; 11(5):R94.
13. Unger JM, Schuchmann GG, Grossman JE, Pellett JR. Tears of the trachea and main bronchi caused by blunt trauma: radiologic findings. AJR Am J

Roentgenol. 1989;153(6):1175–80.
14. Tack D, Defrance P, Delcour C, Gevenois PA. The CT fallen-lung sign. Eur Radiol. 2000;10(5):719–21.
15. Wong EH, Knight S. Tracheobronchial injuries from blunt trauma. ANZ J Surg. 2006;76(5):414–5.
16. Khan SA, Ekeoduru RA, Tariq S. Traumatic tracheobronchial laceration causing complete tracheal resection: challenges of anesthetic management. A A Pract. 2018;11(4):109–11.
17. Barbetakis N, Samanidis G, Paliouras D, Tsilikas C. Tracheal laceration following double-lumen intubation during Ivor Lewis esophagogastrectomy. Interact Cardiovasc Thorac Surg. 2008;7(5):866–8.
18. Antonacci F, De Tisi C, Donadoni I, Maurelli M, Iotti G, Taccone FS, Orlandoni G, Pellegrini C, Belliato M. Veno-venous ECMO during surgical repair of tracheal perforation: a case report. Int J Surg Case Rep. 2018; 42:64–6.
19. Sian K, McAllister B, Brady P. The use of extracorporeal membrane oxygenation therapy in the delayed surgical repair of a tracheal injury. Ann Thorac Surg. 2014;97:338–40.

21

Comparison of the impact of propofol versus sevoflurane on early postoperative recovery in living donors after laparoscopic donor nephrectomy

Sangbin Han[1], Jaesik Park[2], Sang Hyun Hong[2], Soojin Lim[2], Yong Hyun Park[3] and Min Suk Chae[2*]

Abstract

Background: Enhancing postoperative recovery of the donor is important to encourage living kidney donation. We investigated the effects of anesthetic agents (intravenous [IV] propofol versus inhaled [IH] sevoflurane) on the quality of early recovery of healthy living kidney donors after hand-assisted laparoscopic nephrectomy (HALN) under analgesic intrathecal morphine injection.

Methods: This single-center, prospective randomized controlled study enrolled 80 living donors undergoing HALN from October 2019 to June 2020 at Seoul St. Mary's Hospital. Donors were randomly assigned to the IV propofol group or IH sevoflurane group. To measure the quality of recovery, we used the Korean version of the Quality of Recovery-40 questionnaire (QoR-40 K) on postoperative day (POD) 1, and ambulation (success rate, number of footsteps) 6–12 h after surgery and on POD 1. The pain score for the wound site, IV opioid requirement, postoperative complications including incidences of nausea/vomiting, and length of in-hospital stay were also assessed.

Results: The global QoR-40 K score and all subscale scores (physical comfort, emotional state, physical independence, psychological support, and pain) were significantly higher in the IV propofol group than in the IH sevoflurane group. The numbers of footsteps at all time points were also higher in the IV propofol group. Donors in the IV propofol group had a lower incidence of nausea/vomiting, and a shorter hospitalization period.

Conclusions: Total IV anesthesia with propofol led to better early postoperative recovery than that associated with IH sevoflurane.
Keywords: Propofol, Sevoflurane, Quality of recovery-40, Early ambulation, Living kidney donors

* Correspondence: shscms@gmail.com
[2]Department of anesthesiology and Pain medicine, Seoul St. Mary's Hospital, College of Medicine, The Catholic University of Korea, 222, Banpo-daero, Seocho-gu, Seoul 06591, Republic of Korea

Background

In patients with end-stage renal disease, kidney transplantation (KT) is beneficial in terms of quality of life, and also lowers morbidity and mortality rates relative to dialysis [1, 2]. According to the annual report of the Korean Network for Organ Sharing (2018), the requirement for KT has been increasing: 22,620 patients were on the waiting list in 2018, which was almost double that in 2011 [3]. One of the best solutions to satisfy the increasing need for KT is living kidney donation. However, the rate of KT has only increased by 3.25% [4]. Given the lack of organ donors, it is important to improve the experience of living donors and minimize the disincentives related to the procedure, such as postoperative pain/discomfort, prolonged hospital stay and time off work [5] as potential living donors' concerns about the length of hospital stay, and time away from daily activities and work seem to affect their willingness to donate. Additionally, financial losses including direct out-of-pocket expanses along with indirect loss of wages from time off work and reduced productivity are important concerns to some potential living donors [6, 7].

The anesthetic agent is a clinically modifiable factor that can affect the quality of postoperative patient recovery in various surgical settings. Among intravenous (IV) and inhalational (IH) anesthetics, propofol and sevoflurane have been widely used as they offer safe and satisfactory anesthesia. However, these two drugs have different clinical features: IV propofol is associated with a lower incidence of postoperative nausea and vomiting (PONV) [8], a better sense of well-being [9], less postoperative pain [10, 11], but existence of pain on injection, and greater depressive effects on the cardiovascular and respiratory systems [12], while IH sevoflurane has good hemodynamic stability, organ-protective effects including a cardioprotective effect, but a high incidence of PONV [13].

Improving the quality of recovery would lead to a more favorable experience among living donors: i.e., shortened hospital stay, faster return to activities of daily living, improved satisfaction and reduced financial losses [7, 14]. The quality of recovery can be assessed based on Quality of Recovery-40 questionnaire (QoR-40) scores and postoperative ambulation. The QoR-40 is a validated instrument that is widely used to evaluate the quality of postoperative recovery. It is a self-rated questionnaire scored along the following sub-dimensions: physical comfort, emotional state, physical independence, psychological support and pain [14]. The QoR-40 K, which is the Korean version of the QoR-40, has been shown to have acceptable validity, reliability and feasibility [15]. Furthermore, many studies have suggested the importance of early ambulation for preventing postoperative complications [16–20]. The distance ambulated may be an objective indicator of functional status in the recovery period, but no universally accepted instruments are currently used to assess postoperative recovery based on the level of ambulation. Therefore, we used the ambulation success rate and number of steps to evaluate the quality of functional recovery in this study.

To our knowledge, few studies have investigated the effects of anesthetics on the early postoperative recovery of healthy living donors. Therefore, this study investigated the effects of anesthetics (i.e., IV propofol and IH sevoflurane) on the quality of early recovery based on the QoR-40 K scores and ambulation outcomes of healthy living donors undergoing hand-assisted laparoscopic nephrectomy (HALN).

Methods

Ethical considerations

This single-center, prospective randomized controlled study was conducted at Seoul St. Mary's Hospital. Ethical approval was obtained from the Institutional Review Board and Ethics Committee of Seoul St. Mary's Hospital (approval number: KC19MESI0573) on October 7, 2019. The trial was performed according to the Declaration of Helsinki. The protocol was prospectively registered at a publicly accessible clinical trial database recognized by the International Committee of Medical Journal Editors (Clinical Research Information Service, Republic of Korea; approval number: KCT0004351) on October 18, 2019. Written informed consent was obtained from all patients registered in the trial between October 2019 and June 2020. Our study complies with the Consolidated Standards of Reporting Trials (CONSORT) guidelines (CONSORT Checklist); a CONSORT flow chart is presented in Fig. 1 and a summary of the study protocol is presented in Supplemental File 1.

Study population

Adult donors (aged≥19 years) with an American Society of Anesthesiologists physical status (ASA-PS) I or II, who were suitable for kidney donation according to the clinical practice guidelines [21] and were undergoing elective HALN at our hospital, were recruited into the study. We excluded patients who refused to participate or met the following exclusion criteria: emergency case, age < 19 years, ASA-PS III or IV, intraoperative hemodynamic instability (massive hemorrhage, requirement for fluid resuscitation with colloid solution, blood product transfusion and/or infusion of strong inotropic drugs), or not appropriate for intrathecal intervention (bleeding diathesis, neurological dysfunction, history of lumbar spine surgery, recent systemic or local infection or drug allergy).

Among the 84 living donors registered in this trial, four were excluded based on the exclusion criteria: two had a history of spinal surgery and two refused to participate. Consequently, 80 living donors were included in the final analysis.

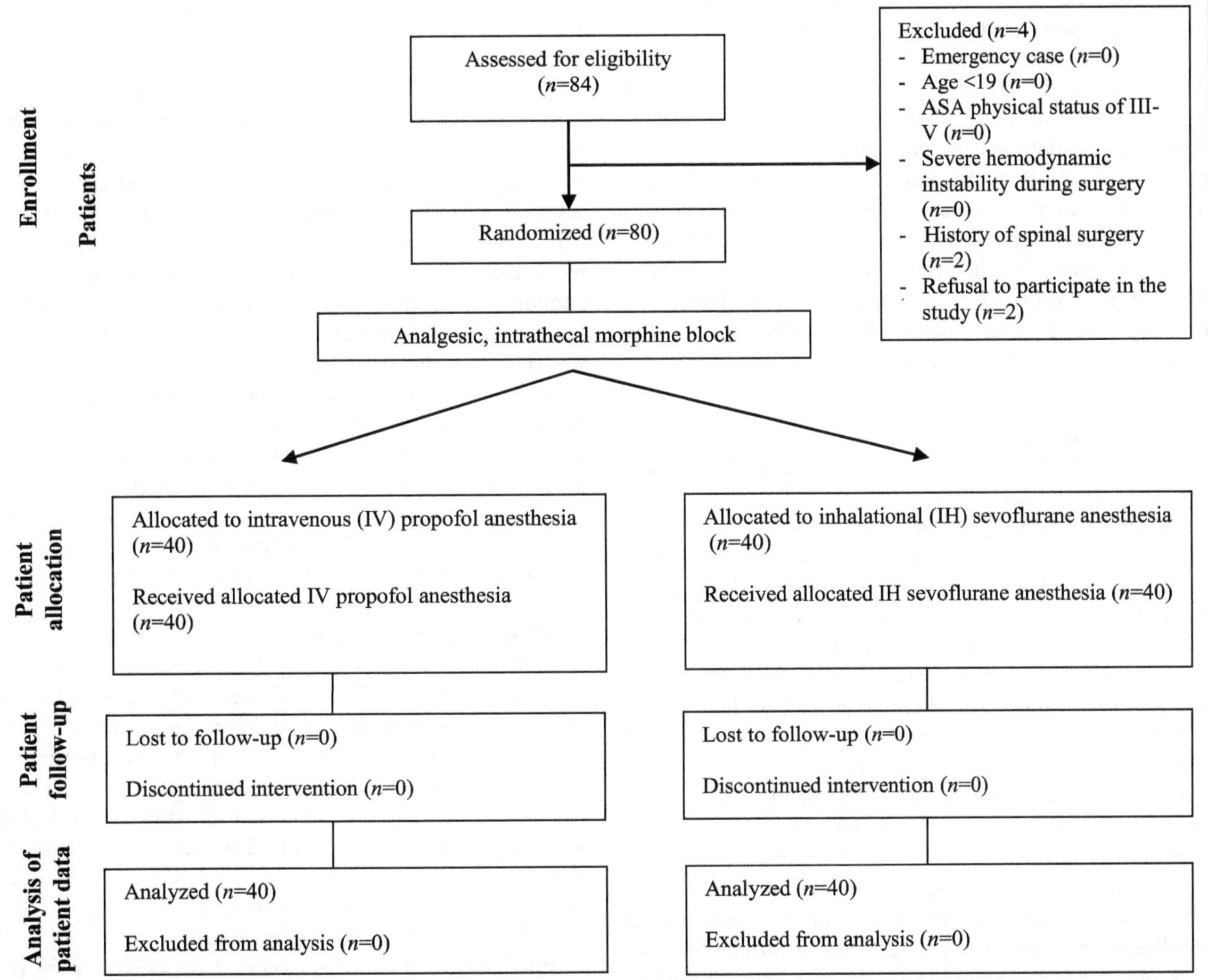

Fig. 1 Consolidated Standards of Reporting Trials (CONSORT) flow chart

Randomization

Living donors were randomly classified into two groups: an IV propofol group ($n = 40$) and an IH sevoflurane group ($n = 40$). We used sealed opaque envelopes to randomly assign the living donors to the groups. The envelopes were divided into groups of 10 and each group contained equal numbers of IV propofol and IH sevoflurane group allocations. A colleague not otherwise involved in this study randomly shuffled and stored the envelopes. When a participating donor entered the preoperative holding area, the uppermost envelope was opened by the attending anesthesiologist who was not a member of the investigational team and the patient was provided the anesthetic management described therein.

The attending anesthesiologist and nurses were aware of the group allocations, but were not involved in patient care after surgery. To prevent their further involvement, nurses from the postanesthetic care unit (PACU) were supervised by a member of the research team who was blinded to the group allocation. The patients, surgical team, physicians, PACU and ward nurses, and all researchers were blinded to the group allocation.

Surgery and anesthesia

HALN, which was comprehensively described in a previous article [22], was performed in all of the patients in both groups by one experienced urological surgeon (Y.H.P). Patients were provided balanced anesthesia by the experienced attending anesthesiologist. Induction of anesthesia was achieved using 1–2 mg kg^{-1} propofol (Fresenius Kabi, Bad Homburg, Germany) and 0.6 mg kg^{-1} rocuronium (Merck Sharp & Dohme Corp., Kenilworth, NJ, USA). Anesthesia in the IV propofol group was maintained by infusing propofol and remifentanil (Hanlim Pharm. Co., Ltd., Seoul, Republic of Korea) according to the effect-site concentration using a target-controlled infusion pump (Orchestra® Workstation; Fresenius Kabi). Schneider's and Minto's pharmacokinetic models were used for propofol and remifentanil, respectively. Anesthesia in the IH sevoflurane group was maintained using sevoflurane (Hana Pharm.) combined with medical air/oxygen. In both groups, anesthetic agents were titrated to maintain the bispectral index (BIS) at 40–60. Neuromuscular blockade was maintained by additional bolus injection of rocuronium. The timing and dosage of injection were determined by the attending anesthesiologist. After the surgical procedure, neuromuscular blockade was reversed with 4 mg kg^{-1} sugammadex (MSD Korea Ltd., Seoul, Republic of Korea) in both groups.

Pain management

All participants received intrathecal morphine (ITM) injection and intravenous patient-controlled analgesia (IV-PCA) for postoperative analgesia. Informed consent for ITM was acquired on the day before the surgery. The ITM injection was administered before the induction of general anesthesia without any sedative. The intrathecal space was approached through the L3–4 interspace. Once free flow of cerebrospinal fluid had been observed, a single bolus of 0.2 mg (0.2 ml) morphine sulfate (BCWorld Pharm. Co., Ltd., Seoul, Republic of Korea) mixed with 0.9% saline (1 ml) to a total volume of 1.2 ml was injected slowly.

All living donors were provided with the IV-PCA device (AutoMed 3200; Ace Medical, Seoul, Republic of Korea) containing 1000 μg of fentanyl (Dai Han Pharm.) and 0.3 mg of ramosetron (Boryung Co., Ltd., Seoul, Republic of Korea) in a total volume of 100 ml. No other local anesthetic or opioid was added to the solution. The IV-PCA device was programmed as follows: no basal infusion, 1 ml bolus injection, and a lockout time of 10 min. If the numerical rating scale (NRS) pain score was ≥7 despite ITM and IV-PCA, a rescue IV opioid was administered on approval by the attending physician in the PACU or ward.

Quality of early postoperative recovery outcomes

The quality of early postoperative recovery was evaluated using the QoR-40 K questionnaire, which consists of the following five subscales: physical comfort (12 items), emotional state (9 items), physical independence (5 items), psychological support (7 items), and pain (7 items). All items are rated on a 5-point Likert scale, where scores range from 1 ("none of the time") to 5 ("all of the time") for positive questions; the anchor points are reversed for negative questions. The total score can range from 40 to 200 and is calculated by summing the scores for all items. Better-quality recovery corresponds to a higher score [14]. In this study, we compared the global and all subdimensional scores of QoR-40 K between IV propofol and IH sevoflurane groups. Donors were asked to complete the QoR-40 K questionnaire on postoperative day (POD) 1.

We assessed functional recovery using the objective measurements of ambulation success rate and number of steps. Donors were advised to attempt sitting, standing and walking only after at least 6 h postoperatively, and only under the guidance of an attending physician. Ambulation was assessed at 6–12 h after surgery and on POD 1, at least 24 h after surgery. Successful ambulation was defined as walking more than 10 steps without any adverse event (nausea, vomiting, or pain) or physical support from the attending physician. Ambulation at the former and latter time points was classed as successful early and late ambulation, respectively. The number of steps was counted using the EI-AN900 activity tracker (Samsung Electronics, Suwon, Republic of Korea). We compared the rate of successful ambulation at early and late postoperative time points between IV propofol and IH sevoflurane groups. The numbers of steps during early and late ambulation and the total footsteps were also compared between the two groups.

Postoperative complications

An NRS was used to evaluate the intensity of postoperative pain at the wound site. Pain severity was measured at 6 h and 24 h after surgery, and during every nursing shift as a part of standard patient care. For each measurement, donors were asked to report the intensity of pain at rest and while coughing. We collected all pain scores during the initial 24 h after surgery, and the highest NRS scores at rest and during coughing were analyzed. Total IV-PCA use and number of rescue IV opioids used during the first 24 h after surgery were also documented.

Other complications that occurred on POD 1 were recorded, including nausea/vomiting, headache, shivering, respiratory depression and pruritus. Adverse events related to the surgery were graded using the Clavien–Dindo classification, which is used to evaluate the severity of postoperative complications after many surgeries [23]. The length of hospital stay after surgery was compared between donors in the IV propofol and IH sevoflurane groups.

Clinical variables

Preoperative findings included demographic and laboratory variables. Intraoperative findings included hemodynamic variables and total surgical duration. Laboratory variables were measured on POD 1.

Statistical analysis

The required sample size was determined based on an unpublished retrospective pilot study conducted at Seoul St. Mary's Hospital including 20 patients. The parameter used for the calculation of effective size was global QoR-40 K score. The number of patients needed in each group for a statistical power of 0.8 at a significance level of 5% was 36, when the standard deviation (SD) and the mean difference between groups were 30 and 20, respectively. We enrolled 40 subjects in each group assuming a dropout rate of 10%.

We used the Shapiro–Wilk test to verify the normality of the data distribution. Normally distributed data were compared using the unpaired *t*-test, while non-normally distributed data were analyzed using the Mann–Whitney *U* test. Categorical data were analyzed using Pearson's χ^2 test or Fisher's exact test, as appropriate. Data are presented as mean ± SD, median and interquartile range, or number (%), as appropriate. All tests were two-sided. To control the overall family-wise error rate, p-value < 0.005 was taken to indicate statistical significance of primary outcomes. In other analyses, p-value < 0.05 was taken to indicate statistical significance. All statistical analyses were performed using SPSS for Windows (ver. 24.0; IBM Corp., Armonk, NY, USA) and MedCalc for Windows (ver. 11.0; MedCalc Software, Ostend, Belgium).

Results

Pre- and intraoperative living donor characteristics

The study population consisted of 32 (40%) male and 48 (60%) female subjects, with a mean age of 47 ± 13 years and a mean body mass index (BMI) of 23.9 ± 3.4 kg/m^2. All living donors were in a clinically acceptable condition (ASA-PS I or II) with controlled comorbidities: two donors had a history of hypertension, but no other systemic diseases were present in the study population.

The pre- and intraoperative donor characteristics were similar between the two groups (Table 1).

QoR-40 K scores and ambulation

The global and subscale scores (i.e., physical comfort, emotional state, psychological support, physical independence, and pain) were significantly higher in the IV propofol group than in the IH sevoflurane group (Table 2). Specifically, the global QoR-40 K score was 169 (162–179) in the IV propofol group and 142 (131–154) in the IH sevoflurane group. Sub-dimension scores in the IV propofol group were 51 (47–54) for physical comfort, 41 (38–43) for emotional state, 32 (29–35) for psychological support, 17 (13–20) for physical independence and 31 (28–33) for pain while these scores in the IH sevoflurane group were 44 (38–47), 36 (32–38), 28 (25–30), 10 (8–13) and 27 (24–29), respectively.

The success rate of early ambulation was marginally higher in the IV propofol group (40 [100%] in the IV propofol group vs. 35 [87.5%] in the IH sevoflurane group; $p = 0.055$); however, all of the donors could ambulate on POD 1 (Table 3). The numbers of steps during the early and late postoperative periods, and the total steps on POD 1, were significantly higher in the IV propofol group than in the IH sevoflurane group. Specifically, the numbers of steps in the IV propofol group were 364 (137–516) for early ambulation, 4086 (1659–4533) for late ambulation and the total number of steps was 4449 (2179–5144), while these numbers in the IH sevoflurane group were 111 (22–398), 1730 (571–3253) and 1970 (639–3649), respectively.

Clinical and laboratory variables during the initial 24 h postoperatively

Nausea and vomiting was the only clinical variable that differed significantly between the two groups (Table 4). Donors in the IV propofol group had a lower incidence of nausea and vomiting than those in the IH sevoflurane group. Pain at the wound site, total IV-PCA use, rescue IV opioid use, and other clinical variables (headache, shivering, and pruritus) were similar between the groups. There were no cases of post-dural puncture headache or respiratory depression.

No significant differences were noted in laboratory variables between the groups on POD 1 (Table 5).

Surgical complications and length of hospital stay

All donors were classified as Clavien–Dindo grade 1 and discharge was uneventful in all cases. The length of hospital stay after surgery was significantly shorter in the IV propofol group than in the IH sevoflurane group (3 [3, 4] days in the IV propofol group versus 4 [3–5] days in the IH sevoflurane group; $p = 0.013$).

Discussion

The main finding of our study was that the global QoR-40 K score was significantly higher in donors receiving IV propofol than in those receiving IH sevoflurane; this tendency was also observed for the physical comfort, emotional state, physical independence, psychological support and pain subscale scores. The numbers of steps during early and late ambulation, and the total number of steps (which was taken to reflect physical capability) were also higher in the IV propofol group than in the IH sevoflurane group. Moreover, the length of hospital stay was shorter in the IV propofol group than in the IH sevoflurane group.

The better recovery outcomes (higher QoR-40 K score and physical capability) observed in the IV propofol group could be explained by differences in characteristics between the two anesthetic agents. First, propofol has anxiolytic effects and produces a general sense of well-being, or even euphoria, after general anesthesia [9, 24, 25]. The anxiolytic effect is related to potentiation of $GABA_A$ receptors and inhibition of the serotonergic system, while the euphoric mood is associated with the stimulation of dopaminergic neurons in the ventral tegmental area [24, 26]. These effects of propofol on patient mood may have contributed to the higher scores on the emotional subscales of the QoR-40 K, considering that some donors

Table 1 Comparison of pre- and intraoperative clinical findings between the IV propofol and IH sevoflurane groups

Group	IV propofol	IH sevoflurane	*p*
n	40	40	
Preoperative findings			
Gender (male)	18 (45.0%)	14 (35.0%)	0.361
Age (years)	50 (40–58)	49 (36–56)	0.371
Height (cm)	162.5 (156.0–170.0)	166.5 (162.0–171.5)	0.167
Weight (kg)	64.0 (54.3–71.5)	64.5 (58.0–68.8)	0.795
Body mass index (kg/m2)	24.5 (21.1–26.5)	23.4 (21.6–25.5)	0.7
ASA physical status			> 0.999
Status 1	32 (80.0%)	32 (80.0%)	
Status 2	8 (20.0%)	8 (20.0%)	
Comorbidity			
Hypertension	2 (5.0%)	0 (0.0%)	0.494
Vital sign			
Systolic blood pressure (mmHg)	120 (111–132)	120 (111–130)	0.742
Diastolic blood pressure (mmHg)	79 (71–80)	76 (69–80)	0.13
Heart rate (beats/min)	76 (71–85)	76 (68–82)	0.623
Laboratory variables			
WBC count (× 109/L)	5.6 (4.8–6.7)	5.3 (4.3–6.2)	0.163
Hemoglobin (g/dL)	13.9 (12.8–15.1)	13.9 (12.6–15.1)	0.715
Platelet count (× 109/L)	244.5 (213.5–282.3)	234.0 (215.5–280.8)	0.832
Creatinine (mg/dL)	0.77 (0.66–0.86)	0.75 (0.66–0.94)	0.647
Albumin (g/dL)	4.5 (4.3–4.7)	4.4 (4.3–4.6)	0.603
Sodium (mEq/L)	142 (141–144)	142 (141–143)	0.476
Potassium (mEq/L)	4.2 (4.0–4.4)	4.2 (4.1–4.3)	0.658
Chloride (mEq/L)	105 (103–106)	104 (103–106)	0.733
International normalized ratio	0.98 (0.95–1.02)	0.98 (0.96–1.04)	0.612
aPTT (sec)	27.2 (26.3–28.2)	26.9 (26.0–28.2)	0.56
Intraoperative findings			
Total surgical duration (min)	138 (125–154)	145 (126–160)	0.289
Side of procured kidney			0.531
Left	33 (82.5%)	35 (87.5%)	
Right	7 (17.5%)	5 (12.5%)	
Average of vital signs[a]			
Systolic blood pressure (mmHg)	118 (106–124)	114 (108–123)	0.476
Diastolic blood pressure (mmHg)	76 (71–83)	74 (67–79)	0.167
Heart rate (beats/min)	66 (61–74)	66 (61–76)	0.836
Hypotension event[b]	0 (0.0%)	2 (5.0%)	0.494
Total remifentanil infusion (mg)	0.5 (0.4–0.7)	0.5 (0.3–0.7)	0.154
Total amount (mL) of			
Fluid input	500 (400–765)	576 (400–750)	0.379
Urine output	185 (100–200)	200 (100–300)	0.115
Hemorrhage	50 (50–100)	100 (50–100)	0.229

Abbreviations: *IV* Intravenous, *IH* Inhalational, *aPTT* Activated partial thrombin time
Average of vital signs[a] were mean of values measured at three time points during surgery: immediately after induction of anesthesia, at the onset of renal arterial clamping and at the end of surgical procedure
Hypotension event[b] was defined as systolic blood pressure < 90 mmHg over 5 min
NOTE: Values are expressed as mean median (interquartile) and number (proportion)

Table 2 Comparison of scores in the QoR-40 K questionnaire on POD 1 between the IV propofol and IH sevoflurane groups

Group	IV propofol	IH sevoflurane	*p*
n	40	40	
Global QoR-40 K score (point)	169 (162–179)	142 (131–154)	< 0.001
Sub-dimension score (point)			
Physical comfort	51 (47–54)	44 (38–47)	< 0.001
Emotional state	41 (38–43)	36 (32–38)	< 0.001
Psychological support	32 (29–35)	28 (25–30)	< 0.001
Physical independence	17 (13–20)	10 (8–13)	< 0.001
Pain	31 (28–33)	27 (24–29)	< 0.001

NOTE: Values are expressed as median and interquartile
Abbreviations: *IV* Intravenous, *IH* Inhalational, *QoR-40 K* Quality of Recovery-40 questionnaire, *POD* Postoperative day

have been reported to experience short-term mood changes after organ donation [27]. Second, many previous studies have demonstrated that propofol has analgesic and antinociceptive effects [24]. The analgesic effect of sevoflurane is also widely known, but which agent provides superior postoperative analgesic effects remains controversial, with equivocal results among studies [10, 11]. In the present trial, a higher pain score on the QoR-40 K, indicating less pain, was observed in the IV propofol group. However, as the pain subscale of the QoR-40 K subsumes extra-surgical pain, such as muscle pain, headache and backache, it is unclear whether the IV propofol actually provided better postoperative analgesia at the wound site. In this trial, the highest NRS pain score for the wound site was slightly, but non-significantly, lower in the IV propofol group, both during coughing and at rest. Third, propofol significantly reduces PONV compared with inhalational anesthetics [28]. The antiemetic effect of propofol is associated with inhibition of the 5-hydroxytryptamine-3 (5-HT) receptors in the serotonergic system, dopaminergic (D2) receptors in the chemoreceptor trigger zone, and the limbic system [24, 29]. PONV is not only covered by a separate item in the QoR-40 K questionnaire, but also affects the overall sense of physical comfort [30]. This is consistent with our findings of a significantly lower incidence of PONV and higher physical comfort scores in the IV propofol group. Fourth, sevoflurane leads to a greater decrease of bronchial mucus transport relative to propofol. Impaired bronchociliary clearance may have resulted in the retention of secretions, which can cause discomfort while breathing after surgery, as well as a higher risk of pulmonary complications [31]. Finally, a modulatory effect on surgical stress of propofol, as well as anti-inflammatory effects, have been demonstrated in previous studies [32–34]. It is well known that surgical injury triggers the systemic inflammatory response (SIR), where an excessive SIR is assumed to contribute to delayed recovery after surgery and postoperative complications [35, 36]. SIR may have played a role in the better recovery of our donors who received IV propofol.

Table 3 Comparison of postoperative ambulation between the IV propofol and IH sevoflurane groups

Group	IV propofol	IH sevoflurane	*p*
n	40	40	
Successful ambulation			
Early ambulation	40 (100.0%)	35 (87.5%)	0.055
Late ambulation	40 (100.0%)	40 (100.0%)	–
Ambulation (foot-steps)			
Total ambulation	4449 (2179–5144)	1970 (639–3649)	0.001
Early ambulation	364 (137–516)	111 (22–398)	0.004
Late ambulation	4086 (1659–4533)	1730 (571–3253)	0.001

Total ambulation was defined as sum of early and late ambulation
Early ambulation was defined as steps on the day after surgery
Late ambulation was defined as steps on postoperative day 1
NOTE: Values are expressed as number (proportion) and median (interquartile)
Abbreviations: *IV* Intravenous, *IH* Inhalational

However, some recent studies have reported no differences in the effects of propofol and sevoflurane on postoperative recovery outcomes, namely the QoR-40 scores, postoperative pain, length of PACU stay, and complications, including PONV [37–39]. Possible explanations for this discrepancy between our results and those of previous studies include different study population characteristics, surgical etiologies and analgesic regimens. The donors in our study were healthier; most had no comorbidities, except for two with controlled hypertension. Although other studies have enrolled patients with ASA-PS of I or II, they did not investigate comorbidities, and the patients were undergoing surgery due to their illness. Differences in underlying health conditions among study populations could confound comparison of postoperative recovery. In one recent study, higher level of physical activity in the pre-donation period was positively associated with the occurrence of chronic postsurgical pain, indicating that donors involved in vigorous physical activities may be more sensitive to postoperative pain or discomfort than stationary donors [40]. Additionally, pain threshold tends to be lower in healthy living donors than in patients undergoing a similar surgical procedure for health reasons, which could also have affected the results [41]. We used ITM as the analgesic in this study, which offers superior analgesia compared with IV opioid, IV-PCA, and continuous wound infusion, for example [42]. Better pain control, and subsequently reduced IV opioid consumption and PONV incidence, may facilitate ambulation, improve physical capability, and prevent severe wound pain,

Table 4 Comparison of clinical variables during 24 h postoperatively between the IV propofol and IH sevoflurane groups

Group	IV propofol	IH sevoflurane	p
n	40	40	
Peak NRS score on wound site			
At rest			0.606
Mild pain (0 to 3 points)	31 (77.5%)	29 (72.5%)	
Moderate pain (4 to 6 points)	9 (22.5%)	11 (27.5%)	
Severe pain (7 to 10 points)	0 (0.0%)	0 (0.0%)	
At cough			0.612
Mild pain (0 to 3 points)	8 (20.0%)	5 (12.5%)	
Moderate pain (4 to 6 points)	18 (45.0%)	18 (45.0%)	
Severe pain (7 to 10 points)	14 (35.0%)	17 (42.5%)	
Requirement of IV opioid			
Total amount of IV-PCA infusion (mL)	13.5 (9.3–23.8)	16.0 (7.0–37.3)	0.522
Rescue IV opioid	2 (5.0%)	3 (7.5%)	> 0.999
Nausea/vomiting	12 (30.0%)	26 (65.0%)	0.002
Headache	3 (7.5%)	5 (12.5%)	0.712
Shivering	5 (12.5%)	10 (25.0%)	0.152
Respiration depression	0 (0.0%)	0 (0.0%)	–
Pruritus	11 (27.5%)	13 (32.5%)	0.626

NOTE: Values are expressed as median (interquartile) and number (proportion)
Abbreviations: *IV* Intravenous, *IH* Inhalational, *NRS* Numeric rating scale, *IV-PCA* Intravenous patient-controlled analgesia

thus resulting in a shorter hospitalization period [43, 44].

Several limitations of this study should be discussed. First, the specific mechanisms underlying the differences in recovery were not determined. Second, we calculated the sample size required to detect group differences in the QoR-40 K scores, rather than in subscale scores or other clinical variables. Third, as this study was performed in healthy donors undergoing HALN in the setting of ITM, the results may not be generalizable to other patient populations, surgeries, or analgesic strategies. Finally, no long-term follow-up was performed.

Table 5 Comparison of laboratory variables on POD 1 between the IV propofol and IH sevoflurane groups

Group	IV propofol	IH sevoflurane	p
n	40	40	
WBC count (× 109/L)	9.5 (8.4–12.1)	9.8 (8.4–10.8)	0.788
Neutrophil (%)	76.8 (72.9–80.5)	77.7 (75.1–81.5)	0.351
Lymphocyte (%)	16.5 (11.7–20.2)	14.4 (11.3–17.3)	0.142
Hemoglobin (g/dL)	11.8 (10.7–12.8)	11.6 (10.9–13.1)	0.758
Platelet count (× 109/L)	201.0 (168.3–233.5)	197.0 (165.0–237.0)	0.627
Creatinine (mg/dL)	1.3 (1.1–1.5)	1.25 (1.11–1.61)	0.988
Albumin (g/dL)	3.4 (3.3–3.6)	3.3 (3.1–3.5)	0.081
Sodium (mEq/L)	139 (138–140)	138 (137–140)	0.072
Potassium (mEq/L)	3.9 (3.8–4.3)	3.9 (3.7–4.2)	0.706
Chloride (mEq/L)	104 (103–106)	104.0 (102.0–105.8)	0.402

NOTE: Median and interquartile
Abbreviations: *WBC* White blood cell, *IV* Intravenous, *IH* Inhalationalm, *POD* Postoperative day

Conclusions

The choice of anesthetic drug may affect the quality of early postoperative recovery in healthy living donors undergoing HALN. IV propofol seems to be a better option with respect to postoperative recovery than IH sevoflurane under appropriate analgesia, such as ITM.

Abbreviations

KT: Kidney transplantation; IV: Intravenous; IH: Inhalational; PONV: Postoperative nausea and vomiting; QoR-40: Quality of Recovery-40; QoR-40 K: The Korean version of the QoR-40; CONSORT: Consolidated Standards of Reporting Trials; HALN: Hand-assisted laparoscopic nephrectomy; ASA-PS: American Society of Anesthesiologists physical status; PACU: Post-anesthetic care unit; BIS: Bispectral index; ITM: Intrathecal morphine; IV-PCA: Intravenous patient-controlled analgesia; NRS: Numerical rating scale; POD: Postoperative day; SD: Standard deviation; BMI: Body mass index; 5-HT: 5-hydroxy tryptamine-3; IL: Interleukin; SIR: Systemic inflammatory response

Acknowledgments

None

Authors' contributions

M.S.C. were responsible for the study concept and design. S.H. and M.S.C. wrote the manuscript. S. H, J.P., S.L., Y.H.P., J.W.S., H.M.L., Y.S.K., Y.E.M., S.H.H. and M.S.C. participated in the collection and interpretation of the data. All authors approved the final version of the manuscript.

Author details
[1]Department of Emergency medicine, Cheongyang Health Center County Hospital, Chungcheongnam-do, Republic of Korea. [2]Department of anesthesiology and Pain medicine, Seoul St. Mary's Hospital, College of Medicine, The Catholic University of Korea, 222, Banpo-daero, Seocho-gu, Seoul 06591, Republic of Korea. [3]Department of Urology, Seoul St. Mary's Hospital, College of Medicine, The Catholic University of Korea, Seoul, Republic of Korea.

References

1. Hart A, Smith J, Skeans M, Gustafson S, Wilk A, Castro S, et al. OPTN/SRTR 2018 annual data report: kidney. Am J Transplant. 2020;20:20–130.
2. Rose C, Gill J, Gill JS. Association of Kidney Transplantation with survival in patients with long dialysis exposure. Clin J Am Soc Nephrol. 2017;12(12): 2024–31.
3. Korean Network for Organ Sharing (KONOS). Organ transplantation and donation of human tissue statistical yearbook 2018. Seoul: KONOS; 2019. p. 258. p. Report No.: 11–1351155–000001-01.
4. Rege A, Leraas H, Vikraman D, Ravindra K, Brennan T, Miller T, et al. Could the use of an enhanced recovery protocol in laparoscopic donor nephrectomy be an incentive for live kidney donation? Cureus. 2016;8(11): e889.
5. Ashcraft EE, Baillie GM, Shafizadeh SF, McEvoy JR, Mohamed HK, Lin A, et al. Further improvements in laparoscopic donor nephrectomy: decreased pain and accelerated recovery. Clin Transpl. 2001;15(Suppl 6):59–61.
6. Boulware LE, Ratner LE, Sosa JA, Tu AH, Nagula S, Simpkins CE, et al. The general Public's concerns about clinical risk in live kidney donation. Am J Transplant. 2002;2(2):186–93.
7. Klarenbach S, Gill J, Knoll G, Caulfield T, Boudville N, Prasad G, et al. Economic consequences incurred by living kidney donors: a Canadian multi-center prospective study. Am J Transplant. 2014;14(4):916–22.
8. Kumar G, Stendall C, Mistry R, Gurusamy K, Walker D. A comparison of total intravenous anesthesia using propofol with sevoflurane or desflurane in ambulatory surgery: systematic review and meta-analysis. Anesthesia. 2014; 69(10):1138–50.
9. Hofer CK, Zollinger A, Buchi S, Klaghofer R, Serafino D, Buhlmann S, et al. Patient well-being after general anesthesia: a prospective, randomized, controlled multi-Centre trial comparing intravenous and inhalation anesthesia. Br J Anaesth. 2003;91(5):631–7.
10. Fassoulaki A, Melemeni A, Paraskeva A, Siafaka I, Sarantopoulos C. Postoperative pain and analgesic requirements after anesthesia with sevoflurane, desflurane or propofol. Anesth Analg. 2008;107(5):1715–9.
11. Li M, Mei W, Wang P, Yu Y, Qian W, Zhang ZG, et al. Propofol reduces early post-operative pain after gynecological laparoscopy. Acta Anaesthesiol Scand. 2012;56(3):368–75.
12. Fredman B, Nathanson MH, Smith I, Wang J, Klein K, White P. Sevoflurane for outpatient anesthesia: a comparison with Propofol. Anesth Analg. 1995; 81(4):823–8.
13. Brioni JD, Varughese S, Ahmed R, Bein B. A clinical review of inhalation anesthesia with sevoflurane: from early research to emerging topics. J Anesth. 2017;31(5):764–78.
14. Myles PS, Weitkamp B, Jones K, Melick J, Hensen S. Validity and reliability of a postoperative quality of recovery score: the QoR-40. Br J Anaesth. 2000; 84(1):11–5.
15. Lee JH, Kim D, Seo D, Son JS, Kim DC. Validity and reliability of the Korean version of the quality of Recovery-40 questionnaire. Korean J Anesthesiol. 2018;71(6):467–75.
16. Cassidy MR, Rosenkranz P, McAneny D. Reducing postoperative venous thromboembolism complications with a standardized risk-stratified prophylaxis protocol and mobilization program. J Am Coll Surg. 2014;218(6): 1095–104.
17. Haines KJ, Skinner EH, Berney S, Investigators AHPS. Association of postoperative pulmonary complications with delayed mobilisation following major abdominal surgery: an observational cohort study. Physiotherapy. 2013;99(2):119–25.
18. Wenger N. The physiologic basis for early ambulation after myocardial infarction. Cardiovasc Clin. 1978;9(3):107–15.
19. Parker HG, Reitman HK. Changing patterns in fracture management emphasizing early motion and function. Surg Clin N Am. 1976;56(3):667–72.
20. Lee T-G, Kang S-B, Kim D-W, Hong S, Heo SC, Park KJ. Comparison of early mobilization and diet rehabilitation program with conventional care after laparoscopic colon surgery: a prospective randomized controlled trial. Dis Colon Rectum. 2011;54(1):21–8.
21. Mandelbrot DA, Reese PP, Garg N, Thomas CP, Rodrigue JR, Schinstock C, et al. KDOQI US commentary on the 2017 KDIGO clinical practice guideline on the evaluation and Care of Living Kidney Donors. Am J Kidney Dis. 2020; 75(3):299–316.
22. Seo SI, Kim JC, Hwangbo K, Park YH, Hwang TK. Comparison of hand-assisted laparoscopic and open donor nephrectomy: a single-center experience from South Korea. J Endourol. 2005;19(1):58–62.
23. Dindo D, Demartines N, Clavien PA. Classification of surgical complications: a new proposal with evaluation in a cohort of 6336 patients and results of a survey. Ann Surg. 2004;240(2):205–13.
24. Vasileiou I, Xanthos T, Koudouna E, Perrea D, Klonaris C, Katsargyris A, et al. Propofol: a review of its non-anaesthetic effects. Eur J Pharmacol. 2009; 605(1–3):1–8.
25. Brechmann T, Maier C, Kaisler M, Vollert J, Schmiegel W, Pak S, et al. Propofol sedation during gastrointestinal endoscopy arouses euphoria in a large subset of patients. United European Gastroenterol J. 2018;6(4):536–46.
26. Li KY, Xiao C, Xiong M, Delphin E, Ye JH. Nanomolar propofol stimulates glutamate transmission to dopamine neurons: a possible mechanism of abuse potential? J Pharmacol Exp Ther. 2008;325(1):165–74.
27. Jowsey SG, Jacobs C, Gross CR, Hong BA, Messersmith EE, Gillespie BW, et al. Emotional well-being of living kidney donors: findings from the RELIVE study. Am J Transplant Off J Am Soc Transplant Am Soc Transplant Surg. 2014;14(11):2535–44.
28. Yoo YC, Bai SJ, Lee KY, Shin S, Choi EK, Lee JW. Total intravenous anesthesia with propofol reduces postoperative nausea and vomiting in patients undergoing robot-assisted laparoscopic radical prostatectomy: a prospective randomized trial. Yonsei Med J. 2012;53(6):1197–202.
29. Barann M, Göthert M, Fink K, Bönisch H. Inhibition by anaesthetics of 14 C-guanidinium flux through the voltage-gated sodium channel and the cation channel of the 5-HT 3 receptor of N1E-115 neuroblastoma cells. Naunyn Schmiedeberg's Arch Pharmacol. 1993;347(2):125–32.
30. Lee WK, Kim MS, Kang SW, Kim S, Lee JR. Type of anaesthesia and patient quality of recovery: a randomized trial comparing propofol-remifentanil total i.v. anaesthesia with desflurane anaesthesia. Br J Anaesth. 2015;114(4): 663–8.
31. Ledowski T, Paech MJ, Patel B, Schug SA. Bronchial mucus transport velocity in patients receiving propofol and remifentanil versus sevoflurane and remifentanil anesthesia. Anesth Analg. 2006;102(5):1427–30.
32. Gilliland HE, Armstrong MA, Carabine U, McMurray TJ. The choice of anesthetic maintenance technique influences the antiinflammatory cytokine response to abdominal surgery. Anesth Analg. 1997;85(6):1394–8.
33. Ke J, Zhan J, Feng X, Wu Y, Rao Y, Wang Y. A comparison of the effect of total intravenous anesthesia with propofol and remifentanil and inhalational anesthesia with isoflurane on the release of pro-and anti-inflammatory cytokines in patients undergoing open cholecystectomy. Anesthesia Intensive Care. 2008;36(1):74–8.
34. Kotani N, Hashimoto H, Sessler DI, Yasuda T, Ebina T, Muraoka M, et al. Expression of genes for proinflammatory cytokines in alveolar macrophages during propofol and isoflurane anesthesia. Anesth Analg. 1999;89(5):1250–6.
35. Crippa J, Mari GM, Miranda A, Costanzi AT, Maggioni D. Surgical stress response and enhanced recovery after laparoscopic surgery - a systematic review. Chirurgia (Bucur). 2018;113(4):455–63.
36. Watt DG, Horgan PG, McMillan DC. Routine clinical markers of the magnitude of the systemic inflammatory response after elective operation: a systematic review. Surgery. 2015;157(2):362–80.
37. Carli D, Meletti JFA, Neto NEU, Martinez G, Kim ALC, de Camargo RPS. General anesthesia technique and perception of quality of postoperative recovery in women undergoing cholecystectomy: a randomized, double-blinded clinical trial. PLoS One. 2020;15(2):e0228805.
38. De Oliveira GS, Jr., Bialek J, Rodes ME, Kendall MC, McCarthy RJ. The effect of sevoflurane compared to propofol maintenance on post-surgical quality of recovery in patients undergoing an ambulatory gynecological surgery: a prospective, randomized, double-blinded, controlled, clinical trial. J Clin Anesth. 2017;43:70–4.
39. Moro ET, Leme FC, Noronha BR, Saraiva GF, de Matos Leite NV, Navarro LH. Quality of recovery from anesthesia of patients undergoing balanced or total intravenous general anesthesia. Prospective randomized clinical trial. J Clin Anesth. 2016;35:369–75.

40. Fleishman A, Khwaja K, Schold JD, Comer CD, Morrissey P, Whiting J, et al. Pain expectancy, prevalence, severity, and patterns following donor nephrectomy: findings from the KDOC study. Am J Transplant. 2020;20(9): 2522–9.
41. Cywinski JB, Parker BM, Xu M, Irefin SA. A comparison of postoperative pain control in patients after right lobe donor hepatectomy and major hepatic resection for tumor. Anesth Analg. 2004;99(6):1747–52.
42. Tang JZJ, Weinberg L. A Literature Review of Intrathecal Morphine Analgesia in Patients Undergoing Major Open Hepato-Pancreatic-Biliary (HPB) Surgery. Anesthesiol Pain Med. 2019;9(6):e94441.
43. Dichtwald S, Ben-Haim M, Papismedov L, Hazan S, Cattan A, Matot I. Intrathecal morphine versus intravenous opioid administration to impact postoperative analgesia in hepato-pancreatic surgery: a randomized controlled trial. J Anesth. 2017;31(2):237–45.
44. Cheah JW, Sing DC, Hansen EN, Aleshi P, Vail TP. Does intrathecal morphine in spinal anesthesia have a role in modern multimodal analgesia for primary Total joint arthroplasty? J Arthroplast. 2018;33(6):1693–8.

22

Perioperative anaesthetic management of patients with or at risk of acute distress respiratory syndrome undergoing emergency surgery

Denise Battaglini[1,2], Chiara Robba[1], Patricia Rieken Macêdo Rocco[3], Marcelo Gama De Abreu[4], Paolo Pelosi[1,2*] and Lorenzo Ball[1,2]

Abstract

Patients undergoing emergency surgery may present with the acute respiratory distress syndrome (ARDS) or develop this syndrome postoperatively. The incidence of ARDS in the postoperative period is relatively low, but the impact of ARDS on patient outcomes and healthcare costs is relevant Aakre et.al (Mayo Clin Proc 89:181-9, 2014). The development of ARDS as a postoperative pulmonary complication (PPC) is associated with prolonged hospitalisation, longer duration of mechanical ventilation, increased intensive care unit length of stay and high morbidity and mortality Ball et.al (Curr Opin Crit Care 22:379-85, 2016). In order to mitigate the risk of ARDS after surgery, the anaesthetic management and protective mechanical ventilation strategies play an important role. In particular, a careful integration of general anaesthesia with neuraxial or locoregional techniques might promote faster recovery and reduce opioid consumption. In addition, the use of low tidal volume, minimising plateau pressure and titrating a low-moderate PEEP level based on the patient's need can improve outcome and reduce intraoperative adverse events. Moreover, perioperative management of ARDS patients includes specific anaesthesia and ventilator settings, hemodynamic monitoring, moderately restrictive fluid administration and pain control. The aim of this review is to provide an overview and evidence- and opinion-based recommendations concerning the management of patients at risk of and with ARDS who undergo emergency surgical procedures.

Keywords: Acute distress respiratory syndrome, Perioperative management, Protective ventilation, Emergency surgery

Background

Acute respiratory distress syndrome (ARDS) is a life-threatening condition characterized by hypoxemic respiratory failure and reduced lung compliance [1–3], with parenchymal heterogenicity as demonstrated by CT scan images [4]. ARDS can result from several causes associated with a direct damage to the lung, such as pneumonia, chest trauma with pulmonary contusions, fat embolism, aspiration, and indirect causes, such as: sepsis, pancreatitis, blood transfusions and extra-thoracic trauma [5]. ARDS represents the most severe pulmonary complication after surgery, and is associated mortality rates in the range of 40 to 50% at 30 days from hospitalisation [6]. The incidence of new onset-ARDS in the postoperative period is relatively low, but its impact on patient outcomes is extremely relevant.

* Correspondence: ppelosi@hotmail.com
[1]Anaesthesia and Intensive Care, IRCCS for Oncology and Neurosciences, San Martino Policlinico Hospital, Genoa, Italy
[2]Department of Surgical Sciences and Integrated Diagnostics, University of Genoa, Genoa, Italy

Perioperative management of patients undergoing emergency surgery

Patients at risk of and with ARDS must to be promptly identified and managed with specific intraoperative strategies including protective ventilator settings, together with haemodynamic monitorization, the use of specific type of fluids, as well as pain management. Figure 1 summarises an overview of recommendations concerning the perioperative management of these patients.

Preoperative management

Patient and surgical-related risk identification

Over the last decade, several scores predicting PPCs and ARDS after surgery have been developed [4–7], but still poorly implemented in the clinical practice [8]. To prevent postoperative ARDS, our ability to identify the surgical population that is at high risk of ARDS is an essential first step. Moreover, delayed recognition of predictive factors for the development of postoperative pulmonary complications is associated with worse outcome [9]. High-risk patients, when correctly identified, require additional monitoring, less invasive surgical procedures, lower risk anaesthesia techniques such as regional anaesthesia when feasible and early planning of intensive care unit (ICU) admission. Preoperative assessment should take into account patient's basal functional state, comorbidities and the complexity of surgery to minimise the risk of postoperative complications [10, 11]. Centre-specific treatment guidelines may reduce risks and should be discussed with a multidisciplinary team.

The occurrence of PPCs is related to different causes and insults occurring throughout the perioperative period, comprising preoperative patients' conditions and intraoperative complications [12]. The interaction between predisposing risk factors and surgical and anaesthesiologic management can lead to organ damage translating into postoperative complications. Moreover, during the perioperative period respiratory complications can be further exacerbated by the administration of sedatives, opioids and prolonged supine position. Among others, mechanical ventilation settings and perioperative ventilator management are important parameters linked to the development of PPCs [12–14]. Postoperative respiratory complications increase healthcare costs, because of longer hospital length of stay, unplanned admission to intensive care, hospital readmission and adverse discharge to a nursing home [11].

Scores have been specifically developed to identify patients at risk of ARDS or severe PPCs [83], including the surgical lung injury prediction 2 model (SLIP-2) [15] and the lung injury prediction score (LIPS) [16]. Other scores were generically developed for predicting all-types PPCs [7, 17–19, 83, 84]. It must be underlined that, in the emergency setting, patients who do not have increased risk of PPC when evaluated preoperatively may develop ARDS if desaturation or hemodynamic problems occur during the intraoperative period. Therefore, scores which include intraoperative factors could be more adequate, such as the LAS VEGAS score (Table 1) [18]. The most common complication during surgery is related to the need of hemodynamic support, by the use of vasoactive drugs or increased fluid administration (almost in 30% of patients and more frequently in high risk surgery), followed by respiratory problems, and desaturation [10].

A simpler stratification tool feasible at the bedside before emergency surgery is the early calculation of the SpO_2/ FiO_2 ratio within 6 h from hospital admission, which has shown to be independently correlated with ARDS development in patients at risk [20]. Several preventive strategies have been proposed to reduce the perioperative risk in patients undergoing non-urgent surgical procedures, such as smoking cessation and physical therapy [21]. However, these strategies cannot be applied to patients that require emergency procedures; therefore, risk stratification is essential in these patients. We believe and suggest that scores should be adopted and included in local hospital guidelines in the evaluation of the patient before surgical intervention to optimize the clinical and organizational pathways in the postoperative period.

Surgical procedure and timing

Emergency surgical procedures are by definition characterized by an elevated number of unpredictable factors that might precipitate patient's conditions. Therefore, modifiable risk factors should be identified and managed appropriately, including timing and choice of interventions [22].

Several surgical procedures and techniques are at higher risk, such as open versus laparoscopic, upper abdominal incision, longer procedures and those requiring general anaesthesia and neuromuscular blockade [7, 17, 23]. In a large cohort of surgical patients, emergency procedures performed during night-time were independently associated with higher incidence of intraoperative adverse events and PPCs [24]: this might suggest that delaying interventions when feasible might improve surgical outcomes.

While the choice of surgical procedure and timing is typically perceived as an exclusive prerogative of the surgeon, we recommend that these factors should be discussed in team, possibly opting for less invasive and shorter duration procedures and procrastinating non-emergency procedures [25].

Intraoperative management

Anaesthesia strategies in patients at risk of developing ARDS

No clear evidence is available concerning the ability of specific anaesthesia techniques to prevent the development of postoperative ARDS.

In 2016, a meta-analysis reported a non-significant trend towards less PPCs and complications in patients undergoing volatile general anaesthesia for non-cardiac surgery, as

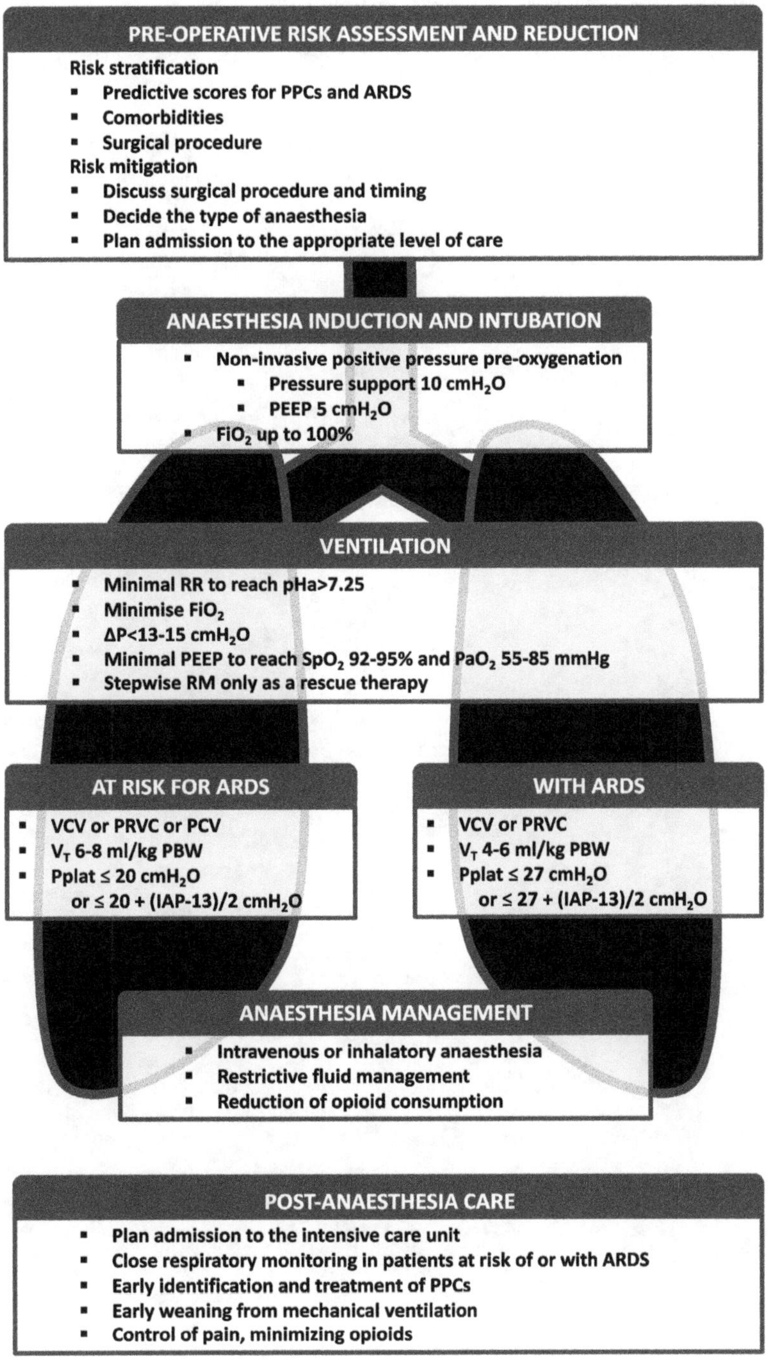

Fig. 1 summarises an overview of recommendations concerning the perioperative management of patients at risk of and with ARDS

compared with intravenous anaesthesia [26]. From a theoretical point of view, volatile agents can reduce pulmonary vasoconstriction, and carry a protective effect on ischaemia-reperfusion injury [27]. On the other hand, they can potentially reduce arterial oxygenation by causing myocardial depression and low cardiac output [28]. Therefore, we cannot conclude that volatile anaesthesia is associated with less PPC than intravenous anaesthesia.

The use of locoregional anaesthesia techniques is often advocated, based on the rationale that sparing sedative drugs avoids impairment of the respiratory function; however, this concept has been challenged in specific surgical populations [29]. Moreover, these techniques can rarely be used in emergency setting. Nonetheless, a potential beneficial effect on the incidence of postoperative pneumonia and respiratory failure has been shown

Table 1 resumes the principal scores used to predict postoperative respiratory complications

Clinical Variable	Canet J et al. 2010	Gupta H et al. 2011	Arozullah AM et al. 2000	LAS VEGAS investig. 2017	Bauman ZM et al. 2015 [16]	Kor DJ et al. 2011 [15]
Patient dependent						
Age	Yes	Yes	Yes	Yes	No	Yes
Dependent functional status	No	Yes	Yes	No	No	No
ASA score	No	Yes	No	Yes	No	No
Chronic obstructive pulmonary disease	No	Yes	Yes	No	No	Yes
Impaired sensorium	No	No	Yes	No	No	No
Cerebrovascular accident	No	No	Yes	No	No	No
Preoperative SpO_2	Yes	No	No	Yes	No	No
Transfusion > 4 units prior surgery	No	No	Yes	No	Yes	No
Significant weight loss	No	No	Yes	No	No	No
Preoperative sepsis	No	Yes	No	No	No	No
Preoperative anaemia	Yes	No	No	Yes	Yes	No
Blood urea nitrogen level	No	No	Yes	No	No	No
Recent respiratory infection	Yes	No	No	No	No	No
Relevant alcohol intake	No	No	Yes	No	Yes	Yes
Smoking before operation	No	Yes	Yes	No	Yes	Yes
Chronic steroid use	No	No	Yes	No	No	No
Cancer	No	No	No	Yes	No	No
Obstructive sleep apnoea	No	No	No	Yes	No	No
Hypoalbuminemia	No	No	No	No	No	No
Chemotherapy	No	No	No	No	Yes	Yes
Diabetes mellitus	No	No	No	No	Yes	Yes
Acidosis	No	No	No	No	Yes	No
Obesity	No	No	No	No	Yes	Yes
$FiO_2 > 0.35$ (or > 4 L/min)	No	No	No	No	Yes	No
Tachypnoea	No	No	No	No	Yes	No
Sepsis	No	No	No	No	Yes	No
Aspiration	No	No	No	No	Yes	No
Shock	No	No	No	No	Yes	No
High risk trauma	No	No	No	No	Yes	No
BMI	No	No	No	No	Yes	No
Amiodarone	No	No	No	No	Yes	Yes
Statins	No	No	No	No	No	Yes
ACE-I/ARB	No	No	No	No	No	Yes
Sex	No	No	No	No	No	Yes
Restrictive lung disease	No	No	No	No	No	Yes
GERD	No	No	No	No	No	Yes
Cirrhosis	No	No	No	No	No	Yes
Procedure dependent						
Elective or emergency procedure	Yes	Yes	Yes	Yes	No	No
Duration of surgery	Yes	Yes	Yes	Yes	No	No
Type of surgical procedure	Yes	Yes	Yes	No	Yes	Yes
Type of anaesthesia	No	No	No	Yes	No	No
Use of supraglottic device	No	No	No	Yes	No	No
Desaturation	No	No	No	Yes	No	No
Need of vasoactive drugs	No	No	No	Yes	No	No
Mechanical ventilation characteristics	No	No	No	Yes	No	No
Validation						
Prospective external validation	Yes	No	No	Yes	No	Yes

ASA American Society of Anesthesiologists, *BMI* Body mass index, *ACE-I* Angiotensin converting enzyme inhibitors, *ARB* Angiotensin receptor blockers, *GERD* Gastro-esophageal reflux disease when general anaesthesia plus neuraxial blockade techniques are used in conjunction, especially in thoracic, abdominal and lower-limb procedures and in patients with pre-existing pulmonary disease [30]. There is a rationale suggesting the use of a peripheral nerve block when possible, thus avoiding the use of general anaesthesia and opioid consumption. Therefore, PPC may reduce, however further studies are required to corroborate these data [31]. Phrenic nerve palsy and pneumothorax are a rare but important side effects of upper-limb locoregional approaches, thus limiting their use in in frail patients [32]. In short, we cannot conclude that regional anaesthesia may result in less complications than general anaesthesia [29]. In patients with established ARDS admitted to the ICU who require emergency surgery, the same sedative drugs used for sedation in the ICU can be maintained as well as mechanical ventilation strategies, increasing the dose of narcotics and analgesics during the surgical procedure [33].

We recommend careful choice of anaesthesia technique in all patients undergoing emergency surgery, avoiding general anaesthesia if possible.

Intubation for general anaesthesia

Patients with established ARDS often come to the operating room already intubated and mechanically ventilated. However, the anaesthesiologist might face the challenge of managing the airway of critically ill patients also in the operating room. The team must be prepared for gas exchange impairment during induction: the intubation procedure must be performed swiftly, with readily available second choice and emergency devices. Video-laryngoscope might offer some advantage as first-choice device, but requires specific training [34]. Haemodynamic impairment should also be expected in critically ill patients, therefore, invasive monitoring, fluids and vasoactive drugs should be readily available [35].

Preoxygenation with non-invasive positive pressure improves end-expiratory lung volume and gas-exchange, allowing more time for a safe airway management procedure [36]. Before intubation, a brief period of pre-oxygenation, using pressure support of 10 cmH_2O and PEEP of 5 cmH_2O, as initial parameters, have been suggested. Moreover, in the emergency setting, FiO_2 levels dispensed to the patients during pre-oxygenation should be up to 100%, especially in those with impaired respiratory function [37]: in this setting, the potential harms of hyperoxia are largely overwhelmed by the advantages of increasing the time-to-desaturation [38]. In all patients, orotracheal intubation should be performed using an endotracheal tube of the largest possible diameter according to the gender and size of the patient, to decrease the resistance of the airway and favour secretions management [39]. Respiratory outcome may also be negatively influenced by inadequate airway secretion clearance and aspiration of pharyngeal or gastric secretions, especially in the emergency setting [40].

Intraoperative mechanical ventilation in patients with or at risk of ARDS

There is lack of evidence regarding the best ventilator settings in patients with or at risk of ARDS in the specific setting of emergency surgery. However, optimization of mechanical ventilation with the use of protective ventilation is important to minimize VILI and improve outcome in patients with ARDS [41] and those at risk of ARDS undergoing surgical procedures [42].

While tidal volume (V_T) size reduction is a widely accepted strategy to reduce VILI in ARDS [43] and surgical [44] patients, other ventilation parameters are under debate. There are controversies concerning the use of high PEEP levels [45] to open the lungs based on findings of physiological [46] and clinical studies [47]. In fact, authors question the beneficial effects of lung recruitment in both ARDS patients [48] and those at risk of ARDS [49]. They suggested keeping lung resting if atelectasis is tolerated and oxygenation is kept under acceptable values.

Ventilation modes and spontaneous breathing

Volume- (VCV) or pressure-controlled (PCV) mode can be applied unrestrictedly in ARDS patients with no influence on outcome [50], and no clear advantage in surgical patients [42]. However, observational data concerning patients at risk of developing PPCs showed that, during surgery, VCV might offer more benefits than PCV [51]. Alternative modes of mechanical ventilation include airway pressure release ventilation and high frequency ventilation, but the lack of outcome data preclude a recommendation on their routine use [35]. While spontaneous breathing activity should be suppressed in severe ARDS, it might have a protective role in mild ARDS [52] and high risk of ARDS surgical patients.

Tidal volume and plateau pressure during surgery

Over the last years, the concept of protective mechanical ventilation-including the use of low V_T to minimize barotrauma and lung injury and maintain low plateau pressure (Pplat), lower driving pressure (ΔP) with moderate levels of PEEP and the use of recruitment manoeuvres (RM) has gained particular attention, showing a positive effect on the reduction of PPCs as well as improvement outcome in ARDS patients [53] and those at risk of ARDS undergoing surgical procedures [44].

In patients with ARDS, it is recommended to maintain V_T of 6 ml/kg predicted body weight (PBW) [53]. However, V_T as low as 4–5 ml/kg, could be preferable if an adequate gas exchange is ensured, and does not increase the risk of atelectasis [54]. In fact, a small RCT showed that atelectasis do not increase with low tidal volumes and without PEEP during surgery [55]. On the other hand, a recent clinical trial comparing 4–6 ml/kg to 8–10 ml/kg PBW, and keeping a plateau pressure below 21 cmH_2O found no benefit from lower V_T, in terms of ventilator-free days, hospital stay and mortality in critically ill patients without ARDS [56]. Nonetheless, tidal volume is considered the main determinant of ventilator-induced lung injury and should be targeted to maintain plateau pressure < 30 cmH_2O and low $\Delta P < 15$ cmH_2O. In patients with increased intra-abdominal pressure, higher values might be tolerated, correcting the upper thresholds as $P_{plat\ target,\ corrected} = Pplat_{target} + (IAP - 13)/2$ [57].

A recent experimental study in rats, investigating the impact of different V_T levels and respiratory rates on lung function, found that V_T was able to predict important increase in the alveolar inflammatory markers, and even maintaining low mechanical power, high V_T resulted in VILI [58].

In surgical patients at risk of ARDS, higher thresholds of V_T and lower ΔP are often considered acceptable compared to ARDS patients [42], but we recommend using the lowest pressures and volumes able to keep gas-exchange in a safe range.

Inspired fraction of oxygen

Inspired fraction of oxygen should aim to maintain SpO_2 between 88 and 95% in ARDS [59] and above 92% in at risk of ARDS surgical patients [42]: higher thresholds might result in hyperoxia especially in at risk of ARDS patients, with potential detrimental effects on alveolar damage, endothelial inflammation and mitochondrial dysfunction through increasing oxidative stress and direct lung injury [60, 61]. If during surgery hypoxemia develops, FiO_2 should be increased, followed by increase of PEEP and then stepwise recruitment manoeuvres. However, high oxygen levels during surgery can cause high risk of major respiratory complications.

Although further research on the effects of hyperoxia is needed, we suggest to target FiO_2 levels to normoxaemia in all surgical patients undergoing emergency procedures [60].

PEEP titration in patients with or at risk of ARDS undergoing emergency surgery

Level of PEEP is another relevant component of lung protective ventilation. In patients with ARDS undergoing surgery, PEEP choice should be guided by the ARDS network low PEEP table [43], while latest clinical trials performed in at risk of ARDS surgical patients demonstrated that the application of low tidal volume (6–8 ml/kg) and low PEEP (< 2 cmH_2O) reduce the risk of developing PPCs and of haemodynamic impairment [62]. No strategy for PEEP titration was demonstrated to be superior to the low PEEP ARDS network table, and experts recently made a recommendation for high PEEP (≥15 cmH_2O) only in patients with moderate to severe ARDS, as rescue strategy [48, 53]. In this context, recruiting the alveoli de-recruits the capillaries. Thus, at higher PEEP hemodynamic is impaired and vasoactive drugs and/or more fluids are needed, which can promote further lung injury in patients at risk and worsen lung function in ARDS patients.

Patients with established ARDS previously admitted to the ICU should continue the protective ventilation received in the intensive care setting, a strategy now made feasible by modern anaesthesia machines [63]. Therefore, we suggest that PEEP should be considered as a tool to maintain oxygenation between 88 and 95%. We recommend using the minimal PEEP level ensuring adequate gas-exchange in all patients undergoing emergency surgery, considering higher PEEP levels only as rescue therapy in severe ARDS.

Recruitment manoeuvres

The effects of recruitment manoeuvres on clinical outcomes in patients with ARDS remain uncertain. Recruitment manoeuvres have received a conditional recommendation in patients with ARDS [53]; among them, stepwise manoeuvres are recommended [64]. However, the Alveolar Recruitment for ARDS trial (ART) comparing lung recruitment and titrated positive end-expiratory pressure compared with low PEEP in patients with ARDS showed an increased 28-day all-cause mortality in the maximal recruitment strategy [47]. In surgical patients without ARDS, recruitment manoeuvres reduced the incidence of PPCs only when combined with V_T reduction [62, 65], and in a recent report in obese patients [66] their use performed by squeezing the anaesthesia bag was associated with an increased incidence of PPCs. However, during laparoscopic surgery alveolar recruitment manoeuvres followed by positive end-expiratory pressure improved lung function and reduced postoperative pain [67].

We do not recommend a routine use of recruitment manoeuvres in patients with and without ARDS undergoing emergency surgical procedures, considering them only as a rescue strategy in the presence of refractory gas-exchange impairment.

Haemodynamic and fluid management

In patients at risk of developing ARDS, maintenance of an adequate tissue perfusion often requires a huge amount of fluids. However, fluid overload and positive balance in patients with ARDS increase extravascular lung water level and mortality [68]. Moreover, blood products transfusions can further increase the risk of ARDS and worsen endothelial lung damage. A restrictive fluid strategy should be therefore applied with haemoglobin trigger for transfusion of > 7 g/dl [69]. Albumin can be used to reduce fluid leakage from the capillary into the alveolus mediated by increased intravascular oncotic pressure. Moreover, in a state of shock, vasopressor could be considered to optimize mean arterial pressure avoiding fluid overload [70], in order to maintain a mean arterial pressure value greater than 65–70 mmHg, that is essential in patients with shock to provide organ perfusion. However, in ARDS patients this might be challenging because of the haemodynamic instability which often occurs during anaesthesia in this subgroup of patients. In addition, haemodynamic instability can be related to increased hypoxic pulmonary vascular resistance or due to the pathology itself. Systemic inflammation can have a direct negative effect on cardiac contractility and function, thus resulting in left ventricle impairment. Right heart failure is common, and its function could be further impaired by the application of mechanical ventilation with high PEEP and intrathoracic pressure with reduced preload. Moreover, right heart dilation could impair left ventricular filling and preload. Left ventricular dysfunction further increase pulmonary capillary hydrostatic pressure and subsequent extravascular lung water extravasation [68].

We recommend using a conservative fluid strategy and conservative transfusion threshold in both ARDS patients and those at risk of ARDS during emergency surgery. Patients with ARDS frequently have hemodynamic impairment requiring specific monitoring to target fluid, vasoconstrictors and inotropes administration. While pulmonary artery catheter (PAC) is the gold standard, its use in the ICU has dramatically decreased over the last decades; the use in the OR is limited to very specific settings, such as cardiac surgery or surgery in patients already admitted to the ICU with a PAC previous placed. Although PAC has been almost abandoned both in OR and ICU, it remains an excellent instrument for the diagnosis and management of several critically illness like pulmonary hypertension, cardiogenic shock and unexplained dyspnea [71].

Modern minimally invasive monitoring systems have replaced its use, but have several limitations [72]. Basic monitoring requires an arterial line, while more critical patients might benefit from non-calibrated or calibrated pulse contour monitors, to estimate cardiac output and vascular resistances. Chest ultrasound can investigate both the lungs and the cardiac function, and is increasingly being used in the emergency setting [73], helping to discriminate between respiratory and cardiac causes of gas exchange impairment, and to detect pulmonary hypertension or right ventricular failure, often reported in ARDS patients [74].

Pharmacologic strategies

Regarding the pharmacological intraoperative management, neuromuscular blocking agents should be used cautiously in patients who can be extubated after surgery, because if not appropriately reversed could result in postoperative residual curarisation and increased incidence of PPCs [2]. Furthermore, Kirmeier E. et al. found that the association between the use of neuromuscular blocking agents and PPCs is probably dose-independent, and even a single dose such as that used for intubation could promote respiratory function impairment [23]. Avoidance or limited use of opioids is feasible in most surgical procedures, and might offer benefits in particular in patients at high risk but planned for extubation after surgery [75], in obese patients and those with suspected or confirmed obstructive sleep apnoea syndrome [76].

Postoperative management

Planned ICU admission is suggested after emergency surgery that is associated to higher risk of complications, but criteria are poorly standardised and planned ICU admission was not associated with better outcome in elective surgery [77]. While ICU admission is obvious for ARDS patients, criteria for planned or unplanned admission in subjects at risk of ARDS undergoing emergency surgery are less clear. Specific indications to ICU admission could be based on clinical reasoning, mechanical ventilation requirement, need for respiratory and cardiac monitoring, difficult glycaemic control, intraoperative surgical or anaesthetic complications and organ failure [78].

To decrease the risk of respiratory complications, there are several postoperative strategies that could be adopted: head-up or sitting position, encouragement of deep breathing exercises, early mobilization, intensive physiotherapy, incentive spirometry [79], airway toilette careful fluid management and an adequate opioid-sparing analgesia. However, high-quality evidence for these strategies is lacking in both elective and emergency surgery. Non-invasive positive pressure ventilation can be used to treat early mild ARDS, but its role as prophylactic measure in patients with previously healthy lungs at risk of ARDS is unclear [80].

Pulmonary infections and pneumonia are the most common cause of pulmonary ARDS [81]. Early recognition of underlying respiratory infections and pneumonia should include the identification of the causative pathogens, with eventually early empiric antibiotic therapy and subsequent de-escalation to directed therapy in patients with sepsis [82]. They may need intensive treatments that require the critical care setting.

When ARDS is established, it should be managed according to international guidelines, and while treating the underlying conditions, when identifiable. Continuous monitoring of vital parameters after surgery allows prompt identification of complications at their earlier stage, in particular pulse oximetry which is still underused [23].

Conclusions

ARDS is a life-threatening condition, which can occur in the perioperative period in the critically ill surgical patients. Early recognition and treatment are necessary in this context to reduce mortality and morbidity. Specific intraoperative anaesthesiologic management and in particular the use of lung protective ventilation are first line strategies to meet the goals of alveolar protection and avoid further lung damage. Preventive strategies including a careful risk stratification of the patients and preoperative optimization of the clinical conditions, can significantly reduce the occurrence of pulmonary complications and prevent the development of ARDS. Patients at high risk or already affected by ARDS should be managed in the intensive care unit in the postoperative phase.

Abbreviation

ARDS: Acute respiratory distress syndrome; DP: Driving pressure; ICU: Intensive care unit; LIP: Lung injury prediction score; PBW: Predicted body weight; PCV: Pressure-controlled ventilation; PEEP: Positive end-expiratory pressure; PPC: Postoperative pulmonary complication; Pplat: Plateau pressure; RM: Recruitment manoeuvre; SLIP-2: Surgical lung injury prediction 2 model; VCV: Volume-controlled ventilation; VILI: Ventilator-induced lung injury; V_T: Tidal volume

Acknowledgements

None

Authors' contributions

PP, CR, LB designed this review. CR, LB, DB drafted the manuscript. PP, MGA, PR revised the manuscript. All the authors approved the final version of this manuscript.

Author details

[1]Anaesthesia and Intensive Care, IRCCS for Oncology and Neurosciences, San Martino Policlinico Hospital, Genoa, Italy. [2]Department of Surgical Sciences and Integrated Diagnostics, University of Genoa, Genoa, Italy. [3]Laboratory of Pulmonary Investigation, Carlos Chagas Filho Institute of Biophysics, Federal University of Rio de Janeiro, Rio de Janeiro, Brazil. [4]Department of Anaesthesiology and Intensive Care Medicine, Pulmonary Engineering Group, University Hospital Carl Gustav Carus, Technische Universität Dresden, Dresden, Germany.

References

1. Aakre BM, Efem RI, Wilson GA, Kor DJ, Eisenach JH. Postoperative acute respiratory distress syndrome in patients with previous exposure to bleomycin. Mayo Clin Proc. 2014;89:181–9.
2. Ball L, Battaglini D, Pelosi P. Postoperative respiratory disorders. Curr Opin Crit Care. 2016;22:379–85.
3. The ARDS Definition Task Force, Ranieri V, Rubenfeld G, Thompson B, Ferguson N, Caldwell E, et al. ARDS Guidelines JAMA 2012-ARDS the Berlin definition. Jama. 2012;307:1.
4. Gattinoni L, Pelosi P, Pesenti A, Brazzi L, Vitale G, Moretto A, et al. CT scan in ARDS: clinical and physiopathological insights. Acta Anaesthesiol Scand. 1991;35:87–96.
5. Wheeler AP, Bernard GR. Acute lung injury and the acute respiratory distress syndrome : a clinical review. Lancet. 2007;369:1553–65.
6. Neto AS, Hemmes SNT, Barbas CSV, Beiderlinden M, Fernandez-bustamante A, Futier E, et al. Incidence of mortality and morbidity related to postoperative lung injury in patients who have undergone abdominal or thoracic surgery : a systematic review and meta-analysis. Lancet Respir. 2014;2:1007–15.
7. Neto AS, da Costa LGV, Hemmes SNT, Canet J, Hedenstierna G, Jaber S, et al. The LAS VEGAS risk score for prediction of postoperative pulmonary complications: an observational study. Eur J Anaesthesiol. 2018;35:691–701.
8. Pickering BW, Dong Y, Ahmed A, Giri J, Kilickaya O, Gupta A, et al. The implementation of clinician designed , human-centered electronic medical record viewer in the intensive care unit : A pilot step-wedge cluster randomized trial. Int J Med Inform. 2015;84:299–307.
9. Ahmed AH, Thongprayoon C, Schenck LA, Malinchoc M, Konvalinová A, Keegan MT, et al. Adverse in-hospital events are associated with increased in-hospital mortality and length of stay in patients with or at risk of acute respiratory distress syndrome. Mayo Clin Proc. 2015;90:321–8.
10. Nightingale CE, Margarson MP, Shearer E, Redman WJ, Lucas DN, Cousin JM, et al. Peri-operative management of the obese surgical patient 2015. Anaesthesia. 2015;70:859–76.
11. Eikermann M, Santer P, Pandit J, Dahan A. Recent advances in understanding and managing postoperative respiratory problems. F1000Res. 2019;18:1–9.
12. Ball L, Hemmes SNT, Serpa Neto A, Bluth T, Canet J, Hiesmayr M, et al. Intraoperative ventilation settings and their associations with postoperative pulmonary complications in obese patients. Br J Anaesth. 2018;121(4):899–908.
13. Ball L. Best Practice & Research Clinical Anaesthesiology Monitoring respiration : what the clinician needs to know. Best Pract Res Clin Anaesthesiol. 2013;27:209–23.
14. Schultz MJ, Hemmes SNT, Neto AS, Binnekade JM, Canet J, Hedenstierna G, et al. Epidemiology, practice of ventilation and outcome for patients at increased risk of postoperative pulmonary complications: LAS VEGAS - an observational study in 29 countries. Eur J Anaesthesiol. 2017;34:492–507.
15. Kor DJ, Warner DO, Alsara A, Fernandez-Perez ER, Malinchoc M, Kashyap R, et al. Derivation and diagnostic accuracy of the surgical lung injury prediction model. Anesthesiology. 2011;115:117–28.
16. Bauman ZM, Gassner MY, Coughlin MA, Mahan M, Watras J. Lung injury prediction score is useful in predicting acute respiratory distress syndrome and mortality in surgical critical care patients. Crit Care Res Pract. 2015;2015: 157408.
17. Canet J, Hardman J, Sabaté S, Langeron O, De Abreu MG, Gallart L, et al. PERISCOPE study: predicting post-operative pulmonary complications in Europe. Eur J Anaesthesiol. 2011;28:459–61.
18. Mazo V, Sabaté S, Canet J, Gallart L, De Abreu MG, Belda J, et al. Prospective external validation of a predictive score for postoperative pulmonary complications. Anesthesiology. 2014;121:219–31.
19. Arozullah AM, Khuri SF, Henderson WG, Daley J. Development and validation of a multifactorial risk index for predicting postoperative pneumonia after major noncardiac surgery. Ann Intern Med. 2001;135: 847–57.
20. Festic E, Banscal V, Kor DJ, Gajic O. US critical illness and injury trials group: lung injury prevention study investigators (USCIITG–LIPS). SpO 2 /FiO 2 ratio on hospital admission is an Indicator of early acute respiratory distress syndrome development among patients at risk. J Intensive Care Med. 2015; 30:209–16.
21. Boden I, Skinner EH, Browning L, Reeve J, Anderson L, Hill C, et al. Preoperative physiotherapy for the prevention of respiratory complications after upper abdominal surgery: pragmatic, double blinded, multicentre randomised controlled trial. BMJ. 2018;360:j5916.
22. Mullen MG, Michaels AD, Mehaffey JH, Guidry CA, Turrentine FE, Hedrick TL, et al. Risk associated with complications and mortality after urgent surgery vs elective and emergency surgery: implications for defining "quality" and reporting outcomes for urgent surgery. JAMA Surg. 2017;152:768–74.
23. Kirmeier E, Eriksson LI, Lewald H, Jonsson Fagerlund M, Hoeft A, Hollmann M, et al. Post-anaesthesia pulmonary complications after use of muscle relaxants (POPULAR): a multicentre, prospective observational study. Lancet Respir Med. 2018;7(2):129–40.
24. Cortegiani A, Gregoretti C, Neto AS, Hemmes SNT, Ball L, Canet J, et al. Association between night-time surgery and occurrence of intraoperative adverse events and postoperative pulmonary complications. Br J Anaesth.

2019;122:361–9.
25. Pelosi P, Ball L, Schultz MJ. How to optimize critical care resources in surgical patients : intensive care without physical borders. Curr Opin Crit Care. 2018;6:581–7.
26. Uhlig C, Bluth T, Schwarz K, Deckert S, Heinrich L, De Hert S, et al. Effects of volatile anesthetics on mortality and postoperative pulmonary and other complications in patients undergoing surgery. Anesthesiology. 2016;124: 1230–45.
27. Erturk E. Ischemia-reperfusion injury and volatile anesthetics. Biomed Res Int. 2014;2014.
28. Fujinaga T, Nakamura T, Fukuse T, Chen F, Zhang J, Ueda S, et al. Isoflurane inhalation after circulatory arrest protects against warm ischemia reperfusion injury of the lungs. Transplantation. 2006;82:1168–74.
29. Macfarlane AJR, Prasad GA, Chan VWS, Brull R. Does regional anaesthesia improve outcome after total hip arthroplasty ? A systematic review. Br J Anaesth. 2009;103:335–45.
30. Pöpping DM, Elia N, Marret E, Remy C, Tramèr MR. Protective effects of epidural analgesia on pulmonary complications after abdominal and thoracic surgery: a meta-analysis. Arch Surg. 2008;143:990–9.
31. Mills GH. Respiratory complications of anaesthesia. Anaesthesia. 2018;73:25–33.
32. Brull MHR, Macfarlane AJR. Regional anaesthesia and outcomes. BJA Educ. 2018;18:52–6.
33. Van Woerden G, Van Den Brand CL, Den Hartog CF, Idenburg FJ, Grootendorst DC, Van Der Linden MC. Increased analgesia administration in emergency medicine after implementation of revised guidelines. Int J Emerg Med. 2016;9:4.
34. Lewis SR, Butler AR, Parker J, Cook TM, Smith AF. Videolaryngoscopy versus direct laryngoscopy for adult patients requiring tracheal intubation. Cochrane Database Syst Rev. 2016;2016:CD011136.
35. Michard F, Giglio MT, Brienza N. Perioperative goal-directed therapy with uncalibrated pulse contour methods: impact on fluid management and postoperative outcome. Br J Anaesth. 2017;119:22–30.
36. Futier E, Constantin JM, Pelosi P, Chanques G, Massone A, Petit A, et al. Noninvasive ventilation and alveolar recruitment maneuver improve respiratory function during and after intubation of morbidly obese patients: a randomized controlled study. Anesthesiology. 2011;114:1354–63.
37. Wetterslev J, Meyhoff CS, Jørgensen LN, Gluud C, Lindschou J, Rasmussen LS. The effects of high perioperative inspiratory oxygen fraction for adult surgical patients. In: Cochrane database of systematic reviews. Wiley: Chichester, UK; 2015.
38. De Jong A, Futier E, Millot A, Coisel Y, Jung B, Chanques G, et al. How to preoxygenate in operative room: Healthy subjects and situations "at risk". Ann Fr Anesth Reanim. 2014;33:453–6.
39. Papazian L, Forel JM, Gacouin A, Penot-Ragon C, Perrin G, Loundou A, et al. Neuromuscular blockers in early acute respiratory distress syndrome. N Engl J Med. 2010;363:1107–16.
40. Miskovic A, Lumb AB. Postoperative pulmonary complications. Br J Anaesth. 2017;118:317–34.
41. Fan E, Del Sorbo L, Goligher EC, Hodgson CL, Munshi L, Walkey AJ, et al. An official American Thoracic Society/European society of intensive care medicine/society of critical care medicine clinical practice guideline: mechanical ventilation in adult patients with acute respiratory distress syndrome. Am J Respir Crit Care Med. 2017;195:1253–63.
42. Ball L, Costantino F, Orefice G, Chandrapatham K, Pelosi P. Intraoperative mechanical ventilation: state of the art. Minerva Anestesiol. 2017;83:1075–88.
43. Acute Respiratory Distress Syndrome Network, Brower RG, Matthay MA, Morris A, Schoenfeld D, Thompson BT, et al. Ventilation with lower tidal volumes as compared with traditional tidal volumes for acute lung injury and the acute respiratory distress syndrome. N Engl J Med. 2000;342:1301–8.
44. Serpa Neto A, Hemmes SNT, Barbas CSV, Beiderlinden M, Biehl M, Binnekade JM, et al. Protective versus conventional ventilation for surgery. Anesthesiology. 2015;123:66–78.
45. Lachmann B. Open up the lung and keep the lung open. Intensive Care Med. 1992;18:319–21.
46. Cressoni M, Chiumello D, Algieri I, Brioni M, Chiurazzi C, Colombo AA, et al. Opening pressures and atelectrauma in acute respiratory distress syndrome. Intensive Care Med. 2017;43:603–11.
47. Cavalcanti AB, Suzumura ÉA, Laranjeira LN, De Moraes PD, Damiani LP, Guimarães HP, et al. Effect of lung recruitment and titrated positive end-expiratory pressure (PEEP) vs low PEEP on mortality in patients with acute respiratory distress syndrome - a randomized clinical trial. JAMA. 2017;318: 1335–45.
48. Pelosi P, Rocco PRM, De Abreu MG. Close down the lungs and keep them resting to minimize ventilator-induced lung injury. Crit Care. 2018;22:72.
49. Pelosi P, Ball L, de Abreu MG, Rocco PRM. General anesthesia closes the lungs: keep them resting. Turk Anesteziyoloji ve Reanimasyon Dern Derg. 2016;44:163–4.
50. Chacko B, Peter JV, Tharyan P, John G, Jeyaseelan L. Pressure-controlled versus volume-controlled ventilation for acute respiratory failure due to acute lung injury (ALI) or acute respiratory distress syndrome (ARDS). Cochrane Database Syst Rev. 2015;1:CD008807.
51. Bagchi A, Rudolph MI, Ng PY, Timm FP, Long DR, Shaefi S, et al. The association of postoperative pulmonary complications in 109,360 patients with pressure-controlled or volume-controlled ventilation. Anaesthesia. 2017;72:1334–43.
52. Gama de Abreu M, Güldner A, Pelosi P. Spontaneous breathing activity in acute lung injury and acute respiratory distress syndrome. Curr Opin Anaesthesiol. 2012;25:148–55.
53. Del Sorbo L, Goligher EC, McAuley DF, Rubenfeld GD, Brochard LJ, Gattinoni L, et al. Mechanical ventilation in adults with acute respiratory distress syndrome. Summary of the experimental evidence for the clinical practice guideline. Ann Am Thorac Soc. 2017;14(Supplement_4):S261–70.
54. Güldner A, Kiss T, Serpa Neto A, Hemmes SNT, Canet J, Spieth PM, et al. Intraoperative protective mechanical ventilation for prevention of postoperative pulmonary complications. Anesthesiology. 2015;123:692–713.
55. Cai H, Gong H, Zhang L, Wang Y, Tian Y. Effect of low tidal volume ventilation on atelectasis in patients during general anesthesia: a computed tomographic scan. J Clin Anesth. 2007;19:125–9.
56. Simonis FD, Serpa Neto A, Binnekade JM, Braber A, Bruin KCM, Determann RM, et al. Effect of a low vs intermediate tidal volume strategy on ventilator-free days in intensive care unit patients without ARDS. JAMA. 2018;320:1872.
57. Pelosi P, Quintel M, Malbrain M. Effect of intra-abdominal pressure on respiratory mechanics. Acta Clin Belg. 2007;62(Suppl 1):78–88.
58. Moraes L, Silva PL, Thompson A, Santos CL, Santos RS, Fernandes MVS, et al. Impact of different tidal volume levels at low mechanical power on ventilator-induced lung injury in rats. Front Physiol. 2018;9:318.
59. Travis WD, Costabel U, Hansell DM, King TE, Lynch DA, Nicholson AG, et al. An official American Thoracic Society/European Respiratory Society statement: update of the international multidisciplinary classification of the idiopathic interstitial pneumonias. Am J Respir Crit Care Med. 2013; 188:733–48.
60. Robba C, Ball L, Pelosi P. Between hypoxia or hyperoxia: not perfect but more physiologic. J Thorac Dis. 2018;10(Suppl 17):S2052–4.
61. Staehr-Rye AK, Meyhoff CS, Scheffenbichler FT, Vidal Melo MF, Gätke MR, Walsh JL, et al. High intraoperative inspiratory oxygen fraction and risk of major respiratory complication. Br J Anaesth. 2017;1:140–9.
62. PROVE Network Investigators for the Clinical Trial Network of the European Society of Anaesthesiology, SNT H, Gama de Abreu M, Pelosi P, Schultz MJ. High versus low positive end-expiratory pressure during general anaesthesia for open abdominal surgery (PROVHILO trial): a multicentre randomised controlled trial. Lancet. 2014;384:495–503.
63. Ball L, Dameri M, Pelosi P. Modes of mechanical ventilation for the operating room. Best Pract Res Clin Anaesthesiol. 2015;29:285–99.
64. Santos RS, Silva PL, Pelosi P, Rocco PR. Recruitment maneuvers in acute respiratory distress syndrome: the safe way is the best way. World J Crit Care Med. 2015;4:278.
65. Futier E, Constantin J-M, Paugam-Burtz C, Pascal J, Eurin M, Neuschwander A, et al. A trial of intraoperative low-tidal-volume ventilation in abdominal surgery. N Engl J Med. 2013;369:428–37.
66. Ball L, Hemmes SNT, Neto AS, Bluth T, Canet J, Hiesmayr M, et al. Intraoperative ventilation settings and their associations with postoperative pulmonary complications in obese patients investigators 14, the PROVE Network 14, the Clinical Trial Network of the; 2018. p. 899–908.
67. Pasquier EK, Andersson E, Ph D. Pulmonary recruitment maneuver reduces pain after laparoscopic bariatric surgery: a randomized controlled clinical trial. Surg Obes Relat Dis. 2017:1–7.
68. Gattinoni L, Cressoni M, Brazzi L. Fluids in ARDS. Curr Opin Crit Care. 2014; 20:373–7.
69. Serpa Neto A, Juffermans NP, Hemmes SNT, Barbas CSV, Beiderlinden M, Biehl M, et al. Interaction between peri-operative blood transfusion, tidal volume, airway pressure and postoperative ARDS: an individual patient data meta-analysis. Ann Transl Med. 2018;6:23.

70. Uhlig C, Silva PL, Deckert S, Schmitt J, de Abreu MG. Albumin versus crystalloid solutions in patients with the acute respiratory distress syndrome: a systematic review and meta-analysis. Crit Care. 2014;18:R10.
71. Rapoport J, Teres D, Steingrub J, Higgins T, McGee W, Lemeshow S. Patient characteristics and ICU organizational factors that influence frequency of pulmonary artery catheterization. JAMA. 2000;283:2559–67.
72. Watson X, Cecconi M. Haemodynamic monitoring in the peri-operative period: the past, the present and the future. Anaesthesia. 2017;72:7–15.
73. Ball L, Vercesi V, Costantino F, Chandrapatham K, Pelosi P. Lung imaging: how to get better look inside the lung. Ann Transl Med. 2017;5:294.
74. Price S, Platz E, Cullen L, Tavazzi G, Christ M, Cowie MR, et al. Expert consensus document: echocardiography and lung ultrasonography for the assessment and management of acute heart failure. Nat Rev Cardiol. 2017; 14:427–40.
75. Sultana A, Torres D, Schumann R. Special indications for opioid free Anaesthesia and analgesia, patient and procedure related: including obesity, sleep apnoea, chronic obstructive pulmonary disease, complex regional pain syndromes, opioid addiction and cancer surgery. Best Pract Res Clin Anaesthesiol. 2017;31:547–60.
76. Beloeil H, Laviolle B, Menard C, Paugam-Burtz C, Garot M, Asehnoune K, et al. POFA trial study protocol: a multicentre, double-blind, randomised, controlled clinical trial comparing opioid-free versus opioid anaesthesia on postoperative opioid-related adverse events after major or intermediate non-cardiac surgery. BMJ Open. 2018;8:e020873.
77. Kahan BC, Koulenti D, Arvaniti K, Beavis V, Campbell D, Chan M, et al. Critical care admission following elective surgery was not associated with survival benefit: prospective analysis of data from 27 countries. Intensive Care Med. 2017;43:971–9.
78. Wang D, Carrano FM, Fisichella PM, Desiato V, Newman E, Berman R, et al. A quest for optimization of postoperative triage after major surgery. J Laparoendosc Adv Surg Tech. 2019;29:203–5.
79. do Nascimento Junior P, NSP M, Andrade S, MMF G, Braz LG, El Dib R. Incentive spirometry for prevention of postoperative pulmonary complications in upper abdominal surgery. Cochrane Database Syst Rev. 2014;2014:CD006058.
80. Ireland CJ, Chapman TM, Mathew SF, Herbison GP, Zacharias M. Continuous positive airway pressure (CPAP) during the postoperative period for prevention of postoperative morbidity and mortality following major abdominal surgery. Cochrane Database Syst Rev. 2014;2014:CD008930.
81. Rezoagli E, Fumagalli R, Bellani G. Definition and epidemiology of acute respiratory distress syndrome. Ann Transl Med. 2017;5:282.
82. Torres A, Niederman MS, Chastre J, Ewig S, Fernandez-Vandellos P, Hanberger H, et al. International ERS/ESICM/ESCMID/ALAT guidelines for the management of hospital-acquired pneumonia and ventilator-associated pneumonia. Eur Respir J. 2017;50:1700582.
83. Gajic O, Dabbagh O, Park PK, Adesanya A, Chang SY, Hou P, et al. Early Identification of Patients at Risk of Acute Lung Injury. Am J Respir Crit Care Med. 2011;183:462–70.
84. Gupta H, Gupta PK, Fang X, Miller WJ, Cemaj S, Forse RA, Morrow LE. Development and Validation of a Risk Calculator Predicting Postoperative Respiratory Failure. Chest. 2011;140(5):1207–15.

Comparison of surgical field visibility during propofol or desflurane anesthesia for middle ear microsurgery

Xia Yuan[†], Tingjie Liu[†], Chunbo Hu and Xia Shen[*]

Abstract

Background: To compare surgical field visibility between patients given propofol/remifentanil (PR) or desflurane/remifentanil (DR) anesthesia.

Methods: A total of 80 adult patients undergoing middle ear microsurgery due to cholesteatoma otitis media with American Society of Anesthesiologists physical status I and II were randomly assigned to the PR or DR groups. The depth of anesthesia was titrated to maintain a Bispectral index (BIS) between 40 and 50. Remifentanil was titrated to maintain the mean blood pressure within ±30% change of the pre-induction value. Surgical field visibility was rated at several timepoints by the surgeons using the Boezaart scores.

Results: Average Boezaart scores for surgical field visibility at different time points were < 2 in both PR and DR groups. Surgical field visibility score was lower in the PR group than in the DR group. Requirement for remifentanil was higher in the PR group (850 (488/1330) μg) than in the DR group (258 (143/399) μg, $P < 0.0001$). The site effect concentration of remifentanil was higher in the PR group (3.6(2.8/5.0)ng/ml) than in the DR group (1.7 (1.0/1.6) ng/ml, $P < 0.0001$). Hemodynamic profile (i.e., heart rate and mean blood pressure) was similar between groups ($P > 0.05$). Extubation time (PR group, 21 min vs. DR group, 19 min; $P = 0.199$) and post-anesthesia care unit time (PR group, 37 min vs. DR group, 34 min; $P = 0.324$) were comparable between groups.

Conclusion: Although PR anesthesia resulted in lower surgical field visibility scores than DR anesthesia, both groups had scores < 2, meaning no clinical differences between the two groups. DR provided acceptable operative conditions as well, albeit more remifentanil consumption was noted in the DR group.

Keywords: Anesthetics, inhalation, Desflurane, Anesthetics, intravenous, Propofol, Hypotension, controlled, Surgery, Otolaryngology

Background

Optimizing the visualization of anatomy during middle ear microsurgery can decrease the duration of surgery, reduce blood loss, and improve surgical outcomes [1]. Therefore, several procedures including head-up tilt maneuver, locally applied vasoconstriction, controlled hypotension [2], pharmacological agents [3], and manipulation of general anesthesia [4] have been employed to improve the visual quality of the surgical field.

Anesthetic agents can influence surgical field visibility and the amount of blood loss through pharmacological effects on vasodilation and heart rate. There is consensus that anesthesia with propofol provides better surgical field visibility and less blood loss than anesthesia with isoflurane or desflurane [5, 6]. Consistent with findings that surgical conditions are correlated with intraoperative heart rate rather than mean blood pressure [6–8], propofol anesthesia is associated with a lower intraoperative heart

* Correspondence: zlsx@yahoo.com
[†]Xia Yuan and Tingjie Liu contributed equally to this work.
Department of Anesthesiology, The Eye, Ear, Nose and Throat Hospital, Fudan University, 83 fenyang road, Shanghai 200031, China

rate and has been found to result in better surgical field visibility than inhalation anesthesia [6].

Desflurane possesses a very low blood-gas partition coefficient (0.45), allowing fast awakening and recovery [9]. It is commonly used during clinical practice to ensure efficient operating room management. However, desflurane tends to stimulate circulation (i.e., increase heart rate) and thus may not be appropriate for middle ear surgery, which demands optimal surgical field visibility. However, in our otology surgical center, desflurane is widely used with little complaint from surgeons regarding impaired surgical field visibility. To our knowledge, few studies have compared middle ear surgical field visibility between propofol/remifentanil (PR) and desflurane/remifentanil (DR) anesthesia. We hypothesized that propofol/remifentanil anesthesia may provide better surgical condition than desflurane/remifentanil anesthesia during middle ear microsurgery. Therefore, we conducted a double-blind, randomized controlled study to assess the effects of desflurane on surgical field visibility, intraoperative hemodynamic profile, and patient recovery from middle ear microsurgery.

Materials and methods

This study was registered in the Chinese Clinical Trial Registry (ChiCTR1800015537). The Institutional Review Board (Shanghai Eye, Ear, Nose, and Throat Hospital affiliated with Fudan University) approved the study procedures, and each enrolled patient provided written informed consent.

Adult patients with American Society of Anesthesiologists physical status I and II scheduled for middle ear surgery due to cholesteatoma otitis media were consecutively recruited. Patients were randomly assigned to the propofol/remifentanil (PR) or desflurane/remifentanil (DR) group by computer-generated allocation. Patients were excluded if they were receiving cardiovascularly active drugs or drugs related to coagulation (e.g., warferin, heparin, enoxiparin, NSAID or aspirin).

Upon arriving to the operating room, non-invasive monitoring of arterial blood pressure, pulse oximetry, electrocardiography, and bispectral index (BIS) monitoring (BIS VISTA Monitoring System; Aspect Medical Systems, Inc., Norwood, MA, USA) was established. Anesthesia was induced by intravenous 2 mg/kg propofol (Fresenius Kabi, Beijing, China), 0.3 µg/kg remifentanil (Yichang Renfu Pharmaceutical, Yichang, China), and 0.6 mg/kg rocuronium (Hameln Pharmaceuticals GmbH, Hameln, Germany). After flexible laryngeal mask insertion, anesthesia was maintained with propofol/remifentanil (PR) or desflurane/remifentanil (DR). Patients in the PR group received an effect site target-controlled infusion of propofol based on Schnider's pharmacokinetic model [10] and remifentanil based on Minto's model [11], delivered using a commercial pump (Orchestraw Base Primea, Fresenius Vial, Brezins, France). Effect site concentration was 2–6 µg/ml for propofol. For patients in the DR group, anesthesia was maintained with 4–8% desflurane. The effect site concentration of remifentanil was 1–8 ng/ml for both groups. Mean blood pressure was maintained within ±30% change of the pre-induction value. Ephedrine was needed for any decrease in mean blood pressure lower than 30% from the patient's pre-induction value.

Patients received mechanical ventilation in pressure-controlled mode with a tidal volume of 8 ml/kg at a rate of 10 breaths per min to provide an end-tidal CO_2 concentration of 35–45 mmHg. The carrier gas flow for both groups consisted of oxygen and air (FiO_2 0.5) during anesthesia maintenance. Intravenous 1 mg/kg parecoxib (Pfizer Pharmaceuticals, Beijing, China), and 0.01 mg/kg hydromorphone hydrochloride (Yichang Renfu Pharmaceutical) were given at the end of surgery for postoperative analgesia, and 0.15 mg/kg ondansetron hydrochloride and 0.1 mg/kg dexamethasone were given to prevent postoperative nausea and vomiting.

Surgery was performed by one of three surgeons with subspecialty training in otology using a similar stepwise technique. The surgeons were blinded to the anesthesia type by shielding the vaporizer and propofol and remifentanil syrings. Patients' heads were positioned 15° higher than their bodies for the entire procedure. Attending surgeons who were blind to treatment group rated surgical field visibility from 0 to 5 according to the Boezaart grading scale where 0 denotes the best and 5 the worst visibility [12]. Surgical field visibility was recorded at four time points: skin incision, bone drilling, clearance of cholesteatoma, and laying of fascia. Hemodynamic profile was recorded at the following time points: arrival to the operating room, 10 min after skin incision, completion of drilling, completion of clearance of cholesteatoma, completion of laying of fascia, extubation, 10 min after extubation, and post-anesthesia care unit (PACU) discharge.

Anesthesia time was defined as the time from anesthesia induction to anesthetic discontinuation. After surgery, patients were transferred to the PACU for monitoring and management by an attending anesthesiologist who was blinded to the group assignment. This anesthesiologist was blinded to the study, as was the research assistant who recorded extubation time (time from the end of surgery to extubation), PACU time (time between extubation and achieving a modified Aldrete score [13] > 9), postoperative pain (visual analogue scale (VAS) from 0 to 10 with 0 = no pain and 10 = worst pain imaginable), and postoperative nausea and vomiting (PONV) episodes. If VAS score was > 4, a rescue analgesic (intravenous 0.01 mg/kg hydromorphone hydrochloride) was given. Intravenous (10 mg) metoclopramide was given when needed as an antiemetic.

The primary outcome was surgical field visibility. Secondary outcomes were requirement for remifentanil, hemodynamic profile, and recovery time. Based on a pilot study of 10 adult patients receiving DR anesthesia, mean surgical field visibility was 2 (standard deviation, 1) during clearance of the focal lesion during middle ear microsurgery. Based on an estimate of 40% improvement in surgical field visibility, we calculated that 40 patients in each group were needed to provide statistical power of 80% at a 5% significance level. Remifentanil usage is expressed as the median (first/third quartiles) and was analyzed using a Mann-Whitney rank sum test. Other continuous variables are expressed as mean ± standard deviation (SD) and were analyzed using Student's *t*-tests. Categorical data were analyzed using χ^2 tests or Fisher's exact tests. Repeated measures ANOVA was used to analyze changes in hemodynamic profiles (heart rate and mean blood pressure) over time. Statistical significance was set at $P < 0.05$.

Results

Eighty patients were enrolled in and completed the study (Fig. 1). Gender, age, height, weight, body mass index, anesthesia and surgery times, and distribution of the three surgeons were similar between PR and DR groups (Table 1).

Average surgical field visibility score was < 2 for both groups (Fig. 2). The PR group had lower surgical field visibility scores (i.e., better visibility) than the DR group during clearance of the focal lesion (1.22 vs. 1.85, P = 0.001). The surgical field visibility scores were also lower at skin incision, bone drilling, and laying of fascia in PR group, but the differences were not significant ($P > 0.05$).

Regarding hemodynamic profile, mean blood pressure was maintained within ±30% change of pre-induction values. Patients in both groups showed significant decreases in mean blood pressure during surgery (T_1–T_4), but there were no differences between groups ($P > 0.05$; Fig. 3). After surgery (T_5–T_7), mean blood pressure returned to baseline values. Heart rate also decreased during surgery (T_1–T_4) and returned to baseline values after surgery (T_5–T_7), with no differences between groups ($P > 0.05$).

Intraoperative BIS was comparable between groups ($P > 0.05$; Table 2). Patients in the PR group required more remifentanil than patients in the DR group (PR group, 850 (488/1330) μg vs. DR group, 258 (143/399) μg, $P < 0.0001$). The site effect concentration of remifentanil was higher in the PR group (PR group, 3.6(2.8/5.0) ng/ml vs. DR group, 1.7 (1.0/1.6) ng/ml, $P < 0.0001$). The mean propofol site effect concentration was 3.4 μg/ml. The

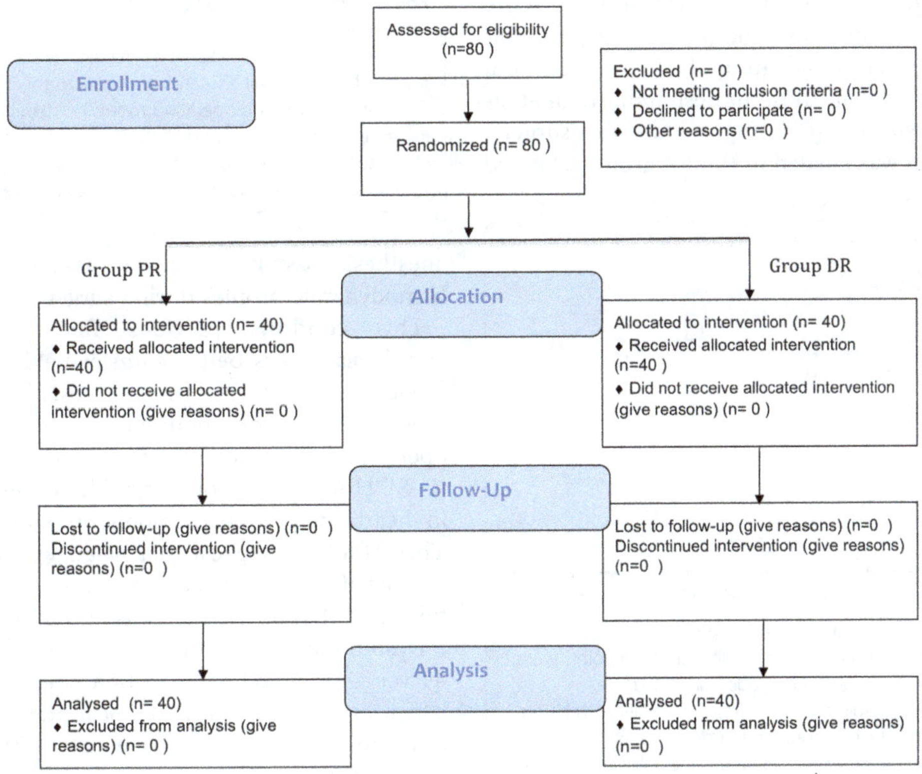

Fig. 1 CONSORT flow diagram. PR, propofol/remifentanil; DR, deflurane/remifentanil

Table 1 Demographic characteristics of patients

	Group PR ($n = 40$)	Group DR ($n = 40$)
Sex (M/F)	21/19	19/21
Age (yr)	43.1 (11.3)	45.7 (11.4)
Weight (kg)	66.4 (11.8)	63.9 (10.2)
Height (cm)	165.2 (7.1)	166.2 (8.0)
Body mass index (kg•m^{-2})	24.2 (3.5)	23.1 (2.8)
ASA classification (I/II)	30/10	32/8
Operator (1/2/3)	16/13/11	14/16/10
Surgery duration (min)	89.1 (34.4)	83.3 (33.0)
Anesthesia duration (min)	103.2 (36.1)	92.5 (31.0)
Baseline BIS value	97 (1)	97 (1)

Values are presented as mean ± standard deviation or number of patients. *PR* propofol/remifentanil, *DR* desflurane/remifentanil, *ASA* American Society of Anesthesiologists, *BIS* bispectral index

mean desflurane MAC was 0.8. Intraoperative ephedrine was required in a similar number of patients in each group ($P > 0.05$). Extubation time (PR group, 21 min vs. DR group, 19 min; $P = 0.199$) and PACU times (PR group, 37 min vs. DR group, 34 min; $P = 0.324$) were comparable between groups. One patient in each group required pain rescue in the PACU, respectively. No patient had PONV episodes in the PACU.

Discussion

We found that the average surgical field visibility score was < 2 for both groups while the patients in propofol/remifentanil (PR) anesthesia group had lower surgical field visibility scores than those in desflurane/remifentanil (DR) anesthesia group during middle ear surgery. More remifentanil was needed in the PR group. The two

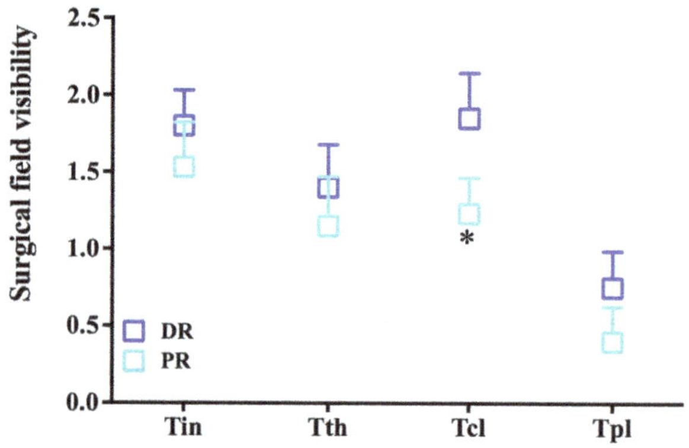

Fig. 2 Surgical field visibility at different time points. Average Boezaart scores for surgical field visibility at different time points were < 2 in both propofol/remifentanil (PR) group and desflurane/remifentanil (DR) group. Surgical field visibility was significantly better in the PR group than in the DR group during clearance of cholesteatoma. T_{in}, at skin incision; T_{dr}, during bone drilling; T_{cl}, during clearance of cholesteatoma; T_{pl}, during laying of fascia. *$P < 0.05$

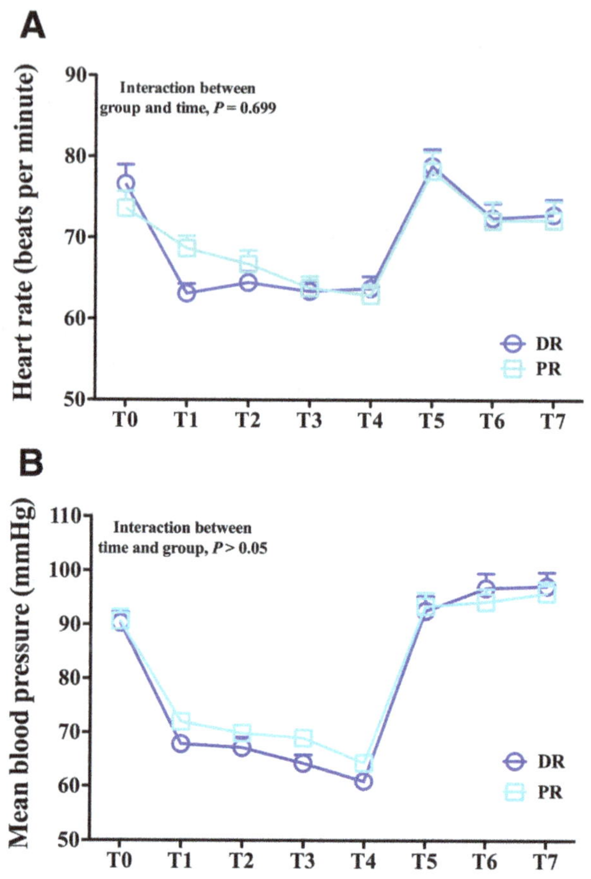

Fig. 3 Hemodynamic profile. Changes in (**a**) heart rate and (**b**) mean blood pressure at different time points. Repeated measures ANOVA showed no differences in hemodynamics over time between the propofol/remifentanil (PR) and desflurane/remifentanil (DR) groups. T_0, upon arrival in the operating room; T_1, 10 min after surgical incision; T_2, completion of drilling; T_3, completion of clearance of cholesteatoma; T_4, completion of laying fascia; T_5, at extubation; T_6, 10 min after extubation; T_7, at PACU discharge

anesthesia techniques were associated with similar hemodynamic profiles during surgery.

This confirms previous findings that propofol anesthesia allows better surgical field visibility and less blood loss than inhalation anesthesia [5, 6]. Some studies report that surgical conditions are correlated with intraoperative heart rate rather than mean blood pressure [6–8]. However, we found no differences between groups in heart rate or mean blood pressure during surgery. These findings suggest that when well controlled, heart rate itself is not the determination of operating conditions and that other mechanisms are in play.

Desflurane allows fast awakening and recovery due to its very low blood-gas partition coefficient (0.45) [9]. It is commonly used during clinical practice to ensure efficient operating room management. Although desflurane has been used for ear, nose, and throat surgery due to its beneficial effect on recovery [14], it tends to increase

Table 2 Perioperative variables

	Group PR ($n = 40$)	Group DR ($n = 40$)	P-value
Intraoperative			
Remifentanil dose (μg)	850 (488/1330)	258 (143/399)	< 0.0001
Remifentanil effect-site concentration (ng/ml)	3.6 (2.8/5.0)	1.7 (1.0/1.6)	< 0.0001
Propofol effect-site concentration (μg/ml)	3.4(0.6)		
Desflurane MAC		0.8 (0.1)	
Intraoperative BIS value	44 (0.3)	43 (0.3)	0.515
Ephedrine usage	9	6	0.568
PACU			
Extubation time (min)	21 ± 11	19 ± 6	0.199
PACU time (min)	37 ± 14	34 ± 8	0.324
Analgesic rescue	1	1	1
PONV episodes	0	0	1

Values are reported as mean ± standard deviation, median (first/third quartiles), or number of patients; *PR* propofol/remifentanil, *DR* desflurane/remifentanil, *BIS* bispectral index, *MAC* minimal alveolar concentration, *PACU* post-anesthesia care unit, *PONV* postoperative nausea and vomiting

heart rate more than 1 minimal alveolar concentration (MAC) [9]. In our study, the mean MAC of desflurane to maintain an appropriate depth of anesthesia (i.e., mean BIS value of 43) was 0.8. We did not observe an increase in heart rate in patients receiving desflurane, perhaps due to remifentanil usage, as opioids can eliminate the stimulatory effect of desflurane on the circulation system [9].

We routinely use remifentanil during middle ear surgery in our clinic because of its analgesic effect and reduction of middle ear blood flow, consistent with Degoute et al. [15, 16]. Degoute et al. found that remifentanil/propofol anesthesia was effective in reducing middle ear blood flow and providing good surgical conditions for adult patients during tympanoplasty in a small sample size study [15]. Later they found that when combined with sevoflurane, an inhalation anesthesia, remifentanil enabled controlled hypotension, reduced middle ear blood flow and provided good surgical conditions for middle ear surgery in children [16]. In our study, although PR anesthesia produced lower surgical field visibility scores than DR anesthesia, average surgical field visibility score was < 2 under DR anesthesia, meaning no clinical difference between the two groups. According to Boezaart grading scale [12], score of 2 means slight bleeding, occasional suctioning required, and surgical field not threatened. These findings suggest that DR anesthesia is applicable for middle ear surgery and can explain why, in our otology surgical center, surgeons seldom complain of impaired surgical visibility during desflurane usage.

It is now well accepted that intraoperative blood pressure may not be correlated with bleeding at the surgical site. Hypotension alone may not improve surgical field visibility [6, 17]. By contrast, hypotension is often associated with peripheral vasodilation, which might increase bleeding and the risk of organ ischemia [12]. Therefore, we maintained mean blood pressure within ±30% change of pre-induction values in both groups. However, patients in the DR group required less remifentanil than those in the PR group, it is more likely that the reduced remifentanil requirement in the desflurane group was due to the far more potent analgesic contribution of desflurane compared with propofol, which has primarily sedative hypnotic (and minimal analgesic) effects.

Our study has some limitations. First, we did not measure blood loss, as middle ear surgery rarely results in massive blood loss. Second, subjective assessment of surgical field visibility makes comparisons to previous studies difficult. Third, we did not measure blood flow in the middle and inner ear during controlled hypotension. However, Degoute et al. [15] reports that remifentanil reduces middle ear blood flow by 25% as measured by laser Doppler flowmetry. Fourth, whether ear infection is present is a major predictor of surgical field visibility. Thus, further studies are needed to understand the effects of anesthetic agents on surgical field visibility in chronic suppurative otitis media patients undergoing middle ear surgery. Finally, due to the study population these results are limited to adults the findings in our study might require further confirmation in children.

Conclusion

Although there is a statistically significant difference between propofol-remifentanil and desflurane-remifentanil groups with regard to surgical field visibility according to the Boezaart grading scale, when remifentanil is used in combination with desflurane, similar operative conditions are achieved. The requirement for remifentanil is greater in the desflurane-remifentanil group.

Abbreviations
BIS: Bispectral index; HR: Heat beat; LOC: Loss of consciosness; MAP: Mean blood pressure; PACU: Post-anesthesia care unit; PONV: Postoperative nausea and vomiting

Acknowledgements
The authors thank the anesthesiologists, surgeons, and anesthesia assistants at The Eye, Ear, Nose and Throat Hospital of Fudan University who participated in this study.

Authors' contributions
YX and LTJ wrote the manuscript and were involved in data gathering, analysis, and interpretation. They made equal contribution. HCB was involved in data gathering. SX conceived of the study, and participated in its design and coordination and the drafting of manuscript. All authors read and approved the final manuscript.

References
1. Richa F, Yazigi A, Sleilaty G, Yazbeck P. Comparison between dexmedetomidine and remifentanil for controlled hypotension during tympanoplasty. Eur J Anaesthesiol. 2008;25(5):369–74.
2. Degoute CS, Dubreuil C, Ray MJ, Guitton J. J, Manchon M, BanssillonV, Saumet JL. Effects of posture, hypotension and locally applied vasoconstriction on the middle ear microcirculation in anaesthetized humans. Eur J Appl Physiol Occup Physiol. 1994;69(5):414–20.
3. Degoute CS. Controlled hypotension: a guide to drug choice. Drugs. 2007;67(7):1053–76.
4. Khosla AJ, Pernas FG, Maeso PA. Meta-analysis and literature review of techniques to achieve hemostasis in endoscopic sinus surgery. Int Forum Allergy Rhinol. 2013;3(6):482–7.
5. Manola M, De Luca E, Moscillo L, Mastella A. Using remifentanil and sufentanil in functional endoscopic sinus surgery to improve surgical conditions. ORL J Otorhinolaryngol Relat Spec. 2005;67(2):83–6.
6. Ahn HJ, Chung SK, Dhong HJ, et al. Comparison of surgical conditions during propofol or sevoflurane anaesthesia for endoscopic sinus surgery. Br J Anaesth. 2008;100(1):50–4.
7. Nair S, Collins M, Hung P, Rees G, Close D, Wormald PJ. The effect of beta-blocker premedication on the surgical field during endoscopic sinus surgery. Laryngoscope. 2004;114(6):1042–6.
8. Eberhart LH, Folz BJ, Wulf H, Geldner G. Intravenous anesthesia provides optimal surgical conditions during microscopic and endoscopic sinus surgery. Laryngoscope. 2003;113(8):1369–73.
9. Pardo MC Jr., Miller RD. Basics of anesthesia. 7th Ed. Chaper 7.:inhaled anesthetics, p83–103. Elsevier publishing.
10. Schnider TW, Minto CF, Shafer SL, Gambers P, Andresen C. The influence of age on propofol pharmacodynamics. Anesthesiology. 1999;90(6):1502–16.
11. Minto CF, Schnider TW, Egan TD, Youngs E, Lemmens HJM. Influence of age and gender on the pharmacokinetics and pharmacodynamics of remifentanil: I. model development. Anesthesiology. 1997;86(1):10–23.
12. Boezaart AP, van der Merwe J, Coetzee A. Comparison of sodium nitroprusside- and esmolol-induced controlled hypotension for functional endoscopic sinus surgery. Can J Anaesth. 1995 (5Pt 1);42:373–6.
13. Aldrete JA. The post-anaesthesia recovery score revisited. J Clin Anesth. 1995;7(1):89–91.
14. Loop T, Priebe HJ. Recovery after anesthesia with remifentanil combined with propofol,desflurane,or sevoflurane for otorhinolaryngeal surgery. Anesth Analg. 2000;91(1):123–9.
15. Degoute CS, Ray MJ, Manchon M, Dubreuil C, Banssillon V. Remifentanil and controlled hypotension; comparison with nitroprusside or esmolol during tym- panoplasty. Can J Anesth. 2001;48:20–7.
16. Degoute CS, Ray MJ, Gueugniaud PY, Dubreuil C. Remifentanil induces consistent and sustained controlled hypotension in children during middle ear surgery. Can J Anesth. 2003;50(3):270–6.
17. Ar K. Anaesthesia with profound hypotension for middle ear surgery. Br J Anaesth. 1977;49(5):447–52.

The effect of 1% glucose loading on metabolism in the elderly patients during remifentanil-induced anesthesia

Kohei Fukuta[1*], Asuka Kasai[1], Noriko Niki[1], Yuki Ishikawa[1], Ryosuke Kawanishi[1], Nami Kakuta[1], Yoko Sakai[1], Yasuo M. Tsutsumi[2] and Katsuya Tanaka[1]

Abstract

Background: Previous studies showed that remifentanil-induced anesthesia can inhibit surgical stress response in non-diabetic adult patients and that low-dose glucose loading during anesthesia may attenuate fat catabolism. However, little is known about the influence of glucose loading on metabolism in elderly patients, whose condition may be influenced by decreased basal metabolism and increased insulin resistance. We hypothesized that, in elderly patients, intraoperative low glucose infusion may attenuate the catabolism of fat without causing harmful hyperglycemia during remifentanil-induced anesthesia.

Methods: Elderly, non-diabetic patients scheduled to undergo elective surgery were enrolled and randomized to receive no glucose (0G group) or low-dose glucose infusion (0.1 g/kg/hr. for 1 h followed by 0.05 g/kg/hr. for 1 h; LG group) during surgery. Glucose, adrenocorticotropic hormone (ACTH), 3-methylhistidine (3-MH), insulin, cortisol, free fatty acid (FFA), creatinine (Cr), and ketone body levels were measured pre-anesthesia, 1 h post-glucose infusion, at the end of surgery, and on the following morning.

Results: A total of 31 patients (aged 75–85) were included (0G, $n = 16$; LG, $n = 15$). ACTH levels during anesthesia decreased significantly in both groups. In the LG group, glucose levels increased significantly after glucose loading but hyperglycemia was not observed. During surgery, ketone bodies and FFA were significantly lower in the LG group than the 0G group. There were no significant differences in insulin, Cr, 3-MH, and 3-MH/Cr between the two groups.

Conclusion: Remifentanil-induced anesthesia inhibited surgical stress response in elderly patients. Intraoperative low-dose glucose infusion attenuated catabolism of fat without inducing hyperglycemia.

Keywords: Glucose, Metabolism, Elderly, Remifentanil

* Correspondence: kouhei_f_1983@yahoo.co.jp
[1]Department of Anesthesiology, Graduate School of Biomedical Sciences, Tokushima University, 3-18-15 Kuramoto, Tokushima 770-8503, Japan

Background

Glucose tolerance is decreased during surgery by catecholamines and stress hormones, such as cortisol and adrenocorticotropic hormone (ACTH) [1–4], and intraoperative hyperglycemia is a risk factor for postoperative complications and mortality [5–7]. Therefore, glucose solution is not generally infused during surgery, despite the fact that an energy deficit may lead to the catabolism of fats and/or proteins. Several studies show that remifentanil reduces the stress response during surgery [8–11]. We previously reported that anesthesia using remifentanil limits the surgical stress response in non-diabetic adult patients and that low-dose glucose loading during anesthesia may attenuate the catabolism of fat [12]. Sawada et al. also showed that intraoperative glucose infusion suppressed lipolysis and proteolysis in patients anesthetized with remifentanil [13].

It is reported that basal energy expenditure (EE) is negatively associated with age in subjects > 52 years old [14]. In addition, many studies have reported that insulin secretion decreasing and resistance increasing with age [15–18]. Elderly patients are, therefore, influenced by a decrease in basal metabolism and an increase in insulin resistance. These studies suggest that, while low-dose glucose loading during remifentanil-induced anesthesia may decrease stress hormone secretion and fat catabolism without causing hyperglycemia in adults, it may induce hyperglycemia in elderly patients. Currently, little is known about the effect of glucose loading on metabolism in elderly patients during remifentanil-induced anesthesia.

Here, we hypothesized that, in elderly patients, intraoperative low glucose infusion during remifentanil-induced anesthesia may attenuate the catabolism of fat without causing harmful hyperglycemia. To test this hypothesis, we examined the effects of glucose infusion on metabolism in elderly patients anesthetized with remifentanil.

Methods

Study design and patient selection

Elderly (aged 75–85 years), non-diabetic patients scheduled to undergo elective surgery in the Tokushima University Hospital between September 2015 and September 2016 were enrolled. Patients were required to have an American Society of Anesthesiologists physical status of 1 or 2 and a scheduled surgery duration of > 1 h. Obese (body mass index [BMI] > 30 kg/m^2) and emaciated (BMI < 17 kg/m^2) patients were excluded, as were those taking steroids or diagnosed with diabetes or thyroid disease. Patients requiring the use of a tourniquet or laparoscopy during surgery were also excluded from the final analysis. Homeostasis Model Assessment Insulin Resistance (HOMA-IR) was calculated by the formula: fasting insulin [μIU/ml] × fasting glucose [mg/dl] / 405. Eligible patients were randomized to receive no glucose (0G group) or a low-dose glucose infusion (0.1 g/kg/hr. for 1 h followed by 0.05 g/kg/hr.; LG group) during surgery.

The study was approved by Clinical Trial Center For Developmental Therapeutics of the Tokushima University Hospital, and the reference number was 2211–1. All participating subjects provided written informed consent. The study was registered with the University hospital Medical Information Network Center (http://www.umin.ac.jp/english/); ID: UMIN000016189.

Anesthesia management and study protocol

Patients were allowed to eat until 00:00 h on the day of surgery. Patients scheduled for surgery in the morning received 250 ml (200 kcal) of Arginaid Water® (Nestle Japan Ltd., Tokyo, Japan), and those scheduled in the afternoon received 500 ml (400 kcal) 2 h before anesthesia. The nutrient profiles of Arginaid Water® are shown in Table 1. No patients were premedicated.

On arrival in the operating room, a 20 G catheter was inserted into the forearm of each patient and bicarbonate Ringer's solution without glucose was infused. General anesthesia was induced by intravenous administration of thiamylal (3 mg/kg) and remifentanil (0.25–0.5 μg/kg/min), and maintained with sevoflurane (end-tidal sevoflurane ≥1.0%) and remifentanil (0.2–0.5 μg/kg/min). Muscle relaxation with 0.7 mg/kg rocuronium bromide was performed to facilitate tracheal intubation. Rocuronium bromide was administered intermittently, if required. All patients were maintenance of the BIS value between 40 to 60 during the surgery.

The study protocol is illustrated in Fig. 1. After tracheal intubation, the heat and moisture exchange filter was equipped with an S/5 compact monitor (GE Healthcare, Helsinki, Finland). The tidal volume was set at 7 ml/kg, the respiratory rate set with the aim of normocapnia, and the O_2/air mixture at FiO_2 0.5. Stable data

Table 1 Major nutrients in Arginaid Water®

Nutrients	Arginaid water 100 mL
Calories (kcal)	80
Moisture (g)	85.6
Arginine (g)	2.0
CHO (g)	18
Fat (g)	0
Sodium (mg)	0
Phosphate (mg)	140
Zinc (mg)	0.8
Copper (mg)	0.8

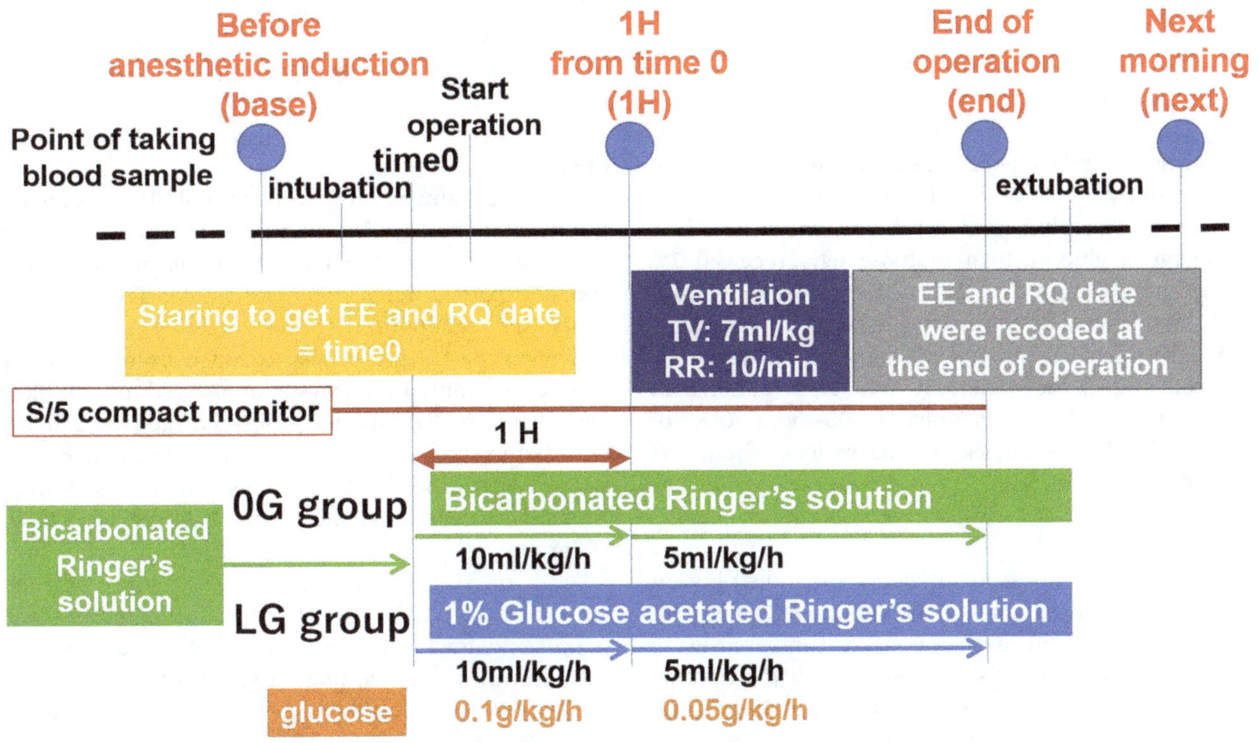

Fig. 1 Study protocol. EE, energy expenditure; RQ, respiratory quotient; TV, tidal volume; RR, respiratory rate

for respiratory quotient (RQ), oxygen consumption ($\dot{V}O_2$), carbon dioxide output ($\dot{V}CO_2$), and EE were obtained from the S/5 compact monitor within approximately 20 min (time 0). In the LG group, the solution was switched to 1% glucose acetated Ringer's solution at time 0, with the solution for both groups being initiated at 10 ml/kg/hr. for 1 h, followed by 5 ml/kg/hr. Therefore, in the LG group, glucose was taken at 0.1 g/kg/hr. for 1 h, followed by 0.05 g/kg/hr.

Measurements

Blood was sampled at baseline (introduction of anesthesia), 1 h after time 0, at the end of surgery, and the next morning. Glucose concentrations were measured using a blood glucose monitor (Medisafe Fit, TERUMO, Tokyo, Japan). Blood glucose concentrations > 200 mg/dl were defined as hyperglycemia in this study. Patients with blood glucose concentrations > 250 mg/dl were intravenously injected with 2 U insulin. Blood samples were centrifuged at 150 g at 4 °C for 10 min (Table Top cooling centrifuge 2800, Kubota, Tokyo, Japan), and plasma and serum samples were stored at − 20 °C until analysis. Plasma concentrations of glucose, ACTH, and 3-methylhistidine (3-MH) and serum concentrations of insulin, cortisol, free fatty acid (FFA), creatinine (Cr), and ketone bodies were analyzed. Plasma glucose was measured using the hexokinase method, plasma ACTH by an electro chemiluminescent immunoassay, and plasma 3-MH by high-performance liquid chromatography. Serum concentrations of FFA, ketone bodies, and Cr were measured enzymatically, serum insulin by a chemiluminescent enzyme immunoassay, and serum cortisol by a radioimmunoassay. RQ, $\dot{V}O_2$, $\dot{V}CO_2$, and EE were measured by the S/5 compact monitor and recorded at 30 min intervals until the end of surgery.

Randomization and blinding

We used a computer-generated distribution (QuickCalcs, GraphPad Inc., La Jolla, CA, USA) for randomly allocation. Anesthesiologists collecting intraoperative data were not blinded to group assignment, however, patients, surgeons and another anesthesiologist evaluating the date were blinded to group assignment.

Endpoints

The primary endpoint in the present study was the concentration of FFA. Secondary endpoints included the concentration of ketone bodies (i.e. lipid metabolism), the value of 3MH/Cr (i.e. protein catabolism), glucose and serum insulin concentrations (i.e. glucose metabolism), ACTH and serum cortisol concentrations (i.e.

stress hormone), and RQ (i.e. the energy source that they used).

Statistical analysis

The primary endpoint was the concentration of FFA. Our previous study reported that the concentration of FFA in adult patients at 2 h after the initiation of infusion was significantly higher in patients who received no intraoperative glucose than in those who received 1% glucose intraoperatively (840 ± 290 versus 510 ± 240 μEq/L, respectively) [12]. Anticipating that the mean difference between the groups during surgery would be 330 ± 260 μEq/L, the minimum number of patients in each group was 12, with an alpha of 0.05 and a power of 80% for FFA. We estimated that 32 patients should be included in this trial, with 16 patients in each group, because of possible dropouts and complications during surgery.

The Shapiro–Wilk test for fit with normal distribution was performed. In parametric data, differences between the time points within each group were compared using repeated-measures analysis of variance with the Bonferroni post hoc test. Parametric data at the same time points between the two groups of variables were analyzed by unpaired t-tests. In nonparametric data, differences between the time points within each group were compared using Friedman's test. Nonparametric data at the same time points between the two groups of variables were analyzed by the Mann–Whitney rank-sum test. Nominal scales were analyzed by the Chi-squared test. $P < 0.05$ was considered to be statistically significant. All statistical analyses were performed with SPSS version 20 (IBM, New York, NY, USA).

Results

Patient recruitment and flow through the protocol is summarized in Fig. 2. Although 34 patients were enrolled, one was excluded due to undiagnosed diabetes and one patient refused to participate. Thirty-two patients were randomized to the 0G and LG groups; one patient in the LG group was excluded from the analysis as a non-permitted fluid was administered to treat bleeding. Therefore, 31 patients completed the trial and were included in the analysis. The patients' demographic data and surgical procedures are shown in Tables 2 and 3. No notable differences were seen between the 0G and LG groups.

Levels of ACTH and cortisol at each study timepoint are shown in Fig. 3. ACTH levels during surgery were significantly lower than baseline in both groups (Fig. 3a).

As shown in Fig. 4a, plasma glucose levels in the LG group were significantly higher than those in the 0G group at 1 h ($P = 0.006$). At 1 h and at the end of surgery, plasma glucose levels were significantly higher than baseline levels in the LG group (1 h vs baseline: $P < 0.001$, the end of surgery vs baseline: $P = 0.043$). However, the highest glucose concentration in the LG group was 156 mg/dl and none of the patients in either group

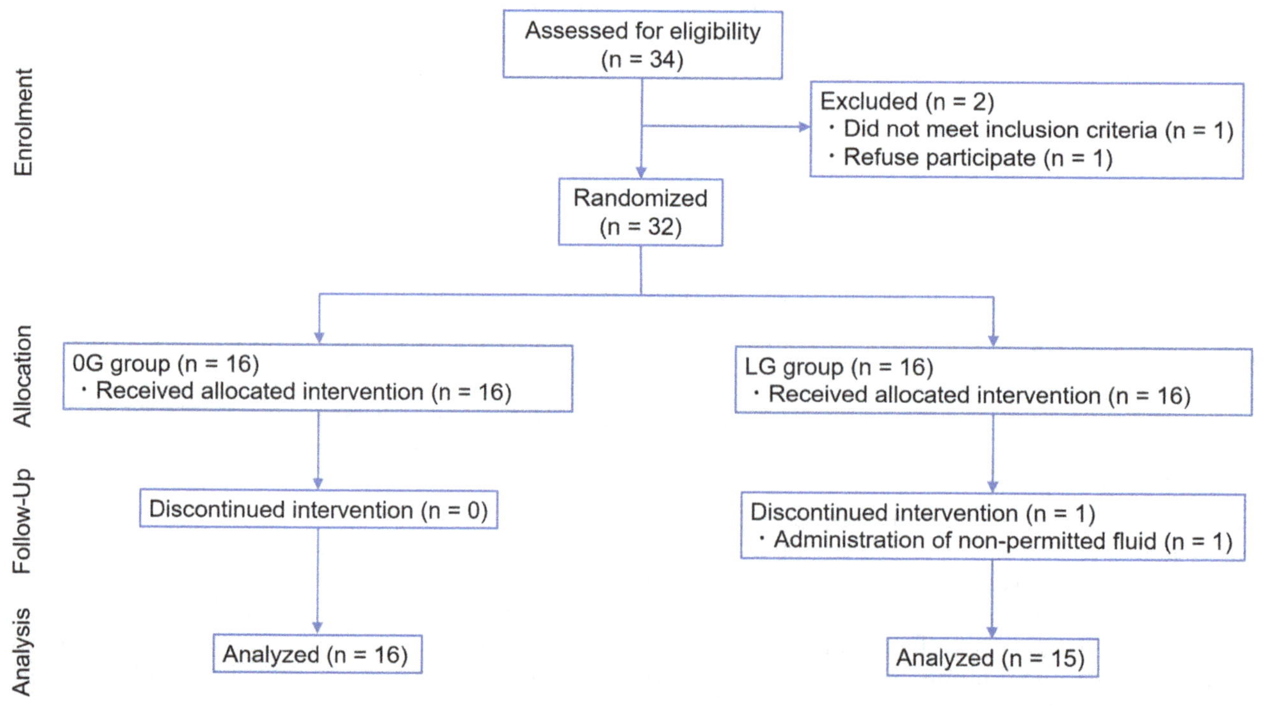

Fig. 2 Study flow diagram

Table 2 Demographic data

	0G group	LG group	*P* value
Male/Female	4/12	7/8	*P* = 0.21
Age (yr)	78.5 ± 2.8	79.0 ± 4.0	*P* = 0.83
Height (cm)	151.0 ± 6.3	157.7 ± 7.6	*P* = 1.0
Weight (kg)	57.3 ± 6.7	58.8 ± 13.1	*P* = 0.70
BMI (kg/m^2)	24.0 ± 2.0	24.2 ± 3.1	*P* = 0.81
HOMA-IR	1.85 ± 0.95	1.61 ± 0.94	*P* = 0.40
APACHE II score	8 ± 4	7 ± 2	*P* = 4.23
Operation time (min)	101.5 ± 35.9	142.0 ± 69.4	*P* = 0.06
Blood loss (ml)	50.0 ± 47.1	90.0 ± 267.5	*P* = 0.57

Data are expressed as the mean ± SD
There were no statistically significant differences between the 2 groups

required intravenous insulin or experienced hypoglycemia (< 70 mg/dl).

FFA levels in the LG group were significantly lower than those seen in the 0G group at 1 h and the end of surgery (1 h: $P = 0.004$, the end of surgery: $P = 0.001$; Fig. 5a). Levels of ketone bodies in the LG group were significantly lower than those in the 0G group at 1 h and at the end of surgery (1 h: $P = 0.037$, the end of surgery: $P = 0.007$; Fig. 5b). Levels of ketone bodies at 1 h were significantly higher than those at baseline in the 0G group ($P = 0.02$; Fig. 5b).

There were no significant differences between the two groups in EE (Fig. 6a), RQ (Fig. 6b), $\dot{V}\,O_2$, $\dot{V}\,CO_2$, insulin (Fig. 4b), Cr, 3-MH, and 3-MH/Cr.

Discussion

In this study of elderly patients, FFA levels in the LG group were significantly lower than those in the 0G group at 1 h and at the end of surgery. Levels of ketone bodies in the LG group were significantly lower than those seen in the 0G group at 1 h and the completion of surgery. In addition, levels at 1 h were significantly higher than those seen at baseline in the 0G group. These results indicate that 1% glucose loading during remifentanil-induced anesthesia attenuated the catabolism of fat in this patient group.

Table 3 Types of surgical procedure performed

0G group		LG group	
Cervical laminoplasty	3	Cervical laminoplasty	1
Lumbar partial laminectomy	1	Microendscopic lunbar laminectomy	1
Discectomy	1	Lumbar posterior fusion	3
Total hip arthroplasty	2	Extreme lateral interbody fusion	1
Mastectomy	3	Total hip arthroplasty	1
Skin malignant tumor resection	1	Mastectomy	1
Scar plasty	1	Patial mastectomy	1
Laryngomicrosurgery	1	Flap surgery	1
Dacryocystorhinostomy	1	Laryngomicrosurgery	1
Perineoplasty	1	Endoscopic sinus surgery	1
Adnexectomy+colpoplasty	1	Dacryocystorhinostomy	1
		Tension-free vaginal tape	1
		Closure of colostomy	1

Our previous study of adult patients demonstrated that ketone levels in subjects with no glucose loading were approximately 300 μmol/L during surgery [12], whereas in the current study of elderly patients, ketone body levels were approximately 500 μmol/L in the 0G group. However, in both studies, ketone body levels during surgery were approximately 200 μmol/L in the LG group. This observation suggests that low-dose glucose loading may be more effective in elderly patients than in adult patients as a whole.

In the present study, all patients were given Arginaid Water® 2 h before anesthesia. Arginaid Water® are carbohydrate with aminoacid solution, and the nutrient profiles are shown in Table 1. In our previous study, we investigated whether the intake of preoperative carbohydrate with aminoacid solution can improve starvation status and lipid catabolism before the induction of anesthesia, and reported that the intake of preoperative carbohydrate with aminoacid solution significantly decrease FFA and ketone bodies at the initiation of anesthesia compared with the control group [19]. Therefore, non-preoperative Arginaid Water® may cause more significantly difference in FFA and ketone bodies between 0G group and LG group.

HOMA-IR has been used widely to measure insulin sensitivity and resistance based on fasting plasma glucose and insulin concentrations [20, 21]. Esteghamati A et al. reported that the 75th percentile of HOMA-IR was 1.6 in healthy Iranians [22]. Beak JH et al. reported that the overall optimal cut-off value of HOMA-IR for identifying dysglycemia was 1.6 in both sex, and that the cut-off values for type 2 diabetes mellitus were 2.87 in men and 2.36 in women [23]. Ascaso JF et al. reported that the 75th percentile value as the cut-off point to define insulin resistance corresponded with a HOMA-IR of 2.6 [24]. In the present study, HOMA-IR did not differ significantly between the two groups (0G group: 1.85 ± 0.95, LG group: 1.61 ± 0.94, $P = 0.40$; Table 2). The highest HOMA-IR in the 0G group was 4.0, and that in the LG group was 4.2. Therefore, in the present study, insulin resistance were increased in both groups.

In the present study, no significant changes in insulin levels were seen. However, our previous study of adult patients showed a significant increase in insulin levels after low-dose glucose loading during surgery [12]. Many studies have reported that insulin secretion decreasing and resistance increasing with age [15–18]. Lozzo et al.

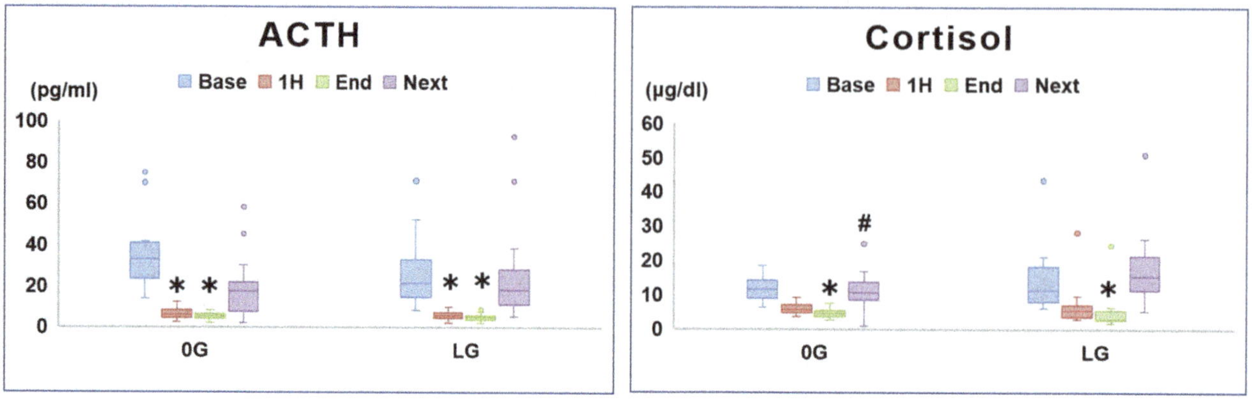

Fig. 3 Plasma ACTH (**a**) and serum cortisol (**b**) concentrations in the 0G and LG groups prior to induction of anesthesia (base), at 1 h (1H) from time 0, at the end of surgery (end), and on the next morning (next). $*P < 0.05$ versus baseline; $\#P < 0.05$ between groups

investigated basal β-cell function in 957 non-diabetic European patients aged 18–85 years, reporting that aging is associated with decreased basal insulin release [15]. Muzumdar et al. studied insulin secretion in rats aged 3–20 months, showing that glucose-stimulated insulin secretion decreased with age in this in vivo model [16]. Reaven et al. studied glucose-stimulated insulin release in β-cells of 2–18-month-old rats, demonstrating that the aging process leads to defects in glucose-stimulated insulin release from β-cells [25]. Therefore, the results seen in our current and previous studies support the data obtained by other groups indicating that aging is associated with impaired glucose-stimulated insulin release.

Parsons et al. reported that acute hyperglycemia adversely affects stroke outcome [26]. In the present study, plasma glucose levels were higher in the LG group than in the 0G group at 1 h and higher at 1 h and at the end of surgery than at baseline in the LG group. However, as the highest concentration of glucose in both groups was 156 mg/dl, none of the patients required intravenous insulin. These results suggest that, even in elderly patients, remifentanil-induced anesthesia may prevent hyperglycemia associated with low-dose glucose infusion.

Remifentanil-induced anesthesia decreases stress hormones, such as ACTH and cortisol, and suppresses the surgical stress response in adults [8–11]. Demirbilek et al. compared the effects of remifentanil and alfentanil as part of total intravenous anesthesia on plasma concentrations of cortisol, insulin, and glucose in patients undergoing abdominal hysterectomy, demonstrating that remifentanil-induced anesthesia was associated with decreased cortisol levels [8]. We previously reported that anesthesia using remifentanil significantly decreases

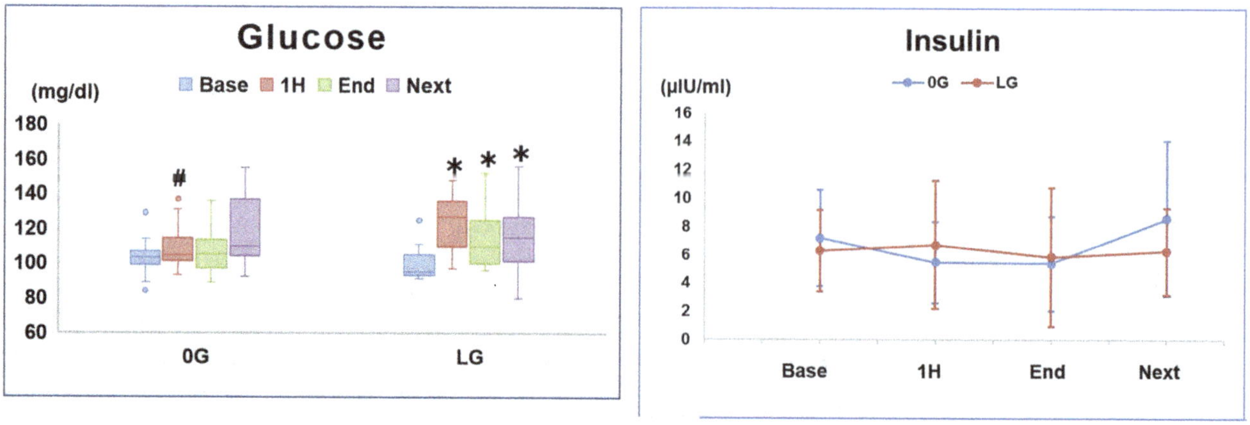

Fig. 4 Plasma glucose (**a**) and serum insulin (**b**) concentrations in the 0G and LG groups prior to induction of anesthesia (base), at 1 h (1H) from time 0, at the end of surgery (end), and on the next morning (next). $*P < 0.05$ versus baseline; $\#P < 0.05$ between groups

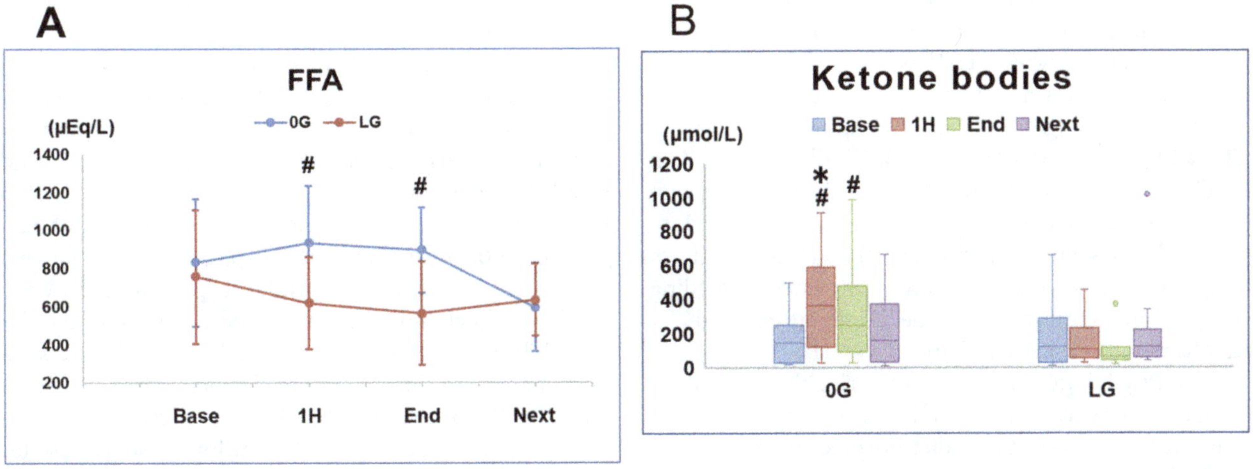

Fig. 5 Serum FFA (**a**) and ketone body (**b**) concentrations in the 0G and LG groups prior to induction of anesthesia (base), at 1 h (1H) from time 0, at the end of surgery (end), and on the next morning (next). *$P < 0.05$ versus baseline; #$P < 0.05$ between groups

ACTH and cortisol levels in adult patients [12]. In the present study, ACTH in both the 0G and LG groups was significantly decreased during remifentanil-induced anesthesia, suggesting that general anesthesia using remifentanil may suppress the stress response in elderly patients.

There were no significant differences in 3-MH/Cre levels in our current or previous studies [12]. In the present study, the surgical procedures were primarily performed on the body surface, rather than being highly invasive, and the surgery time was approximately 2 h. The aim was to exclude the influence of surgical stress in order to observe the effect of aging in the present study. Sawada et al. showed that 3-MH/Cr levels at 6 h were significantly higher than levels prior to anesthesia during major surgery in patients receiving no glucose infusion [13]. This discrepancy suggests that significant surgical stress may induce protein catabolism in the absence of glucose loading.

In the present study, subjects were elderly, but were not obese. It is reported that age per se does not increase HOMA-IR levels and that the changes might be related to higher rates of obesity in older subjects [27]. In addition, it is reported that the deterioration of glucose tolerance in healthy elderly subjects is due to a decrease in insulin secretion and can be explained by the degree of obesity rather than age [28]. Furthermore, one study demonstrated that aging has no effect on insulin sensitivity independent of changes in body composition [29]. These studies show that age itself does not increase insulin resistance and that changes may be related to the development of obesity. The low-dose glucose infusion

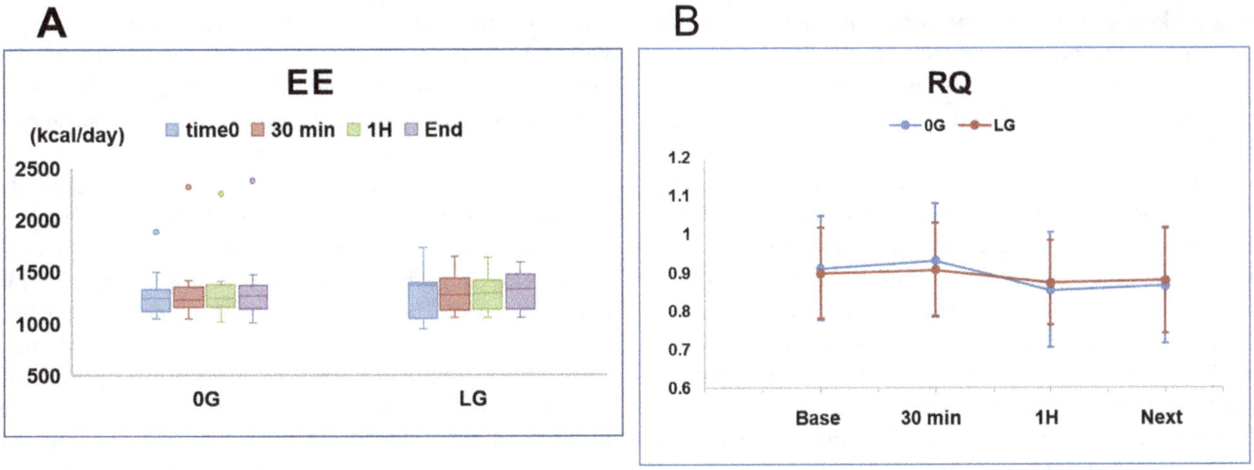

Fig. 6 EE (**a**) and RQ (**b**) in the 0G and LG groups from the time of stabilization (time 0) to the end of surgery (end). EE, energy expenditure; RQ, respiratory quotient

during remifentanil-induced anesthesia in obese patients may, therefore, induce hyperglycemia. In the present study, one patient whose BMI was > 30 kg/m^2 was excluded and BMI did not differ significantly between the two groups (0G group: 24.0 ± 2.0 kg/m^2, LG group: 24.2 ± 3.1 kg/m^2, P = 0.81; Table 2). The highest BMI in the 0G group was 26.9 kg/m^2, and that in the LG group was 29.1 kg/m^2. While further studies are required to evaluate this association further, in the current study of elderly, non-obese patients, low-dose glucose loading during remifentanil-induced anesthesia attenuated fat catabolism without causing hyperglycemia.

Acute Physiology and Chronic Health Evaluation (APACHE) II score is a general measure of severity of disease, has been used to predict hospital mortality [30–32]. We have done analysis to evaluate APACHE II score with preoperative data. Gupta S et al. reported that critically ill patients (CIP) with APACHE II score of ≥15 at admission or within 24 h are at risk for the development of CIP [31]. Joe BH et al. reported that patients with APACHE II score greater than 20 had tendency to expire than the others, and that APACHE II score more than 20, rather than cardiac function, is associated with mortality in patients with stress-induced cardiomyopathy [32]. In present study, APACHE II score did not differ significantly between the two groups (0G group: 8 ± 4, LG group: 7 ± 2, P = 4.23; Table 2). The highest APACHE II score in the 0G group was 12, and that in the LG group was 11. In present study, elderly (75–85 years) were required to have American Society of Anesthesiologists physical status of 1 or 2. Therefore, in present study, there were low severity in both groups.

In the present study, we used sevoflurane, but not propofol, to maintain the general anesthesia in elderly patients. Sevoflurane and propofol are commonly used general anesthetics during surgery. Several clinical studies were tried to see whether the choice of the anesthetic agent make a difference in postoperative delirium or the postoperative cognitive dysfunction (POCD) after noncardiac surgery in elderly patients. Some studies indicated that propofol reduced POCD as compared with sevoflurane [33, 34]. In contrast, it was reported that propofol significantly increased the delirium rating scale on day 2 and 3 after surgery, the time required for emergence from anesthesia as defined by eye opening and the time to tracheal extubation, as compared with sevoflurane [35]. Recent systematic review reported that it was uncertain whether maintenance with propofol or with volatile anesthetics affect incidence of postoperative delirium, mortality, or length hospital stay as certainty of the evidence was very low [36]. Additionally, the authors showed low-certainty evidence that maintenance with propofol may reduce POCD [36]. Thus, there is insufficient evidence to inform the choice of general anesthetic agent with respect to the beneficial effect during surgery in the elderly patients.

It was well known that volatile anesthetics were able to impair insulin secretion and glucose utilization [37]. Our previous studies using patch clamp experiments and intravenous glucose tolerance tests in rabbits indicated that isoflurane-induced inhibition of insulin secretion was mediated by the isoflurane-induced opening of adenosine triphosphate-sensitive potassium (K_{ATP}) channels in pancreatic β-cells, while propofol had no effects on the K_{ATP} channels in pancreatic β-cells, consequently no inhibition of insulin secretion [38, 39]. It is also reported that sevoflurane reduced glucose tolerance compared with propofol [40]. In the present study, we showed in the elderly patients that low-dose glucose load was able to be safe during sevoflurane based anesthesia. These results suggest that low-dose glucose load may be safe during propofol based anesthesia as well.

There were no significant differences in EE and RQ data in the current study of elderly patients or our previous study of adult subjects [12]. The low-dose glucose load may, therefore, not influence EE and RQ, although these parameters may change in patients undergoing major surgery.

This study has several limitations. First, data were obtained over a relatively short period, the final timepoint being the morning of postoperative day 1. Although we did not investigate the influence of glucose on long-term outcomes, there were no significant differences in protein catabolism. Second, in present study, the surgeries were minor surgery, because we want to exclude the influence of surgical stress to see the effect of aging on lipid metabolism in the present study. There may be significantly difference in prolonged and major surgery. Further studies to see the differences of low-dose glucose loading on the lipid metabolism and protein catabolism in the prolonged and major surgery are needed. However, we demonstrated that even in minor surgery with a little stress, low-dose glucose loading to the elderly patients improved lipid metabolism without developing hyperglycemia. Prolonged and major surgery in the absence of glucose loading was shown to induce protein catabolism in adults [13]. These results suggest that in major surgeries and/or prolonged surgeries which induce more remarkable stress, low-dose glucose loading to the elderly patients may control the increase of FFA and the ketone bodies and inhibit protein catabolism, when compared without glucose loading. Third, there were differences in the types of surgical procedures performed on patients in the two groups. These differences, however, were regarded as irrelevant because the concentrations of ACTH and cortisol during surgery were similar in the two groups. Finally, in the present study, the elderly patients who were not diabetes were subject of the study. The effects of low dose glucose infusion on both glucose and fat metabolism on elderly patients with diabetes or acute neurologic insults are not clear from the findings of the present study.

Conclusions

The present study indicates that intraoperative low glucose infusion during remifentanil-induced anesthesia attenuated the catabolism of fat without causing harmful hyperglycemia in this population of elderly patients. These data suggest that low-dose glucose loading may be useful in elderly patients undergoing relatively minor surgical procedures.

Abbreviations

3-MH: 3-methylhistidine; ACTH: adrenocorticotropic hormone; Cr: creatinine; EE: energy expenditure; FFA: free fatty acid; HOMA-IR: Homeostasis Model Assessment Insulin Resistance; RQ: respiratory quotient; $\dot{V}O_2$: oxygen consumption; $\dot{V}CO_2$: carbon dioxide output

Acknowledgments

Not applicable.

Authors' contributions

KF collected date, performed the statistical analysis, and write the manuscript. AK collected date and performed the statistical analysis. NN designed the study and collected date. YI, RK, YS, NK and YMT collected date. KT designed the study, helped the statistical analysis and edited the manuscript. All author read and approved the final manuscript.

Author details

[1]Department of Anesthesiology, Graduate School of Biomedical Sciences, Tokushima University, 3-18-15 Kuramoto, Tokushima 770-8503, Japan. [2]Department of Anesthesiology and Critical Care, Graduate School of Biomedical and Health Sciences, Hiroshima University, 1-2-3 Kasumi Minami, Hiroshima 774-8551, Japan.

References

1. Bower WF, Lee PY, Kong APS, Jiang JY, Underwood MJ, Chan JCN, van Hasselt CA. Peri-operative hyperglycemia: a consideration for general surgery? Am J Surg. 2010;199:240–8.
2. Marana E, Scambia G, Colicci S, Maviglia R, Maussier ML, Marana R, Proietti R. Leptin and perioperative neuroendocrine stress response with two different anaesthetic techniques. Acta Anaesthesiol Scand. 2008;52:541–6.
3. Desborough JP. The stress response to trauma and surgery. Br J Anaesth. 2000;85:109–17.
4. Weissman C. The metabolic response to stress: an overview and update. Anesthesiology. 1990;73:308–27.
5. Ouattara A, Lecomte P, Le Manach Y, Landi M, Jacqueminet S, Platonov I, Bonnet N, Riou B, Coriat P. Poor intraoperative blood glucose control is associated with a worsened hospital outcome after cardiac surgery in diabetic patients. Anesthesiology. 2005;103:687–94.
6. Ascione R, Rogers CA, Rajakaruna C, Angelini GD. Inadequate blood glucose control is associated with in-hospital mortality and morbidity in diabetic and nondiabetic patients undergoing cardiac surgery. Circulation. 2008;118:113–23.
7. Kotagal M, Symons RG, Hirsch IB, Umpierrez GE, Dellinger EP, Farrokhi ET, Flum DR, SCOAPCERTAIN Collaborative. Perioperative hyperglycemia and risk of adverse events among patients with and without diabetes. Ann Surg. 2015;261:97–103.
8. Demirbilek S, Ganidagli S, Aksoy N, Becerik C, Baysal Z. The effects of remifentanil and alfentanil-based total intravenous anesthesia (TIVA) on the endocrine response to abdominal hysterectomy. J Clin Anesth. 2004;16:358–63.
9. Shinoda T, Murakami W, Takamichi Y, Iizuka H, Tanaka M, Kuwasako Y. Effect of remifentanil infusion rate on stress response in orthopedic surgery using a tourniquet application. BMC Anesthesiol. 2013;13:14.
10. Taniguchi H, Sasaki T, Fujita H, Takano O, Hayashi T, Cho H, Yoshikawa T, Tsuburaya A. The effect of intraoperative use of high-dose remifentanil on postoperative insulin resistance and muscle protein catabolism: a randomized controlled study. Int J Med Sci. 2013;10:1099–107.
11. Weale NK, Rogers CA, Cooper R, Nolan J, Wolf AR. Effect of remifentanil infusion rate on stress response to the prebypass phase of paediatric cardiac surgery. Br J Anaesth. 2004;92:187–94.
12. Kambe N, Tanaka K, Kakuta N, Kawanishi R, Tsutsumi YM. The influence of glucose load on metabolism during minor surgery using remifentanil-induced anesthesia. Acta Anaesthesiol Scand. 2014;58:948–54.
13. Sawada A, Kamada Y, Hayashi H, Ichinose H, Sumita S, Yamakage M. Effect of intraoperative glucose infusion on catabolism of adipose tissue and muscle protein in patients anesthetized with remifentanil in combination with sevoflurane during major surgery: a randomized controlled multicenter trial. Anesth Analg. 2016;123:869–76.
14. Speakman JR, Westerterp KR. Associations between energy demands, physical activity, and body composition in adult humans between 18 and 96 y of age. Am J Clin Nutr. 2010;92:826–34.
15. Iozzo P, Beck-Nielsen H, Laakso M, Smith U, YKI-Jarvinen H, Ferrannini E. Independent influence of age on basal insulin secretion in nondiabetic humans. J Clin Endocrinol Metab 1999; 84: 863–868.
16. Muzumdar R, Ma X, Atzmon G, Vuguin P, Yang X, Barzilai N. Decrease in glucose-stimulated insulin secretion with aging is independent of insulin action. Diabetes. 2004;53:441–6.
17. De Tata V. Age-related impairment of pancreatic beta-cell function: pathophysiological and cellular mechanisms. Front Endocrinol (Lausanne). 2014;5:138.
18. Oya J, Nakagami T, Yamamoto Y, Fukushima S, Takeda M, Endo Y, Uchigata Y. Effects of age on insulin resistance and secretion in subjects without diabetes. Intern Med. 2014;53:941–7.
19. Tsutsumi R, Kakuta N, Kadota T, Oyama T, Kume K, Hamaguchi E, Niki N, Tanaka K, Tsutsumi YM. Effects of oral carbohydrate with amino acid solution on the metabolic status of patients in the preoperative period: a randomized, prospective clinical trial. J Anesth. 2016;30:842–9.
20. Matthews DR, Hosker JP, Rudenski AS, Naylor BA, Treacher DF, Turner DC. Homeostasis model assessment: insulin resistance and fl-cell function from fasting plasma glucose and insulin concentrations in man. Diabetologia. 1985;28:412–9.
21. Wallace TM, Levy JC, Matthews DR. Use and abuse of HOMA modeling. Diabetes Care. 2004;27:1487–95.
22. Esteghamati A, Ashraf H, Esteghamati AR, Meysamie A, Khalilzadeh O, Nakhjavani M, Abbasi M. Optimal threshold of homeostasis model assessment for insulin resistance in an Iranian population: the implication of metabolic syndrome to detect insulin resistance. Diabetes Res Clin Pract. 2009;84:279–87.
23. Baek JH, Kim H, Kim KY, Jung J. Insulin resistance and the risk of diabetes and dysglycemia in korean general adult population. Diabetes Metab J. 2018;42:296–307.
24. Ascaso JF, Pardo S, Real JT, Lorente RI, Priego A, Carmena R. Diagnosing insulin resistance by simple quantitative methods in subjects with normal glucose metabolism. Diabetes Care. 2003;26:3320–5.
25. Reaven EP, Gold G, Reaven GM. Effect of age on glucose-stimulated insulin release by the β-cell of the rat. J Clin Invest. 1979;64:591–9.
26. Parsons MW, Barber PA, Desmond PM, Baird TA, Darby DG, Byrnes G, Tress BM, Davis SM. Acute hyperglycemia adversely affects stroke outcome: a magnetic resonance imaging and spectroscopy study. Ann Neurol. 2002;52:20–8.
27. Soriguer F, Colomo N, Valdes S, Goday A, Rubio-Martin E, Esteva I, Castano L, Ruiz de Adana MS, Morcillo S, Calle A, Garcia-Fuentes E, Catala M, Gutie rrez-Repiso C, Delgado E, Gomis R, Ortega E, Rojo-Martinez G. Modifications of the homeostasis model assessment of insulin resistance index with age. Acta Diabetol 2014; 51: 917–925.
28. Basu R, Breda E, Oberg AL, Powell CC, Dalla Man C, Basu A, Vittone JL, Klee GG, Arora P, Jensen MD, Toffolo G, Cobelli C, Rizza RA. Mechanisms of the age-associated deterioration in glucose tolerance: contribution of alterationsin insulin secretion, action, and clearance. Diabetes. 2003;52:1738–48.
29. Szoke M, Shrayyef MZ, Messing S, Woerle HJ, van Haeften TW, Meyer C, Mitrakou A, Pimenta W, Gerich JE. Effect of aging on glucose homeostasis. Diabetes Care. 2008;31:539–43.
30. Argyriou G, Vrettou CS, Filippatos G, Sainis G, Nanas S, Routsi C. Comparative evaluation of acute physiology and chronic health evaluation

II and sequential organ failure assessment scoring systems in patients admitted to the cardiac intensive care unit. J Crit Care. 2015;30:752–7.
31. Gupta S, Mishra M. Acute physiology and chronic health evaluation II score of ≥15: a risk factor for sepsis-induced critical illness polyneuropathy. Neurol India. 2016;64:640–5.
32. Joe BH, Jo U, Kim HS, Park CB, Hwang HJ, Sohn IS, Jin ES, Cho JM, Park JH, Kim CJ. APACHE II score, rather than cardiac function, may predict poor prognosis in patients with stress-induced cardiomyopathy. J Korean Med Sci. 2012;27:52–7.
33. Zhang Y, Shan GJ, Zhang YX, Cao SJ, Zhu SN, Li HJ, Ma D, Wang DX. Propofol compared with sevoflurane general anesthesia is associated with decreased delayed neurocognitive recovery in older adults. Br J Anaesth. 2018;121:595–604.
34. Qiao Y, Feng H, Zhao T, Yan H, Zhang H, Zhao X. Postoperative cognitive dysfunction after inhalational anesthesia in elderly patients undergoing major surgery: the influence of anesthetic technique, cerebral injury and systemic inflammation. BMC Anestheiol. 2015;15:154.
35. Nishikawa K, Nakayama M, Omote K, Namiki A. Recovery characteristics and post-operative delirium after long-duration laparoscope-assisted surgery in elderly patients: propofol-based vs. sevoflurane-based anesthesia. Acta Anaesthesiol Scand. 2004;48:162–8.
36. Millere D, Lewis SR, Pritchard MW, Schofield-Robinson OJ, Shelton CL, Alderson P, Smith AF. Intravenous versus inhalational maintenance of anaesthesia for postoperative cognitive outcomes in elderly people undergoing non-cardiac surgery. Cochrane Database Syst Rev. 2018;8: CD012317.
37. Diltoer M, Camu F. Glucose homeostasis and insulin secretion during isoflurane anesthesia in humans. Anesthesiology. 1988;68:880–6.
38. Tanaka K, Kawano T, Tomino T, Kawano H, Okada T, Oshita S, Takahashi A, Nakaya Y. Mechanisms of impaired glucose tolerance and insulin secretion during isoflurane anesthesia. Anesthesiology. 2009;111:1044–51.
39. Tanaka K, Kawano T, Tsutsumi YM, Kinoshita M, Kakuta N, Hirose K, Kimura M, Oshita S. Differential effects of propofol and isoflurane on glucose utilization and insulin secretion. Life Sci. 2011;88:96–103.
40. Kitamura T, Ogawa M, Kawamura G, Sato K, Yamada Y. The effects of Sevoflurane and Propofol on glucose metabolism under aerobic conditions in fed rats. Anesth Analg. 2009;109:1479–85.

25

Perioperative dexmedetomidine for outpatient cataract surgery

James Harvey Jones* and Robin Aldwinckle

Abstract

Background: Cataract surgery is one of the most common procedures performed worldwide in the elderly. Various medications can provide effective anesthesia and analgesia for cataract surgery, but undesirable side effects limit the utility of each medication or combination of medications. Dexmedetomidine may serve as an anesthesia adjunct for outpatient cataract surgery in the elderly.

Methods: Searches were conducted in Cochrane, Embase, and PubMed for randomized clinical trials investigating the use of dexmedetomidine in adult patients undergoing outpatient, or ambulatory, cataract surgery with sedation and topical or peribulbar block. Ninety-nine publications were identified, of which 15 trials satisfied the inclusion criteria. A total of 914 patients were included in this review. The following data were collected: American Society of Anesthesiologists' (ASA) physical status and age of study patients; method of blinding and randomization; medication doses and routes of administration; and intraoperative levels of sedation. We also recorded statistically significant differences between dexmedetomidine and other study medications or placebo with respect to the following outcomes: hemodynamic and respiratory parameters; pain; sedation; post-operative nausea and vomiting (PONV); discharge from post-anesthesia care unit (PACU) or recovery times; patient satisfaction; surgeon satisfaction; and effects on intraocular pressure (IOP).

Results: Hypotension with or without bradycardia was reported following bolus doses of dexmedetomidine ranging from 0.5–1.0 mcg/kg with or without a continuous dexmedetomidine infusion. Delayed PACU discharge times were associated with the use of dexmedetomidine, but no clear association was identified between delayed recovery and higher levels of intraoperative sedation. Better analgesia and higher patient satisfaction were commonly reported with dexmedetomidine as well as reductions in IOP.

Conclusions: Overall, this review demonstrates better analgesia, higher patient satisfaction, and reduced IOP with dexmedetomidine for outpatient cataract surgery when compared to traditional sedatives, hypnotics, and opioids. These benefits of dexmedetomidine, however, must be weighed against relative cardiovascular depression and delayed PACU discharge or recovery times. Therefore, the utility of dexmedetomidine for outpatient cataract surgery should be considered on a patient-by-patient basis.

Keywords: Dexmedetomidine, Outpatient surgery, Ambulatory surgery, Cataract surgery

* Correspondence: jamesjns137@gmail.com
UC Davis Department of Anesthesiology and Pain Medicine, University of California Davis Medical Center, 4150 V Street, PSSB Suite 1200, Sacramento, CA 95817, USA

Background

Cataract is a leading cause of visual impairment that currently affects almost 25 million Americans and is projected to reach almost 50 million by 2050 [1]. Approximately 2 million cataract operations are performed in the United States each year, and the majority are done in elderly patients [2, 3].

Anesthesia for cataract surgery often includes sedatives and hypnotics (such as propofol, ketamine, or midazolam) with or without opioids, along with topical analgesia or peribulbar block. Propofol and benzodiazepines may induce persistent sedation and respiratory depression, particularly when they are administered in combination with opioids in elderly patients [4]. Opioids may also lead to nausea, vomiting, and perioperative neurocognitive disorders [5].

Ambulatory, or outpatient, cataract surgery demands quick resolution of anesthesia-related effects prior to patient discharge. Postoperative pain, sedation, nausea, vomiting, as well as hemodynamic and respiratory parameters that have not returned to an acceptable percentage of baseline may delay discharge, require additional monitoring, or lead to unexpected hospital admission.

Dexmedetomidine is an alpha-2 agonist with a half-life of approximately 2 h that provides sedation and analgesia without compromising oxygenation and ventilation [6, 7]. However, reported side effects of bradycardia, hypotension, hypertension, and nausea may restrict the use of dexmedetomidine in the ambulatory surgery setting [6–8]. Despite the popularity of cataract surgery and the widespread use of dexmedetomidine in anesthesia, no systematic review is currently available that assembles the evidence regarding dexmedetomidine for outpatient cataract surgery.

This systematic review attempts to synthesize the results from randomized clinical trials investigating the use of dexmedetomidine for sedation in adult patients undergoing outpatient cataract surgery. Our review focuses on patient and surgeon satisfaction as well as factors that impact perioperative outcomes: hemodynamic and respiratory parameters; pain; sedation; postoperative nausea and vomiting (PONV); post-anesthesia care unit (PACU) discharge or recovery times; and intraocular pressure (IOP).

Methods

Literature search

The authors (JHJ and RA) independently performed initial literature searches in PubMed, Embase, and Cochrane databases for articles published before January 1, 2019, using the following key terms in the English language: "dexmedetomidine" and "cataract surgery." Additionally, the bibliographies of recovered publications were screened for relevant titles, which were then also reviewed. Eligible studies included randomized clinical trials of adult patients undergoing outpatient, or ambulatory, cataract surgery with sedation supplemented by topical analgesia or peribulbar block.

Data collection

The following data were collected from each randomized clinical trial: age and American Society of Anesthesiologists' (ASA) physical status of study patients; method of blinding and randomization; medication doses and routes of administration; and intraoperative level of sedation. We also recorded statistically significant differences between dexmedetomidine and other study medications or placebo with respect to the following outcomes: hemodynamic and respiratory parameters; pain; sedation; PONV; discharge from PACU or recovery times; patient satisfaction; surgeon satisfaction; and IOP. The methods by which the studies measured each outcome (such as Visual Analog Score, Numeric Rating Scale, Aldrete's scoring system, and Ramsay Sedation Scale) were also noted. Data regarding outcomes not expected to impact patient discharge from an ambulatory surgery center (such as incidence of dry mouth) were not recorded.

Definitions

Ambulatory surgery was defined as surgery after which the patients were discharged from the PACU to home and was considered synonymous with outpatient surgery for the purposes of this review. Unless the authors specifically stated otherwise, it was assumed that all patients were discharged from the PACU to home. Adverse events were only recorded if they were experienced by dexmedetomidine-treated patients. Adverse events of other study medications were not recorded given the heterogeneity of medications analyzed, and the focus of this review was on the effects of dexmedetomidine.

Assessment of study quality

The quality of each study was assessed with 3 measures and given a score between 0 and 5 [9]. One point was awarded if the study was randomized and another point was awarded if the study utilized a double-blind approach. Additional points were given based on the appropriateness of randomization and blinding and if the study included a clear description of withdrawals or dropouts (or specifically stated that there were none). Points were not awarded for inappropriate randomization or blinding.

Results

Study selection

Literature searches in PubMed, Cochrane, and Embase databases identified 99 articles published prior to January 1, 2019. One additional publication was identified after reviewing the bibliographies of recovered studies. After removing duplicates from database searches, 31 publications were screened and 16 were excluded due to the following reasons: ophthalmic procedures other than cataract surgery included in the study (number (n) = 2), primary outcome regarding the effects of dexmedetomidine on regional anesthesia for ophthalmic surgery (n = 2), outcomes not applicable to this review (n = 4), clinical trials without retrievable results (n = 3), study patients received general anesthesia (n = 2), and pediatric patient population (n = 3). All of the remaining 15 eligible studies were included for qualitative synthesis. The method used to identify and screen publications is displayed in Fig. 1: Identification and Screening of Publications. Additional information regarding study designs and demographic information are shown in Table 1.

Quality of studies

Although each study in this review utilized a randomized design, the method of randomization was frequently inappropriate and led to decreased quality scores. Failure to describe withdrawals and dropouts also accounted for low quality scores as noted in Table 1. Most studies utilized a double-blind approach that was considered appropriate.

Routes of administration, dosing, and titration of medications

Two studies titrated dexmedetomidine, remifentanil, and midazolam to pre-determined target levels of sedation as defined by Bispectral index (BIS) scores 70–80 and > 85 [10, 11]. Of the remaining studies, 7 titrated medications to Ramsay Sedation Scale (RSS) scores of 2 or 3 [12–18]. Two studies administered intramuscular (IM) dexmedetomidine 45 min prior to the regional block [19, 20]. One study employed patient-controlled sedation [21]. Another study utilized target effect site concentrations to titrate remifentanil [22]. Table 2 shows the medication doses, routes of administration, total medication administered, and intraoperative levels of sedation.

Intravenous bolus doses of dexmedetomidine were given over 10–20 min and ranged from 0.5–1.0 mcg/kg [10, 12–16, 18, 21–23]. Continuous infusions of dexmedetomidine ranged from 0.05–0.7 $mcg{\cdot}kg^{-1}{\cdot}hr.^{-1}$ [10–

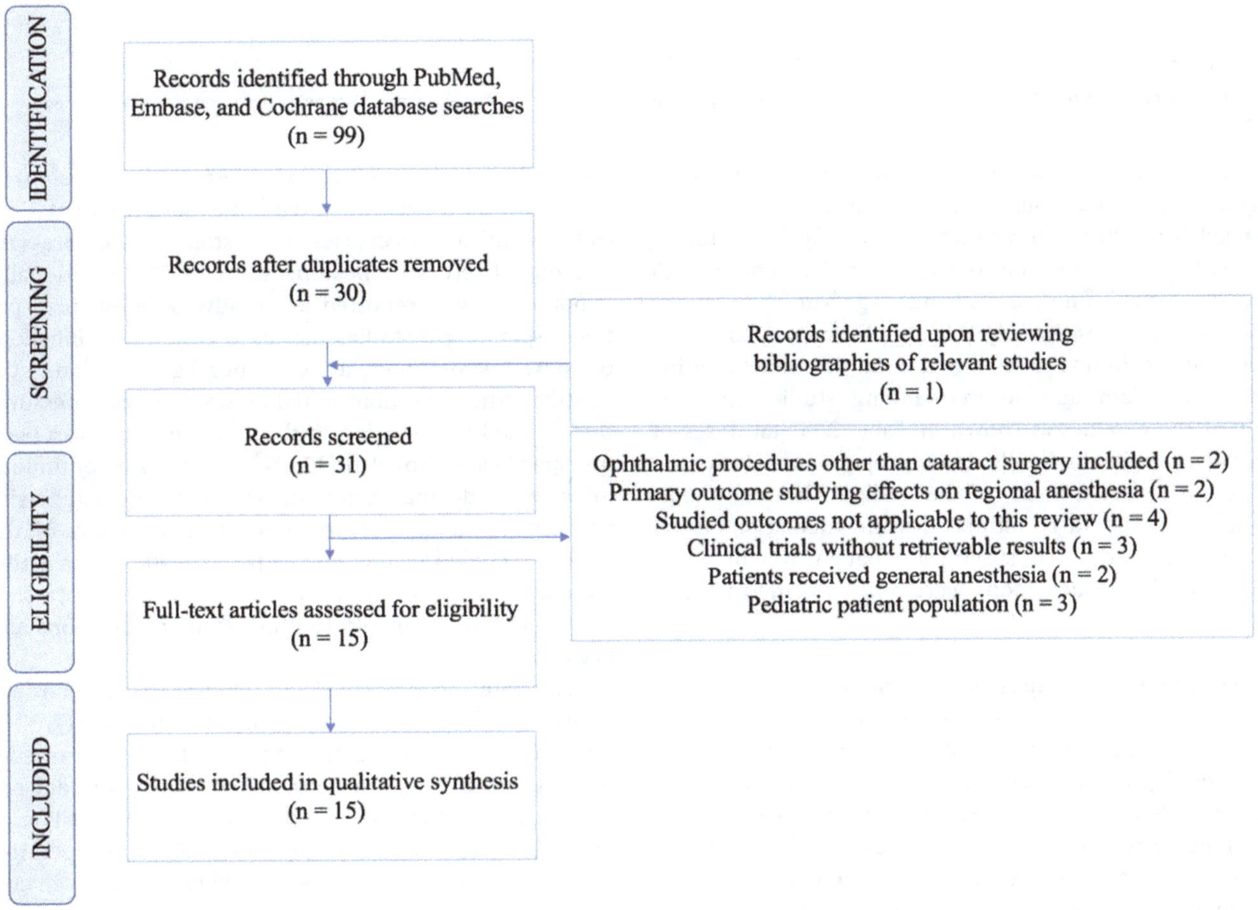

Fig. 1 Identification and Screening of Publications

Table 1 Study Design, Quality Score, and Demographic Data of Included Studies

Study	Quality Score	N[a]	ASA[b]	Age in Dexmedetomidine Group(s)[c]		Age in Other Group(s)[c]	
Abdalla [23]	3	40	–	63 (11)		60 (13)	
Alhashemi [12]	4	44	I-III	61 (34–79)		61 (40–75)	
Altiparmak [24]	5	80	II-III	58 (5.7)		57 (5.8)	
Apan [11]	3	90	I-III	65.7 (11.3)		midazolam	65.8 (11.8)
						saline	66.3 (9.8)
Ayoglu [21]	1	40	I-II	50–75		50–75	
Dogan [13]	4	80	I-II	50–70		50–70	
Erdurmus [14]	3	44	–	67.41 (9.83)		69.46 (9.99)	
Ghodki [15]	4	60	I-II	62.6 (6.5)		61.4 (6.9)	
Kermany [10]	1	100	I-II	50.26 (9.44)		51.9 (10.2)	
Muttu [16]	1	40	–	Unknown		Unknown	
Na [17]	1	31	I-III	60.8 (11.4)		57.4 (13.4)	
Park [22]	0	80	I-III	60–80		60–80	
Virkilla [19]	0	35	I-III	0.25 mcg/kg[d]	69.0 (8.7)	60.8 (12.2)	
				0.5 mcg/kg	70.2 (3.3)		
				0.75 mcg/kg	67.8 (6.7)		
				1.0 mcg/kg	66.6 (15.0)		
				1.5 mcg/kg	71.4 (10.9)		
Virkilla [20]	4	90	I-III	63.3 (11.2)		midazolam	66.2 (9.5)
						placebo	66.6 (10.3)
Yagan [18]	3	60	I-III	68.6 (8.4)		66.4 (6.3)	

[a]*N* number of patients studied, [b]*ASA* American Society of Anesthesiologists' classification of Physical Health score, [c]Data are mean (standard deviation or age range) or age range, [d]*mcg/kg* micrograms per kilogram

14, 16, 17, 22–24]. Variability was also noted in the dosing of midazolam. Bolus doses of intravenous midazolam ranged from 20 to 50 mcg/kg [12, 16, 20]. Two studies titrated continuous infusions of midazolam at 25 mcg•kg^{-1}•hr.$^{-1}$ and 2.5–35.0 mcg•kg^{-1}•hr.$^{-1}$ to BIS > 85 and RSS 2, respectively [11, 16]. There was considerable variety in the total amount of dexmedetomidine and midazolam administered among studies that reported these values as shown in Table 2. Total doses of fentanyl, remifentanil, alfentanil, propofol, and ketamine were not reported in any of the studies. Although medication doses could be estimated from calculations using the average duration of surgery and patient weight, when reported, these calculations were not performed for this review.

Hemodynamic and respiratory parameters

Cardiovascular depression was noted with dexmedetomidine as evidenced by statistically significant decreases in arterial pressure, heart rate, or both. Administration of dexmedetomidine by continuous infusion without initial bolus was not associated with statistically significant decreases in arterial pressure when compared to remifentanil, midazolam, and saline [11, 24]. However, when compared to propofol-alfentanil (combination of propofol and alfentanil), dexmedetomidine infusion titrated to RSS 3 without initial bolus dose led to statistically significant decreases in systolic blood pressure intraoperatively and postoperatively [17]. Additionally, hypotension was reported as an adverse event in 5 patients spanning 2 studies that used continuous infusions of dexmedetomidine at 0.4 mcg•kg^{-1}•hr.$^{-1}$and 0.6 mcg•kg^{-1}•hr.$^{-1}$ without initial boluses; arterial pressures that defined hypotension in these studies, however, were not specifically provided [17, 24]. Omitting a continuous infusion of dexmedetomidine was not associated with preserved arterial pressure or heart rate in any of the studies included in this review [15, 18–20]. Table 3 displays the effects of dexmedetomidine on arterial pressure and heart rate compared to other study medications and placebo.

Heart rate was preserved in 2 studies that did not administer a bolus dose of dexmedetomidine [17, 24]. However, one study comparing the effects of dexmedetomidine to midazolam or saline in 90 patients did not bolus dexmedetomidine, and reported statistically significant decreases in intraoperative and postoperative heart rates [11]. Bradycardia was reported as an adverse event in 5 studies and frequently required atropine treatment [15, 17, 19–21].

Table 2 Route of Administration, Doses, Titration Method, and Total Medication Administered of Included Studies

Study	Route[a]	Dexmedetomidine Bolus Dose(s)[b]	Bolus Duration (mins)[c]	Dexmedetomidine Infusion Rate[d]	Other Treatment Group(s)	Medication Titration	Total Medication Administered[e]
Abdalla [23]	IV	0.5 mcg•kg^{-1}•hr.$^{-1}$	10	0.2 mcg•kg^{-1}•hr.$^{-1}$ over 50 mins	saline	NA	Unknown
Alhashemi [12]	IV	1 mcg/kg	10	0.1–0.7 mcg•kg^{-1}•hr.$^{-1}$	midazolam 20 mcg/kg then 0.5 mg PRN[f]	RSS[g] 3	dexmedetomidine 79.5 (21.7) mcg midazolam 1.5 (0.6) mg
Altiparmak [24]	IV	–	NA	0.4 mcg•kg^{-1}•hr.$^{-1}$	remifentanil 0.05 mcg•kg^{-1}•min^{-1}	Unknown	Unknown
Apan [11]	IV	–	NA	0.25 mcg•kg^{-1}•hr.$^{-1}$	midazolam 25 mcg•kg^{-1}•hr.$^{-1}$ or saline	BIS[h] > 85	dexmedetomidine 18.8 (11.6) mcg midazolam 1.8 (0.6) mg
Ayoglu [21]	IV	1 mcg/kg	10	patient-controlled sedation (5 mcg bolus dose; 10 min lockout)	no sedation	Patient-controlled sedation	dexmedetomidine 66.4 (3.7) mcg
Dogan [13]	IV	0.6 mcg/kg	10	0.1–0.5 mcg•kg^{-1}•hr.$^{-1}$ (and topical analgesia or peribulbar block)	fentanyl 0.5 mcg/kg; and midazolam 20 mcg/kg then 5–15 mcg•kg^{-1}•hr.$^{-1}$ (and topical analgesia or peribulbar block)	RSS 3	Dexmedetomidine infusion: topical analgesia 8.54 mcg; peribulbar block 8.92 mcg midazolam: topical analgesia 213.80 mcg; peribulbar block 226.24 mcg
Erdurmus [14]	IV	1 mcg/kg	10	0.1–0.7 mcg/kg	saline	RSS 3	Unknown
Ghodki [15]	IV	1 mcg/kg	10	–	saline	RSS 3	dexmedetomidine 65.4 (3.6) mcg
Kermany [10]	IV	0.5 mcg/kg	10	0.2 mcg•kg^{-1}•hr.$^{-1}$	remifentanil 0.1 mcg/kg over 5 mins then 0.05 mcg•kg^{-1}•min^{-1}	BIS 70–80	Unknown
Muttu [16]	IV	1 mcg/kg	20	0.05–0.7 mcg•kg^{-1}•hr.$^{-1}$	midazolam 50 mcg/kg then 2.5–35.0 mcg•kg^{-1}•hr.$^{-1}$	RSS 2	Unknown
Na [17]	IV	–	NA	0.6 mcg•kg^{-1}•hr.$^{-1}$	propofol 2 mg•kg^{-1}•hr.$^{-1}$ and alfentanil 20 mcg•kg^{-1}•hr.$^{-1}$	RSS 3	Unknown
Park [22]	IV	0.5 mcg/kg	10	0.2 mcg•kg^{-1}•hr.$^{-1}$	Remifentanil target effect site concentration 1 ng/ml	–	Unknown
Virkilla [19]	IM	0.25 mcg/kg 0.5 mcg/kg 0.75 mcg/kg 1.0 mcg/kg 1.5 mcg/kg	NA	NA	placebo	45 mins before regional block	Unknown
Virkilla [20]	IM	1.0 mcg/kg	NA	NA	midazolam 20 mcg/kg and placebo	45 mins before regional block	Unknown
Yagan [18]	IV	0.5 mcg/kg	10	–	ketofol (200 mg propofol and 100 mg ketamine) 0.125 ml/kg	RSS 3	Unknown

[a]*Route* route of study drug administration, data are, *IV* intravenous or, *IM*, intramuscular, [b]Data are mcg/kg = micrograms per kilogram or mcg•kg^{-1}•hr.$^{-1}$ = micrograms per kilogram per hour; [c]mins = minutes; [d]Data are mcg•kg^{-1}•hr.$^{-1}$ = micrograms per kilogram per hour or mcg•kg^{-1}•min^{-1} = micrograms per kilogram per minute; [e]Data are total medication administered (standard deviation); [f]*PRN* pro re nata, [g]*RSS* Ramsay sedation scale score; [h]*BIS* Bispectral index

Table 3 Effects of Dexmedetomidine on Arterial Pressure, Heart Rate, and Respiratory Parameters

Study	Dexmedetomidine		Other Treatment Group(s)	Arterial Pressure	Heart Rate	Respiratory Parameters
	Bolus	Continuous infusion				
Abdalla [23]	+	+	saline	Decreased SBP[a] at 30 mins after starting infusion [SBP mean (SD[b]): 136.10 (15.24) vs 150.15 (21.73) mm Hg[c], $P = 0.043$]	Decreased at 30 mins after starting infusion [HR[d] mean (SD): 66.90 (5.42) vs 81.20 (7.83), $P = 0.041$] Decreased at 60 mins after starting infusion [HR mean (SD): 63.60 (4.55) vs 79.75 (7.83), $P = 0.049$]	–
Alhashemi [12]	+	+	midazolam	Decreased MAP[e] [MAP (SE[f]): 86 (3) vs 102 (3) mm Hg, $P < 0.05$]	Decreased [HR (SE): 65 (2) vs 72 (2) bpm, $P < 0.05$]	No statistically significant differences reported
Altiparmak [24]	–	+	remifentanil	No statistically significant differences in MAP between groups	No statistically significant differences	Increased oxygen saturation at 1 min [mean SpO_2[g] (SD): 94.97 (2.0) vs 93.56 (2.69), $P = 0.014$], 5 mins [mean SpO_2 (SD): 95.50 vs 92.84 (4.56), $P = 0.001$], 10 mins [mean SpO_2 (SD): 95.52 (2.57) vs 92.65 (3.31), $P = 0.000$], 15 mins [96.02 (2.27) vs 93.34 (4.08), $P = 0.001$], and 20 mins [mean SpO_2 (SD): 95.95 (2.43) vs 92.78 (4.15), $P = 0.000$] after inductionDecreased oxygen at 35 mins [mean SpO_2 (SD): 93.14 (4.71) vs 97.0 (1.63), $P = 0.002$], 40 mins [mean SpO_2 (SD): 94.29 (3.94) vs 97.08 (1.13), $P = 0.027$], and 45 mins [mean SpO_2 (SD): 93.92 (4.17) vs 97.42 (1.51), $P = 0.048$] after induction
Apan [11]	–	+	midazolam and saline	No statistically significant differences in MAP between groups	Decreased 35–50 min after start of surgery and extending to 15 mins postoperatively [data values not reported, $P < 0.05$]	No statistically significant differences in respiratory rate or $ETCO_2$[h] values
Ayoglu [21]	+	+	no sedation	Decreased arterial pressure up to 30 mins after start of surgery [data values not reported, $P < 0.05$]	Decreased intraoperative mean HR up to 50 mins after start of surgery [data values not reported, $P < 0.05$]	No statistically significant differences in SpO_2 or respiratory rate reported
Dogan [13]	+	+	midazolam-fentanyl with topical analgesia or peribulbar block	No statistically significant differences in SBP and DBP[i] between groups	No statistically significant differences	No statistically significant differences in respiratory rate
Erdurmus [14]	+	+	saline	No statistically significant differences in SBP and DBP between groups	No statistically significant differences	No statistically significant differences in SpO_2 between groups
Ghodki [15]	+	–	saline	Decreased MAP after premedication [mean MAP (SD): 86.88 (10.75) vs 99.10 (12.36), $P = 0.005$], intraoperatively [mean MAP (SD): 88.26 (11.03) vs 107.20 (7.90), $P = 0.000$], and postoperatively [mean MAP (SD): 81.02 (11.10) vs 90.03 (9.24), $P = 0.008$]	Decreased after premedication [mean HR (SD): 72.42 (13.25) vs 81.4 (7.36), $P = 0.005$], intraoperatively [mean HR (SD): 76.00 (14.21) vs 89.75 (9.21), $P = 0.000$], and postoperatively [mean HR (SD): 68.50 (11.54) vs 79.50 (15.68), $P = 0.009$]	No statistically significant differences in $ETCO_2$ between groups
Kermany [10]	+	+	remifentanil	Decreased MAP postoperatively [mean MAP (SD): 76.3 (5.4) vs 85.2 (8.6), $P = 0.01$]	Decreased postoperatively [mean HR (SD): 65.4 (7.6) vs 72.1 (4.5), $P = 0.009$]	No statistically significant difference in SpO_2 between groups
Muttu [16]	+	+	midazolam	No statistical analyses provided	No statistical analyses provided	No periods of desaturation in either group

Table 3 Effects of Dexmedetomidine on Arterial Pressure, Heart Rate, and Respiratory Parameters *(Continued)*

Study	Dexmedetomidine		Other Treatment Group(s)	Arterial Pressure	Heart Rate	Respiratory Parameters
	Bolus	Continuous infusion				
Na [17]	–	+	propofol-alfentanil	Decreased SBP at surgery start [SBP (SD): 117 (16) vs 129 (19), P < 0.05], all intraoperative time points [SBP (SD): 117 (17) vs 129 (18), $P < 0.05$; 114 (15) vs 127 (18), P < 0.05; 112 (14) vs 126 (15), $P < 0.05$], and postoperatively [SBP (SD): 107 (15) vs 129 (18), P < 0.05]	No statistically significant differences between groups	No statistically significant difference in respiratory rate or SpO_2 between groups
Park [22]	+	+	remifentanil	Decreased MAP [data values and P values not reported]	No statistically significant differences	Decreased $ETCO_2$ and increased respiratory rate [data values not reported] No statistically significant differences in SpO_2
Virkilla [19]	+	–	placebo	Decreased SBP in 1.5 mcg/kg group compared to placebo [data values not reported, P < 0.001]	Decreased in 1.5 mcg/kg group compared to placebo [data values not reported, $P = 0.004$]	No statistically significant changes in SpO_2
Virkilla [20]	+	–	midazolam and placebo	Decreased SBP and DBP before periocular block compared to placebo [data values not reported, P < 0.001] Decreased SBP [data values not reported, P = 0.003] and DBP [data values not reported, P = 0.009] compared to midazolam before periocular block Decreased mean SBP and DBP compared to midazolam and placebo [data values not reported, $P < 0.001$] Decreased SBP postoperatively compared to midazolam and placebo [data values not reported, P < 0.001]	Decreased intraoperatively compared to placebo [data values not reported, P < 0.001] and midazolam [data values not reported, P = 0.01]Decreased postoperatively compared to placebo [data values not reported, P < 0.001]	Decreased SpO_2 compared to midazolam and placebo before block [data values not reported, P < 0.001]
Yagan [18]	+	–	ketofol[j]	Decreased MAP after drug administration and all time points thereafter compared to baseline and ketofol [data values not reported, P < 0.05]	Decreased after drug administration and all time points thereafter compared to baseline [data values not reported, P < 0.05]	No statistically significant difference in respiratory rate

[a]*SBP* systolic blood pressure, [b]*SD* standard deviation; [c]*mm Hg* millimeters mercury, [d]*HR* heart rate, [e]*MAP* mean arterial pressure, [f]*SE* standard error, [g]*SpO_2* blood oxygen saturation, [h]*$ETCO_2$* end-tidal carbon dioxide, [i]*DBP* diastolic blood pressure, [j]*ketofol* ketamine and propofol

No statistically significant differences in oxygen saturation (SpO_2), end-tidal carbon dioxide ($ETCO_2$) values, or respiratory rates were reported in studies investigating the respiratory effects of dexmedetomidine compared to saline; no sedation; midazolam and fentanyl; propofol and alfentanil; and ketamine and propofol (ketofol) [10–15, 17–19, 21]. However, there were inconsistent results among studies investigating changes in $ETCO_2$ and SpO_2 when comparing dexmedetomidine to midazolam, placebo, and remifentanil [20, 22, 24]. One study demonstrated statistically significant decreases in oxygen saturation with IM dexmedetomidine 1 mcg/kg compared to midazolam 20 mcg/kg and placebo [20]. Better ventilation as evidenced by lower $ETCO_2$ values and increased respiratory rates was noted in dexmedetomidine-treated patients compared to those receiving remifentanil titrated to a target effect site concentration of 1 ng/ml [22]. However, another study comparing dexmedetomidine to remifentanil infusion at 0.05 $mcg \cdot kg^{-1} \cdot min^{-1}$ reported statistically significant decreases in oxygen saturation in dexmedetomidine-treated patients 35–45 min after induction [24].

Analgesia, sedation/cognitive dysfunction, and ponv

There were inconsistent results among studies that investigated pain perception during regional blocks and postoperative analgesia with dexmedetomidine compared to other study medications as shown in Table 4 [11, 13–16, 18, 20, 21, 24]. One study demonstrated better analgesia as measured by Verbal Pain Scale (VPS) score in patients receiving bolus doses of fentanyl 0.5 mcg/kg and midazolam 20 mcg/kg followed by midazolam infusion at 5–15 $mcg \cdot kg^{-1} \cdot hr.^{-1}$ compared to those receiving dexmedetomidine 0.6 mcg/kg followed by continuous dexmedetomidine infusion at 0.1–0.5 $mcg \cdot kg^{-1} \cdot hr.^{-1}$ titrated to RSS 3 [13].

Better cognitive outcomes as measured by performance on Mini-Mental State Examination (MMSE) were noted in a study comparing dexmedetomidine to remifentanil [10]. Increased intraoperative levels of sedation as measured by Observer Assessment of Alertness/Sedation Scale (OAA/S) and BIS were noted when dexmedetomidine was compared to remifentanil [24]. Increased sedation was also noted with dexmedetomidine compared to saline as measured by BIS and RSS [15, 23]. Increased postoperative sedation lasting up to 3 h postoperatively as measured by 4-point sedation score was reported in one study comparing dexmedetomidine to midazolam and saline [11].

Three studies commented on the incidence of PONV [11, 13, 20]. One study found no statistically significant difference in the subjective assessment of nausea in patients receiving IM dexmedetomidine compared to IM midazolam or placebo, but confidence intervals are unknown [20]. Another study comparing dexmedetomidine to midazolam and saline stated that PONV was not experienced by any patients, while another study reported nausea in 2 patients (2.5%) [11, 13].

Pacu discharge and recovery times

Four studies investigated the time necessary to achieve a pre-determined target Aldrete score [12, 13, 15, 18]. One study noted that dexmedetomidine-treated patients required more time to achieve an Aldrete score of 10 when compared to midazolam-treated patients [median interquartile range (IQR): 45 (36–54) vs 21 (10–32) min, $P < 0.01$] [12]. Prolonged PACU discharge times were also noted in a study comparing dexmedetomidine to ketofol [mean time to achieve Aldrete score 9 (standard deviation (SD)): 24.9 (4.5) vs 16.1 (2.1) min, $P < 0.001$] [18]. These findings were not consistent with one study that utilized intravenous dexmedetomidine 1 mcg/kg followed by patient-controlled sedation with dexmedetomidine, which demonstrated no statistically significant differences in Aldrete scores at 30 min postoperatively compared to patients who received no sedation [21]. However, it is not clear from this study if the Aldrete scores achieved in 30 min were acceptable to discharge the patient, such as an Aldrete score 9 or 10 [21].

Intraocular pressure

Seven studies in our review demonstrated significant reductions in IOP [13, 15, 18–21, 23]. One study reported a 3.8 mmHg decrease in IOP compared to control after a 1 mcg/kg bolus of dexmedetomidine [21]. Intramuscular dexmedetomidine was also shown to reduce IOP, and the greatest reductions were noted in patients who received 1 mcg/kg and 1.5 mcg/kg [mean IOP (SD): 6.8 (3.1) and 6.8 (3.0), respectively] [19]. Another study reported statistically significant decreases in IOP for patients who received dexmedetomidine [mean IOP (SD): 17.10 (1.92) to 13.81 (1.63), $P < 0.0001$] compared to those who received saline [mean IOP (SD):16.90 (4.11) to 15.41 (3.93), $P > 0.05$] [15]. Ketofol was also shown to reduce IOP at a rate similar to dexmedetomidine [18].

Preoperative decreases in IOP from dexmedetomidine were not sustained postoperatively. Dogan et al. identified no statistically significant differences in IOP between patients who received dexmedetomidine or the combination of fentanyl and midazolam at 1 h and 24 h following surgery [13]. These findings of non-sustained reductions in IOP are supported by another study comparing the effects of IM dexmedetomidine to IM placebo and IM midazolam, which reported similar mean IOP values in the operated eye in all groups 24 h after surgery [20].

Patient and surgeon satisfaction

Compared to patients who received propofol-alfentanil, patients who received dexmedetomidine reported higher

Table 4 Effects of Dexmedetomidine on Analgesia, Sedation/Cognitive Dysfunction, Nausea/Vomiting, and PACU Discharge/Recovery Time

Study	Other Treatment Group(s)	Analgesia	Sedation or Cognitive Dysfunction	PONV[a]	PACU[b] Discharge or Recovery Time
Abdalla [23]	saline	–	Increased sedation at 60 mins [mean BIS[c] (SD[d]): 78.90 (4.99) vs 96.50 (2.09), $P = 0.008$] and 90 mins after starting infusion [93.00 (3.00) vs 96.35 (1.87), $P = 0.047$]	–	–
Alhashemi [12]	midazolam	–	–	–	Increased recovery time [median time required to achieve Aldrete 10 (IQR[e]) 45 (36–54) mins vs 21 (10–32) mins, $P < 0.01$]
Altiparmak [24]	remifentanil	Better analgesia at 10 mins [mean VRS[f] (SD): 0.67 (0.69) vs 1.78 (1.68), $P = 0.016$], 15 mins [mean VRS (SD): 0.57 (0.59) vs 1.15 (1.0), P = 0.008], 20 mins [mean VRS (SD): 0.52 (0.55) vs 1.16 (1.04), $P = 0.006$], 25 mins [mean VRS (SD): 0.54 (0.60) vs 1.12 (1.02), $P = 0.015$], 30 mins [mean VRS (SD): 0.54 (0.56) vs 1.13 (1.02), $P = 0.023$], and 35 mins [mean VRS (SD): 0.42 (0.50) vs 1.09 (0.99), $P = 0.024$] after start of surgery	Increased sedation at 1 min [mean OAA/S[g] (SD): 3.45 (0.74) vs 3.82 (0.93), $P = 0.012$] and 45 mins [mean OAA/S (SD): 4.00 (0.46) vs 3.30 (1.18), $P = 0.003$] following start of surgery Increased sedation at 1 min [mean BIS (SD): 86.1 (14.07) vs 91.95 (7.72), P = 0.024], 5 mins [mean BIS (SD): 79.92 (8.03) vs 88.76 (7.23), $P = 0.000$], 10 mins [mean BIS (SD): 76.92 (6.30) vs 84.35 (8.59), P = 0.000], 15 mins [mean BIS (SD): 76.77 (5.94) vs 83.39 (7.29), P = 0.000], 20 mins [mean BIS (SD): 76.67 (6.17) vs 82.76 (6.81), P = 0.000], and 45 mins [mean BIS (SD): 87.3 (8.4) vs 94.25 (1.75), $P = 0.017$] after start of surgery	–	–
Apan [11]	midazolam and saline	Better analgesia at 1 h postoperatively compared to midazolam [median VAS[h] (range): 0 (0) vs 0 (13), $P < 0.05$] and saline [median VAS (range): 0 (0) vs 0 (12), P < 0.05] Better analgesia compared to midazolam at 2 h [median VAS (range): 0 (13) vs 8 (32), P < 0.05] and 3 h [median VAS (range): 5 (16) vs 13 (31), P < 0.05] postoperatively	Increased sedation compared to control group at 1 h [median 4-point sedation score (range): 2 (2) vs 1 (1), $P < 0.05$] and 3 h [median 4-point sedation score (range): 1 (1) vs 1 (1), P < 0.05] postoperatively	Not experienced by any patients	–
Ayoglu [21]	no sedation	Lower perception of pain during block [NRS[i] (SD): 1.9 (0.5) vs 3.9 (0.6), P = 0.016]	Higher intraoperative RSS[j] scores [data values not reported, P < 0.05]	–	No statistically significant differences in Aldrete scores
Dogan [13]	midazolam-fentanyl with topical analgesia or peribulbar block	Increased VPS [data values not reported, $P = 0.001$] Increased intraoperative analgesic requirement [data values not reported, P < 0.05]	No statistically significant differences in RSS scores between groups	Nausea and vomiting were observed in 1 patient ineach dexmedetomidine group	Increased time needed to achieve Aldrete 10 [data values not reported, P < 0.05]
Erdurmus [14]	saline	Decreased pain perception [mean VPS[k] (SD): 1.23 (1.72) vs 3.64 (1.43), $P < 0.001$]	–	–	–

Table 4 Effects of Dexmedetomidine on Analgesia, Sedation/Cognitive Dysfunction, Nausea/Vomiting, and PACU Discharge/Recovery Time *(Continued)*

Study	Other Treatment Group(s)	Analgesia	Sedation or Cognitive Dysfunction	PONV[a]	PACU[b] Discharge or Recovery Time
Ghodki [15]	saline	No statistically significant difference (NRS)	Increased [mean RSS (SD): 2.67 (0.48) vs 1.56 (0.44), $P < 0.0001$]	–	No statistically significant difference in time required to achieve Aldrete 10
Kermany [10]	remifentanil	–	Better cognitive outcomes postoperatively for patients younger than 65-years [postoperative MMSE[l]: 26.3 vs 25.5, $P = 0.03$] and older than 65-years [postoperative MMSE: 26.1 vs 24.1, $P = 0.0001$]	–	–
Muttu [16]	midazolam	No statistically significant difference [median VAS: 0.8 vs 1.1, *P* value not provided]	No persistent sedation in either group	–	–
Na [17]	propofol-alfentanil	–	–	–	–
Park [22]	remifentanil	–	No statistically significant differences between groups (BIS) Increased at 10 mins [data values not provided, $P < 0.05$]	–	Increased time needed to achieve RSS 2 [7.0–8.0 mins vs 1.9–1.7 mins, *P* value not provided]
Virkilla [19]	placebo	–	No statistically significant difference between doses (VAS)	–	–
Virkilla [20]	midazolam and placebo	No statistically significant differences in VAS associated with local anesthetic injection between treatment groups	No statistically significant differences compared to midazolam (VAS) Increased VAS compared to placebo [data not reported, $P = 0.03$] No statistically significant differences postoperatively between groups (VAS)	No statistically significant differences in nausea (VAS), and no patients vomited	–
Yagan [18]	ketofol[m]	No statistically significant difference in VAS scores during the block and 1, 2, and 4 h postoperatively	Decreased sedation following drug administration [data not reported, $P < 0.001$] and after block [data not reported, $P < 0.017$]	–	Increased recovery time [mean time to achieve Aldrete 9 (SD): 24.9 (4.5) vs 16.1 (2.1), $P < 0.001$]

[a]*PONV* postoperative nausea and vomiting, [b]*PACU* post-anesthesia care unit, [c]*BIS* bispectral index, [d]*SD* standard deviation, [e]*IQR* interquartile range, [f]*VRS* verbal rating scale, [g]*OAA/S* observer assessment of alertness/sedation, [h]*VAS* visual analog scale, [i]*NRS* numeric rating scale, [j]*RSS* ramsay sedation scale, [k]*VPS* verbal pain scale, [l]*MMSE* mini-mental state examination, [m]*ketofol* ketamine and propofol

satisfaction scores [Iowa Satisfaction with Anesthesia Scale (ISAS) mean (SD): 50.3 (6.2) vs 42.7 (8.7), $P < 0.001$] [17]. Other studies corroborate this finding of higher patient satisfaction with dexmedetomidine compared to no sedation, saline, and midazolam [12, 14, 15, 21]. No statistically significant difference in patient satisfaction was noted when dexmedetomidine was compared to ketofol [mean 7-point Likert-like verbal rating scale (SD): 6.3 (0.5) vs 6.1 (0.7), $P = 0.084$] [18]. Furthermore, no statistically significant difference in patient satisfaction was noted when dexmedetomidine was compared to remifentanil [22].

Surgeon satisfaction was higher in 2 studies comparing dexmedetomidine to saline [14, 15]. There was no statistically significant difference in surgeon satisfaction when comparing dexmedetomidine to the combination of ketamine and propofol, or ketofol, [mean 7-point Likert-like verbal rating scale (SD): 6.4 (0.6) vs 6.2 (0.8), $P = 0.067$] or midazolam [median 7-point Likert-like verbal rating scale (IQR): 5 (4–6) vs 5 (4–6)] [12, 18]. Lower surgeon satisfaction was noted when dexmedetomidine was compared to remifentanil and midazolam-fentanyl [13, 22]. However, reasons for surgeon dissatisfaction were not specifically stated. Table 5 provides study details regarding patient and surgeon satisfaction.

Discussion

There is noteworthy inconsistency in medication classes, doses, routes of administration, and outcomes analyzed in randomized clinical trials investigating the use of dexmedetomidine for sedation in outpatient cataract surgery. Although strict selection criteria could allow for meta-analysis, the number of relevant studies would be substantially reduced. In attempt to capture relevant

Table 5 Effects of Dexmedetomidine on Patient and Surgeon Satisfaction

Study	Other Treatment Group(s)	Patient Satisfaction	Surgeon Satisfaction
Abdalla [23]	saline	–	–
Alhashemi [12]	midazolam	Increased satisfaction with sedation [median 7-point Likert-like verbal rating scale (IQR): 6 (6–7) vs 6 (5–7), $P < 0.05$]	No statistically significant difference (7-point Likert-like verbal rating scale)
Altiparmak [24]	remifentanil	–	–
Apan [11]	midazolam and saline	No statistical analyses of patient comments regarding satisfaction and effectiveness of sedation	No statistically significant difference (4-point scale)
Ayoglu [21]	no sedation	Increased NRS[a] scores [data not reported, $P = 0.001$]	No statistically significant difference (NRS)
Dogan [13]	midazolam-fentanyl with topical analgesia or peribulbar block	Decreased [mean patient satisfaction on 5-point scale: 3.60 and 3.65 for patients receiving midazolam, fentanyl, and topical or peribulbar block, respectively; compared to 3.15 and 2.90 for patients receiving dexmedetomidine and topical or peribulbar block, respectively; $P < 0.05$]	Decreased [mean surgeon satisfaction on 5-point scale: 3.75 and 3.70 for patients receiving midazolam, fentanyl, and topical or peribulbar block, respectively; compared to 3.25 and 3.25 for patients receiving dexmedetomidine and topical or peribulbar block, respectively; P < 0.05]
Erdurmus [14]	saline	Increased score on 5-point scale [no data reported, $P = 0.042$]	Increased [mean surgeon satisfaction score on 5-point scale (SD[b]): 3.41 (0.80) vs 2.36 (1.26), $P = 0.003$]
Ghodki [15]	saline	Increased [mean patient satisfaction score on 10-point scale (range): 9 (8–10) vs 7 (5–8), $P = 0.0001$]	Increased [surgeon satisfaction score (excellent/good): 26/4 vs 13/17, P = 0.0001]
Kermany [10]	remifentanil	–	–
Muttu [16]	midazolam	–	No statistically significant difference on 4-point scale[d]
Na [17]	propofol-alfentanil	Increased [ISAS[c] (SD): 50.3 (6.2) vs 42.7 (8.7), $P < 0.001$; and median ISAS (IQR): 50 (48–55) vs 45.0 (39–49)]	–
Park [22]	remifentanil	No statistically significant difference in 7-point Likert-like verbal rating scale	Decreased [mean 7-point Likert-like verbal rating scale (range): 6.05 (4–7) vs 6.35 (3–7), P < 0.05]
Virkilla [19]	placebo	–	–
Virkilla [20]	midazolam and placebo	–	–
Yagan [18]	ketofol[e]	No statistically significant difference in 7-point Likert-like verbal rating scale	No statistically significant difference in 7-point Likert-like verbal rating scale

[a]*NRS* numeric rating scale, [b]*SD* standard deviation, [c]*ISAS* Iowa Satisfaction with Anesthesia Scale, [d]*4-point scale* poor, acceptable, good, or excellent, [e]*ketofol* ketamine and propofol

outcomes for outpatient cataract surgery, we reviewed the impact of dexmedetomidine on hemodynamic parameters, respiratory parameters, pain, sedation, PONV, PACU discharge times, patient satisfaction, surgeon satisfaction, and IOP.

Safety

Hemodynamic and respiratory parameters

Cardiovascular depression secondary to dexmedetomidine is consistent with the known effects of alpha-2 agonists and, particularly, the perioperative administration of dexmedetomidine [6, 7]. Our review demonstrates statistically significant decreases in arterial pressures and heart rates associated with dexmedetomidine in multiple studies utilizing various medication dosages and titration schemes. However, these decreases in arterial pressures and heart rates may not be clinically significant or negatively impact a patient's perioperative course.

Although there appears to be some association between the bolus administration of dexmedetomidine and decreases in arterial pressures and heart rates, these findings are not supported by all studies. Specific data regarding arterial pressures, heart rates, and associated standard deviations are not retrievable from all publications. Many investigators graphically displayed these data without providing absolute values, thus precluding meta-analyses.

The ability to provide sedation and analgesia while also maintaining oxygenation and spontaneous ventilation is a commonly cited advantage of dexmedetomidine over alternative hypnotics, sedatives, and opioids [6, 7]. Multiple studies in this review demonstrated preserved oxygenation and ventilation [12, 17, 21, 22]. Statistically significant decreases in oxygen saturation in dexmedetomidine-treated patients were noted in two studies [20, 24]. However, the mean oxygen saturation did not fall below 93.14% (± 4.71%) in one study that reported the nadir [24]. Adverse respiratory events, such as the need for emergent intubation, were not reported in any study.

Post-operative cognitive dysfunction and sedation

Dexmedetomidine has been recommended as a safe therapy for reducing the incidence of post-operative delirium in the elderly after non-cardiac surgery in patients admitted to the ICU [25]. POCD and delirium have been associated with inflammatory mediators, which may be suppressed by dexmedetomidine [26, 27]. The incidence of POCD following cataract surgery has been reported at 4.4% and identified risk factors include advanced age and benzodiazepine pre-medication [28]. Overall, the commonest medications resulting in delirium (in the aging brain) include benzodiazepines, morphine, and anti-cholinergics [29]. Mansouri et al. identified no difference in the occurrence of POCD between midazolam and dexmedetomidine following cataract surgery under general anesthesia, although both were superior to placebo [30]. Unfortunately, the studies included in this review primarily focused on intraoperative levels of sedation and cognitive dysfunction, thus limiting our ability to draw conclusions regarding dexmedetomidine and postoperative neurocognitive disorders following cataract surgery.

The studies included in this review attempted to standardize the dosing of medications by targeting specific levels of intraoperative sedation. However, the methods used to assess sedation were variable. One study titrated dexmedetomidine and remifentanil to a BIS of 70–80 and described improved cognitive outcomes with dexmedetomidine as demonstrated by higher performance on MMSE [10]. Another study titrated dexmedetomidine and midazolam to a BIS greater than 85 and described persistent postoperative sedation on a 4-point scale [11]. Inconsistent study methods in assessing sedation preclude meta-analysis of these outcomes.

Nausea

Nausea is a known side effect of dexmedetomidine [6]. Only one study investigated the subjective assessment of nausea utilizing VAS and found no statistically significant difference between IM midazolam, IM dexmedetomidine, and IM placebo; however, the number of patients who experienced nausea was not provided and the confidence intervals for this result are unknown [20]. After combining the number of patients studied in 2 trials that defined nausea as an adverse event, only 2 patients (1.18%) reported nausea [11, 13].

Efficacy

Analgesia

Pain is one of the most powerful predictors of return to normal activity after surgery [31]. Although pain after cataract surgery is often considered minimal, Porela-Tiihonen reported that 34% of patients had some pain and 9% had more than moderate pain (VAS > 4) in the first few hours after cataract surgery [32].

Better analgesia was noted in patients treated with dexmedetomidine compared to remifentanil, midazolam, saline, and placebo in several studies [11, 14, 21, 24]. These findings are consistent with the known pharmacodynamic properties of dexmedetomidine. However, multiple studies reported no statistically significant difference in analgesia when comparing dexmedetomidine to saline, placebo, midazolam, and ketofol [15, 16, 18, 20]. Peribulbar blocks can provide complete analgesia for cataract surgery, which may limit the ability to identify statistically significant differences in analgesia between dexmedetomidine and other medications or placebo in patients following cataract surgery. Most studies did not investigate analgesia beyond 1 h postoperatively, at which time the peribulbar block may start to dissipate and potentially reveal differences in analgesia between study medications or placebo. Only one study compared dexmedetomidine to the common pairing of midazolam and fentanyl, which exhibited better analgesia [13].

Intraocular pressure

Dexmedetomidine reduces intraocular pressure by its central action [33]. Kim et al. reported that dexmedetomidine attenuated the increases in IOP associated with steep Trendelenburg positioning during laparoscopic radical prostatectomy [34]. Reduced eye pressure may improve surgical operating conditions and decrease the risk for elevated IOP following cataract surgery [35].

Multiple studies in our review demonstrated significant reductions in IOP [13, 15, 18–21, 23]. However, these decreases in IOP were not sustained postoperatively. These findings may be related to the relatively short half-life of dexmedetomidine, the short duration of surgery during which dexmedetomidine was infused, or both.

Recovery time

Our review demonstrates a tendency for prolonged recovery in patients who received dexmedetomidine, which may limit its utility in the ambulatory surgery setting. When compared to ketofol or midazolam, patients treated with dexmedetomidine required longer times to achieve an Aldrete score of 9 or 10, respectively [12, 18]. In these studies demonstrating prolonged recovery, medications were titrated to RSS 3, which was a common sedation target of other studies included in this review. These findings may be the clinical manifestations of differences in context-sensitive half-times between medications. Overall, PACU discharge and recovery times were infrequently reported by investigators.

Satisfaction

Patients who received dexmedetomidine generally reported higher satisfaction scores [12, 14, 15, 17, 21]. Each of the articles included in this review studied patients undergoing monitored anesthesia care, a form of anesthesia in which patient cooperation with the surgeon is critical. Therefore, despite unknown validity and reliability, we considered surgeon satisfaction to be a key component in comparing sedative agents. Surgeons most frequently reported no statistically significant difference in satisfaction associated with the administration of dexmedetomidine compared to other agents [11, 12, 16, 18, 21]. However, lower satisfaction was noted by surgeons when dexmedetomidine was compared to remifentanil [22]. The combination of midazolam and fentanyl was the only study medication group other than saline that was associated with higher patient and surgeon satisfaction scores [13]. Specific reasons for patient or surgeon dissatisfaction were not provided, thus limiting our ability to further analyze these outcomes.

Limitations

This systematic review is limited by inconsistent study medications, doses, routes of administration, and primary study outcomes of randomized clinical trials. Additionally, the publications included in this review demonstrate variability in the quality of randomization, double-blinding, and reporting of withdrawals and dropouts. These limitations preclude meta-analyses.

Conclusion

Dexmedetomidine offers several advantages over traditional sedatives, hypnotics, and opioids in adult patients undergoing outpatient cataract surgery, such as better analgesia, preserved respiratory function, reduced intraocular pressure, and higher patient satisfaction. However, dexmedetomidine is frequently associated with cardiovascular depression, particularly when administered in bolus doses ranging from 0.5–1.0 mcg/kg, and may delay PACU discharge. The advantages and disadvantages of perioperative dexmedetomidine for outpatient cataract surgery should be considered on a patient-by-patient basis.

Abbreviations

ASA: American Society of Anesthesiologists'; BIS: Bispectral index; DBP: Diastolic blood pressure; $ETCO_2$: End-tidal carbon dioxide; HR: Heart rate; hr.: hour; IM: Intramuscular; IOP: Intraocular pressure; IQR: Interquartile range; ISAS: Iowa Satisfaction with Anesthesia Scale; IV : Intravenous; ketofol: ketamine-propofol; kg: kilogram; MAP: Mean arterial pressure; mcg: microgram; mcg/kg: micrograms per kilogram; $mcg{\cdot}kg^{-1}{\cdot}hr.^{-1}$: micrograms per kilogram per hour; $mcg{\cdot}kg^{-1}{\cdot}min^{-1}$: micrograms per kilogram per minute; mg: milligrams; min: minute; mm Hg: millimeters of mercury; MMSE: Mini-mental state examination; n: number; NRS: Numeric rating scale; OAA/S: Observer assessment of alertness/sedation scale; PACU: Post-anesthesia care unit; POCD: Postoperative cognitive dysfunction; PONV: Post-operative nausea and vomiting; PRN: Pro re nata; RSS: Ramsay sedation scale; SBP: Systolic blood pressure; SD: Standard deviation; SE: Standard error; SpO_2: Oxygen saturation; VAS: Visual analog scale; VPS: Verbal pain scale; VRS: Verbal rating scale

Acknowledgements

We would like to thank our colleagues within the Department of Anesthesiology and Pain medicine at the UC Davis Medical Center for their help and support.

Authors' contributions

RA helped review the available medical literature on this topic and prepare the manuscript. JHJ helped review the available medical literature on this topic and prepare the manuscript. All authors have read and approved the manuscript, and ensure that this is the case.

References

1. Kauh CY, Blachley TS, Lichter PR, Lee PP, Stein JD. Geographic variation in the rate and timing of cataract surgery among US communities. JAMA Ophthalmol. 2016;134(3):267–76.

2. Liu YC, Wilkins M, Kim T, Malyugin B, Mehta JS. Cataracts. Lancet. 2017; 390(10094):600–12.
3. Cataract Surgery Infographic. https://www.aao.org/eye-health/news/cataract-surgery-infographic. Accessed 24 Sept 2019.
4. Stuth EA, Stucke AG, Zuperku EJ. Effects of anesthetics, sedatives, and opioids on ventilatory control. Compr Physiol. 2012;2(4):2281–367.
5. Benyamin R, Trescot AM, Datta S, Buenaventura R, Adlaka R, Sehgal N, Glaser SE, Vallejo R. Opioid complications and side effects. Pain Physician. 2008; 11(2 Suppl):S105–20.
6. Naaz S, Ozair E. Dexmedetomidine in current anaesthesia practice- a review. J Clin Diagn Res. 2014;8(10):GE01–4.
7. Scott-Warren VLSJ. Dexmedetomidine: its use in intensive care medicine and anaesthesia. BJA Education. 2016;16(7):242–6.
8. Blaudszun G, Lysakowski C, Elia N, Tramer MR. Effect of perioperative systemic alpha2 agonists on postoperative morphine consumption and pain intensity: systematic review and meta-analysis of randomized controlled trials. Anesthesiology. 2012;116(6):1312–22.
9. Jadad AR, Moore RA, Carroll D, Jenkinson C, Reynolds DJ, Gavaghan DJ, McQuay HJ. Assessing the quality of reports of randomized clinical trials: is blinding necessary? Control Clin Trials. 1996;17(1):1–12.
10. Poorzamany Nejat Kermany M, Dahi M, Yamini Sharif R, Radpay B. Comparison of the Effects of Dexmedetomidine and Remifentanil on Cognition State After Cataract Surgery. Anesth Pain Med. 2016;6(3):e33448.
11. Apan A, Doganci N, Ergan A, Buyukkocak U. Bispectral index-guided intraoperative sedation with dexmedetomidine and midazolam infusion in outpatient cataract surgery. Minerva Anestesiol. 2009;75(5):239–44.
12. Alhashemi JA. Dexmedetomidine vs midazolam for monitored anaesthesia care during cataract surgery. Br J Anaesth. 2006;96(6):722–6.
13. Dogan R, Karalezli A, Sahin D, Gumus F. Comparison of sedative drugs under peribulbar or topical anesthesia during phacoemulsification. Ophthalmic Surg Lasers Imaging. 2012;43(2):121–7.
14. Erdurmus M, Aydin B, Usta B, Yagci R, Gozdemir M, Totan Y. Patient comfort and surgeon satisfaction during cataract surgery using topical anesthesia with or without dexmedetomidine sedation. Eur J Ophthalmol. 2008;18(3): 361–7.
15. Ghodki PS, Sardesai SP, Halikar SS. Dexmedetomidine premedication in cataract surgery under topical anaesthesia: to assess patient and surgeon satisfaction. Southern Afr J Anaesthesia Analg. 2015;21(2):35–9.
16. Muttu S, Liu EH, Ang SB, Chew PT, Lee TL, Ti LK. Comparison of dexmedetomidine and midazolam sedation for cataract surgery under topical anesthesia. J Cataract Refract Surg. 2005;31(9):1845–6.
17. Na HS, Song IA, Park HS, Hwang JW, Do SH, Kim CS. Dexmedetomidine is effective for monitored anesthesia care in outpatients undergoing cataract surgery. Korean J Anesthesiol. 2011;61(6):453–9.
18. Yagan O, Karakahya RH, Tas N, Kucuk A. Comparison of Dexmedetomidine versus ketamine-Propofol combination for sedation in cataract surgery. Turk J Anaesthesiol Reanim. 2015;43(2):84–90.
19. Virkkila M, Ali-Melkkila T, Kanto J, Turunen J, Scheinin H. Dexmedetomidine as intramuscular premedication in outpatient cataract surgery. A placebo-controlled dose-ranging study. Anaesthesia. 1993;48(6):482–7.
20. Virkkila M, Ali-Melkkila T, Kanto J, Turunen J, Scheinin H. Dexmedetomidine as intramuscular premedication for day-case cataract surgery. A comparative study of dexmedetomidine, midazolam and placebo. Anaesthesia. 1994; 49(10):853–8.
21. Ayoglu H, Altunkaya H, Ozer Y, Yapakci O, Ozkocak I, Oz O, Alpay A, Ugurbas SH. Dexmedetomidine sedation during cataract surgery under regional anaesthesia. Br J Anaesth. 2007;99(3):448.
22. Park JH, Kwon JY. Remifentanil or dexmedetomidine for monitored anesthesia care during cataract surgery under topical anesthesia. Korean J Anesthesiol. 2012;63(1):92–3.
23. Abdalla MI, Al Mansouri F, Bener A. Dexmedetomidine during local anesthesia. J Anesth. 2006;20(1):54–6.
24. Altiparmak BÇN. Dexmedetomidine versus remifentanil sedation for obese patients undergoing cataract surgery. Int J Clin Exp Med. 2016;9(7):14728–33.
25. Su X, Meng ZT, Wu XH, Cui F, Li HL, Wang DX, Zhu X, Zhu SN, Maze M, Ma D. Dexmedetomidine for prevention of delirium in elderly patients after non-cardiac surgery: a randomised, double-blind, placebo-controlled trial. Lancet. 2016;388(10054):1893–902.
26. Liu X, Yu Y, Zhu S. Inflammatory markers in postoperative delirium (POD) and cognitive dysfunction (POCD): a meta-analysis of observational studies. PLoS One. 2018;13(4):e0195659.
27. Chen W, Liu B, Zhang F, Xue P, Cui R, Lei W. The effects of dexmedetomidine on post-operative cognitive dysfunction and inflammatory factors in senile patients. Int J Clin Exp Med. 2015;8(3):4601–5.
28. Milstein A, Pollack A, Kleinman G, Barak Y. Confusion/delirium following cataract surgery: an incidence study of 1-year duration. Int Psychogeriatr. 2002;14(3):301–6.
29. Young J, Inouye SK. Delirium in older people. BMJ. 2007;334(7598):842–6.
30. Mansouri N, Nasrollahi K, Shetabi H. Prevention of cognitive dysfunction after cataract surgery with intravenous Administration of Midazolam and Dexmedetomidine in elderly patients undergoing cataract surgery. Adv Biomed Res. 2019;8(1):6–6.
31. Fraser RA, Hotz SB, Hurtig JB, Hodges SN, Moher D. The prevalence and impact of pain after day-care tubal ligation surgery. Pain. 1989;39(2):189–201.
32. Porela-Tiihonen S, Kaarniranta K, Kokki H. Postoperative pain after cataract surgery. J Cataract Refract Surg. 2013;39(5):789–98.
33. Bloor BC, Ward DS, Belleville JP, Maze M. Effects of intravenous dexmedetomidine in humans. II Hemodynamic changes. Anesthesiology. 1992;77(6):1134–42.
34. Kim NY, Yoo YC, Park H, Choi YD, Kim CY, Bai SJ. The effect of dexmedetomidine on intraocular pressure increase in patients during robot-assisted laparoscopic radical prostatectomy in the steep Trendelenburg position. J Endourol. 2015;29(3):310–6.
35. Guan H, Mick A, Porco T, Dolan BJ. Preoperative factors associated with IOP reduction after cataract surgery. Optom Vis Sci. 2013;90(2):179–84..

Acceptance of mHealth among health professionals: a case study on anesthesia practitioners

Hugo Carvalho[1*†], Michael Verdonck[1,2†], Patrice Forget[3] and Jan Poelaert[1]

Abstract

Background: mHealth, the practice of medicine aided by mobile devices is a growing market. Although the offer on Anesthesia applications (Apps) is quite prolific, representative formal assessments on the views of anesthesia practitioners on its use and potential place in daily practice is lacking. This survey aimed thus to cross-assess the Belgian anesthesia population on the use of smartphone Apps and peripherals.

Methods: The survey was exclusively distributed as an online anonymous questionnaire. Sharing took place via hyperlink forwarding by the Belgian Society for Anesthesia and Reanimation (BSAR) and by the Belgian Association for Regional Anesthesia (BARA) to all registered members. The first answer took place on 5 September 2018, the last on 22 January 2019.

Results: Three hundred forty-nine answers were obtained (26.9% corresponding to trainees, 73.1% to specialists). Anesthesiologists were positively confident that Apps and peripherals could help improve anesthesia care (57.0 and 47.9%, respectively, scored 4 or 5, in a scale from 0 to 5). Trainees were significantly more confident than specialists on both mobile Apps (71.2% and 51.8%, respectively; $p = 0.001$) and peripherals (77.7% and 45.1%, respectively; $p = 0.09$).
The usefulness of Apps and Peripherals was rated 1 or below (on a 0 to 5 scale), respectively, by 9.5 and 14.6% of the total surveyed population, being specialists proportionally less confident in Smartphone peripherals than trainees ($p = 0.008$). Mobile apps are actively used by a significantly higher proportional number of trainees (67.0% vs. 37.3%, respectively; $p = 0.000001$).
The preferred category of mobile Apps was dose-calculating applications (39.15%), followed by digital books (21.1%) and Apps for active perioperative monitoring (20.0%).

Conclusions: Belgian Anesthesia practitioners show a global positive attitude towards smartphone Apps and Peripherals, with trainees trending to be more confident than specialists.

Keywords: Anesthesia, mHealth, Smartphone application, Smartphone peripherals, Apps

* Correspondence: carvalho.hn@gmail.com
†Hugo Carvalho and Michael Verdonck contributed equally to this work.
[1]Vrije Universiteit Brussel (VUB), Universitair Ziekenhuis Brussel (UZ Brussel), Brussels, Belgium

Background

Smartphones are a ubiquitous phenomenon. The massive production of these multisensory devices has reduced their overall cost and increased their societal penetrance. Their high processing capacity entails a rather useful leverage for healthcare in general, a sector where data is abundant and its processing relevant for clinical decision-making [1, 2]. These advantageous features have been quickly assimilated by anesthesiologists, and dedicated anesthesia applications for various perioperative purposes have been continuously sprouting [3]. Medical device manufacturers have been similarly leveraging on this versatility in order to commercialize smartphone plug-in devices (also known as smartphone peripherals) that can be used for diagnostic purposes. These include, among others, echography probes (Butterfly™, Clarius™, Philips Lumify™), video laryngoscopes (Airtraq™ Phone adapter) and stetoscopes (StethIO™).

Commonly referred to as "mHealth" (abbreviation for Mobile Health), the practice of medicine aided by mobile devices is a growing market. In the United States of America (USA), this sector has been estimated to be worth more than 28 billion dollars in 2018, and predicted to surpass the 100 billion dollar barrier by 2023 [4]. Despite its exponential growth, regulation has been lagging behind and Food and Drug Administration (FDA) data shows that from a pool of more than 150,000 mobile applications (Apps) within the Health/Wellness category, only around 200 (0.1%) had been submitted to standardized governmental validation procedures [5].

Despite the high mobile applications output, formal surveying of the views of anesthesia providers on these applications is scarce [3, 5]. Green et al. have conducted one of the most complete, although non-representative, studies on the pattern of utilization of smartphone applications by anesthesiologists in the USA [3].

The aim of the present survey was to specifically cross-assess the Belgian anesthesia population on this same subject, as well as to discuss the results with respect to the current legal European framework around mHealth.

Methods

The present study was approved by Ethical Committee of the Universitair Ziekenhuis Brussel, Belgium (Reference 2018/435, B.U.N. 143201837927), and registered at the ClinicalTrials.gov database (Identifier: NCT03750084). The survey was specifically developed for the present study and has not been published elsewhere. The targeted population referred to active (practising) Belgian anesthesiologists (both trainees and specialists), and the a priori established aim was the assessment of the confidence level of this population on both smartphone applications and dedicated smartphone peripherals within daily anesthesia practice. Future development expectations/desires were also to be assessed. Assessment of user experience was not within the scope of the present study.

The survey was not piloted and was exclusively distributed as an online anonymous questionnaire (Google™ Forms platform) for traceability purposes. Sharing took place via hyperlink distribution by the Belgian Society for Anaesthesia and Reanimation (BSAR) and by the Belgian Association for Regional Anaesthesia (BARA) to all registered members. The first answer took place on 5 September 2018, the last on 22 January 2019.

The original survey is available as a supplementary file as well as online at: https://goo.gl/forms/7job24qgFOPXpUD12

It was divided in two main sections: one pertaining to Smartphone Applications themselves, another to Smartphone Peripherals. Each section was identically subdivided and sequentially evaluated the following topics:

- Confidence that Smartphone applications / peripherals can help improve Anesthesia care and why.
- Phase of perioperative care in which Smartphone applications / peripherals are most useful.
- Which sort of Smartphone applications appeal the user the most.
- Which Smartphone applications / peripherals the user employs in his/her daily practice.
- What are the user's wishes on the development of future Smartphone applications / peripherals.

The survey has been structured based on the Technology Acceptance Model (TAM), an information systems theory that describes how users come to accept and use new technologies [6, 7]. The model suggests that when users are presented with a new technology, two primary factors influence their decision about how and when they will use it: (1) Perceived ease of use, which is determined by the degree to which a person believes that using a particular technique would be free of effort; and (2) Perceived usefulness, referring to the degree in which a person believes that a technique will be effective in achieving the intended modelling objective. The aforementioned model and associated measures were concordantly translated into the current survey to assess how respondents perceived the acceptance of mobile applications and peripherals within anesthesia. More specifically, participants had to answer several questions – using multiple-item scales with a Likert structure – which measured both the perceived usefulness and perceived ease of use. The reliability and validity of these type assessments has been assessed in several similar research efforts [8–11].

Questions were in their majority presented to the surveyees with a categorical structure. Dichotomous, nominal and contingency questions were used to categorize individuals as well as the contextual use of

Apps and Peripherals. Confidence levels were assessed by a Likert-type scale with balanced keying in order to allow for discrete quantitative comparisons. A score of 3 was considered the positivism transition point (considered to "Improve Anesthesia Care"), and a score of 4 or 5 was considered as positively trending confidence. Optional open text questions were used for detailing the reasons for the selected subjective confidence level.

Data reporting for the total population and for each subgroup (consultants/trainees) was descriptive in nature and precision reported with 95% Confidence Intervals [95%CI]. The inter-group confidence level comparisons based on the multi-point (ordinal) rating scales levels were carried out by means of binary reconversion of the Likert scale into two mutually exclusive intervals (one encompassing the ratings 0 to 3, and the second 4 to 5), and by sequential non-parametric analysis by means of Chi-square testing with a significance cut-off of 0.05. Identical methodology was used for the analysis of inter-group differences in terms of active use of Apps or Peripherals to aid Anesthesia care.

Results

A total of 349 answers were obtained. Ninety-four (26.9%) responses were of Belgian Anesthesia trainees, 255 (73.1%) from Belgian Anesthesia consultants. A majority of the answering specialists (21.7%) had no dedicated subspecialty activities or were all-round specialists (Fig. 1). Anesthesiologists with an orthopedic anesthesia subspecialty accounted for 17.6% of the total, followed by cardio-thoracic anesthesiologists (14.3%), Pediatric Anesthesiologists (13.4%), Pain Clinic specialists (12.8%), Neuro-anesthesiologists (6.5%) and Intensive care specialists (6.0%). The remainder subspecialties were underrepresented (less than 1.8%).

When asked on how confident they were that Smartphone Applications (Apps) or Smartphone Peripherals (Peripherals) could improve anesthesia care, a majority of the Belgian anesthesiologists were positively confident (score of 4 or 5, on a 0 to 5 categorical scale) that these could indeed help improve anesthesia care (57.0% [95%CI: 51.8–62.2%] and 47.9% [95%CI: 42.7–53.1%], respectively, scored 4 or 5) (Fig. 2). When subanalyzing the data per experience group, anesthesia trainees demonstrated a significantly higher degree of optimism (score of 4 or 5, out of 5) on Mobile Apps compared to consultants (71.3% [95%CI: 62.1–80.4%] and 51.8% [95%CI: 45.6 57.9%], respectively) (X^2 [1, $N = 349$] = 10.6696, $p = 0.001$) (Fig. 3). This positivity trend was maintained for Smartphone peripherals (77.7% [95%CI: 69.3–86.1%] and 45.1% [95%CI: 39.0–51.2%], respectively), although no statistical significance was retained (X^2 [1, $N = 349$] = 2.8754, $p = 0.090$) (Fig. 4).

Nine and a half percent [95%CI: 6.4–12.6%] of the surveyees (consultants and trainees combined) rated Apps' usefulness in Anesthesia as 1 or below (on a 0 to 5 scale), and 14.6% [95%CI: 10.9–18.3%] gave the same rating when asked about Peripherals. Inter-group analysis for this rating showed no statistical significance between trainees and consultants for Apps (X^2 [1, $N = 349$] = 2.5711, $p = 0.108833$). On the other hand, smartphone peripherals were significantly more negatively rated by consultants than by trainees (X^2 [1, N = 349] = 6.9839, $p = 0.008225$).

From all the responders, 45. 3% [95%CI: 40.0–50.5%] actively used Apps to aid their anesthesia practice, compared to only 3.2% [95%CI: 1.3–5.0%] that use Peripherals in their daily anesthesia practice. Again, subanalysis of the answers per training group showed that trainees actively use mobile apps in a significantly higher proportion when compared to consultants (67.0% [95%CI:

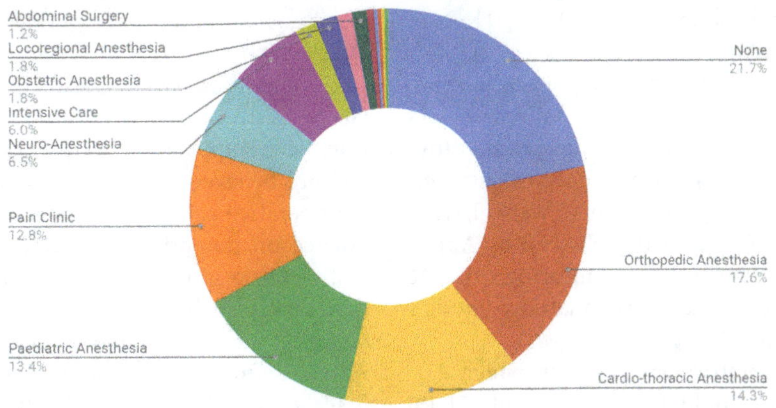

Fig. 1 Subspecialty stacked distribution of responding Anesthesia Specialists (one specialist can be accounted for more than once if he holds multiple subspecialty competences). Percentages represent the total number of surveyees per specific category relative to total number of surveyees

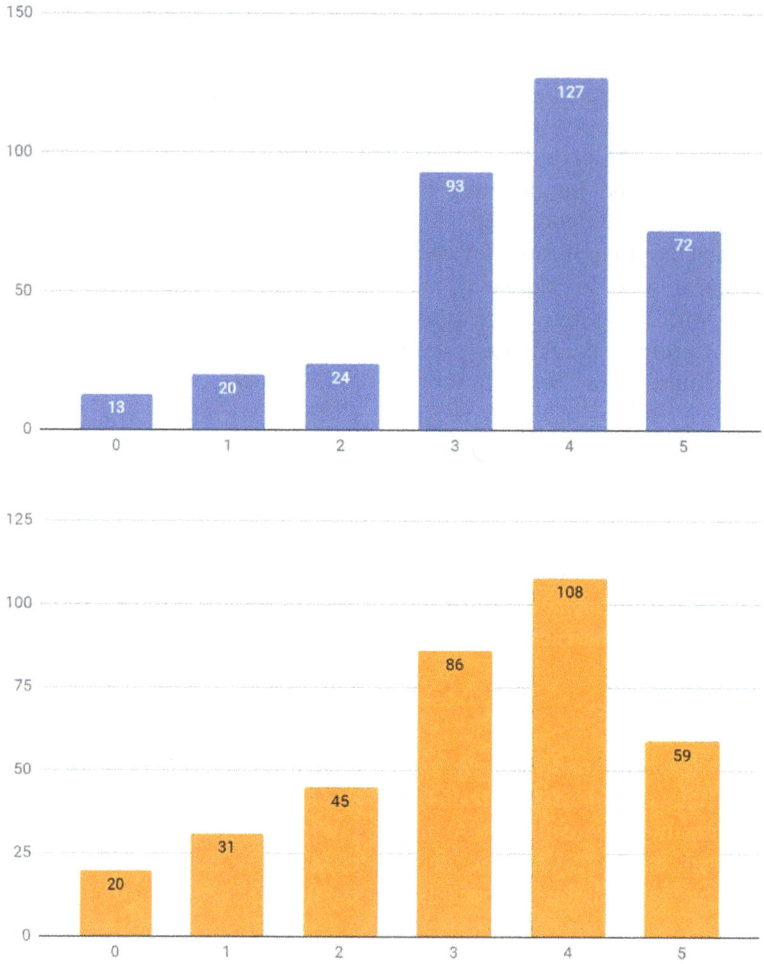

Fig. 2 Apps (left - blue) vs Peripherals (right - orange) - Confidence level (scale: 0 to 5). x axis – Confidence level category, y axis – absolute number of survey answers ("How confident are you that Smartphone Apps can help improve anesthesia care?" / "How confident are you that combining your smartphone with a dedicated monitoring peripheral can help improve anesthesia care?")

57.5–76.5%] and 37.3% [95%CI: 31.3–43.2%], respectively) (X^2 [1, N = 349] = 24.5615, $p = 0.000001$) (Table 1). No statistically significant inter-group difference was found in terms of active peripherals use) (X^2 [1, N = 349] = 0.4421, $p = 0.506108$) (Table 1).

When questioned on which App category was more appealing, 39.15% [95%CI: 34.0–44.3] of total responders gave preference to dose-calculating applications (dynamic [TCI modelling] and static [fixed dose calculation] apps). The next bigger App preference were Digital Books (21.12% [95%CI: 16.8–25.4%]), followed by Applications used for perioperative monitoring (20.0% [95%CI: 15.8–24.2%]) and interactive anatomy models (12.39% [95%CI: 8.9–15.8%]) (Fig. 5).

Concerning the perioperative care phase in which Applications or Peripherals could be more useful, 71.1% [95%CI: 66.3–75.9%] and 57.0% [95%CI: 51.8–62.2%], respectively, considered them to have a potential use in all phases of the perioperative care (Figs. 6 and 7).

The categories in which anesthesiologists would like to see development of smartphone peripheral devices are illustrated in Fig. 8.

Discussion

In general, these survey results agree with the findings of Green et al. on the American anesthesiologists population, where apps enjoy a significant degree of confidence and are believed to have a potential use on all phases of perioperative care [3]. Peripherals also enjoy a high confidence on potential use, rating 47.9% [95%CI: 42.7–53.1%] of the responders their confidence as 80% or higher that these can be useful in Anesthesia care. Nine and a half percent [95%CI: 6.4–12.6%] of the surveyees rated Apps' usefulness in anesthesia as 1 or bellow (on a 0 to 5 scale), and 14.6% [95%CI: 10.9–18.3%] gave the same rating when asked about Peripherals. Thus, Apps enjoy both a greater degree of optimisms as well as a lower degree of disbelief in comparison to Peripherals. The

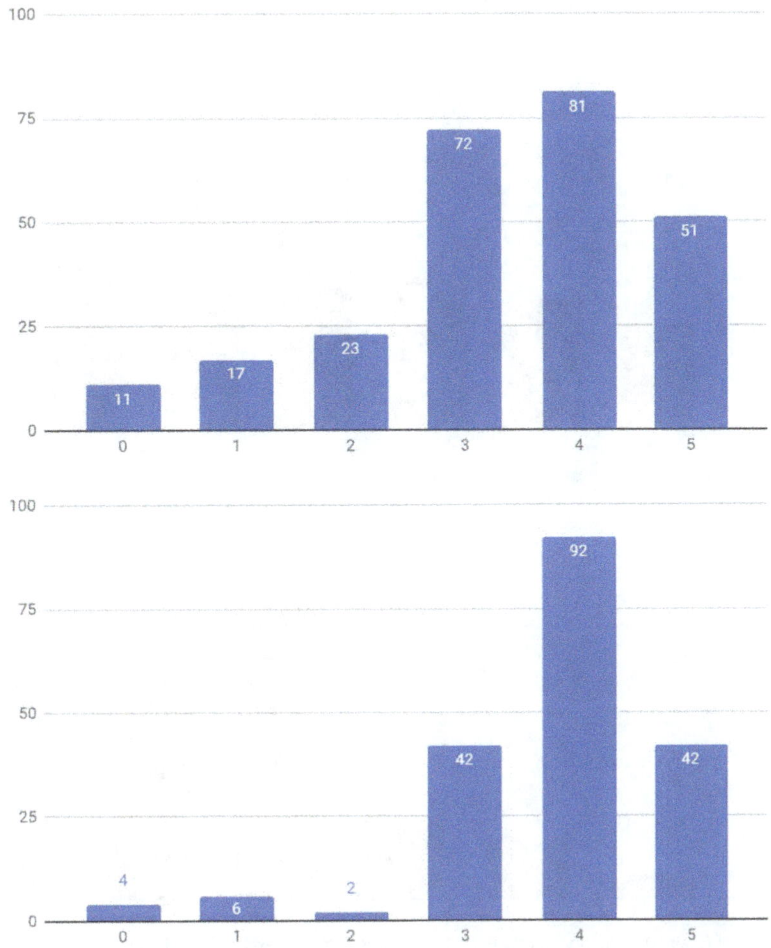

Fig. 3 Apps Confidence level (scale: 0 to 5): Specialists (left) vs Trainees (right). x axis – Confidence level category, y axis – absolute number of survey answers

reasons for this discrepancy were not evaluated by this questionnaire, but one can speculate that the underdeveloped regulated market of smartphone peripherals for diagnostic aid is still not firmly established within today's anesthesia practice. Although the major players have already created a dedicated peripherals market branch (f.e., the Philips Lumifym® portable echography series), convincing of practitioners on their usefulness is still needed. Curiously, when asked on which peripherals they wanted to see developed, 61.7% of the anesthesiologists answered "Echography". This is nonetheless one of the more exploited areas in terms of Anesthesia smartphone peripherals, and has been explored both by the major players in the medical device industry (Philips™, Airtraq™), as well as by less known and upcoming competitors (Clarius™, Butterfly™). From the total of 66 individuals providing a written rationale for their confidence levels on mobile peripheral devices, 6 (9.1%) suggested that although they did know of the existence of such products, they still found them economically inaccessible. Other, however, suggested they had no knowledge of such devices. Another possible reason that might contribute to the greater disbelief possibly relates to the medical use of an originally partially non-medical device. Although it seems logical that controlled CE-labelling (Conformité Européenne) of smartphone peripherals for medical use might help overcome this phenomenon, a subjective factor cannot be underestimated. Just like heavy, well designed and good fitting over-head headphones feel subconsciously better than in-ear equivalents, traditional anesthesia monitors might still convey more confidence [12].

Another curious pattern observed on the surveyees' answers was the fact that although 57.0% [95%CI: 51.8–62.2%] considered Apps useful (classification of 4 or 5 out of 5), only 45.3% [95%CI: 40.0–50.5%] reported actually using them in their daily practice. The gap was proportionally bigger when analysing smartphone peripherals (47.9% [95%CI: 42.7–53.1%], and 3.2% [95%CI: 1.3–5.0%], respectively), although the latter easier to justify in light of the underdeveloped smartphone peripherals

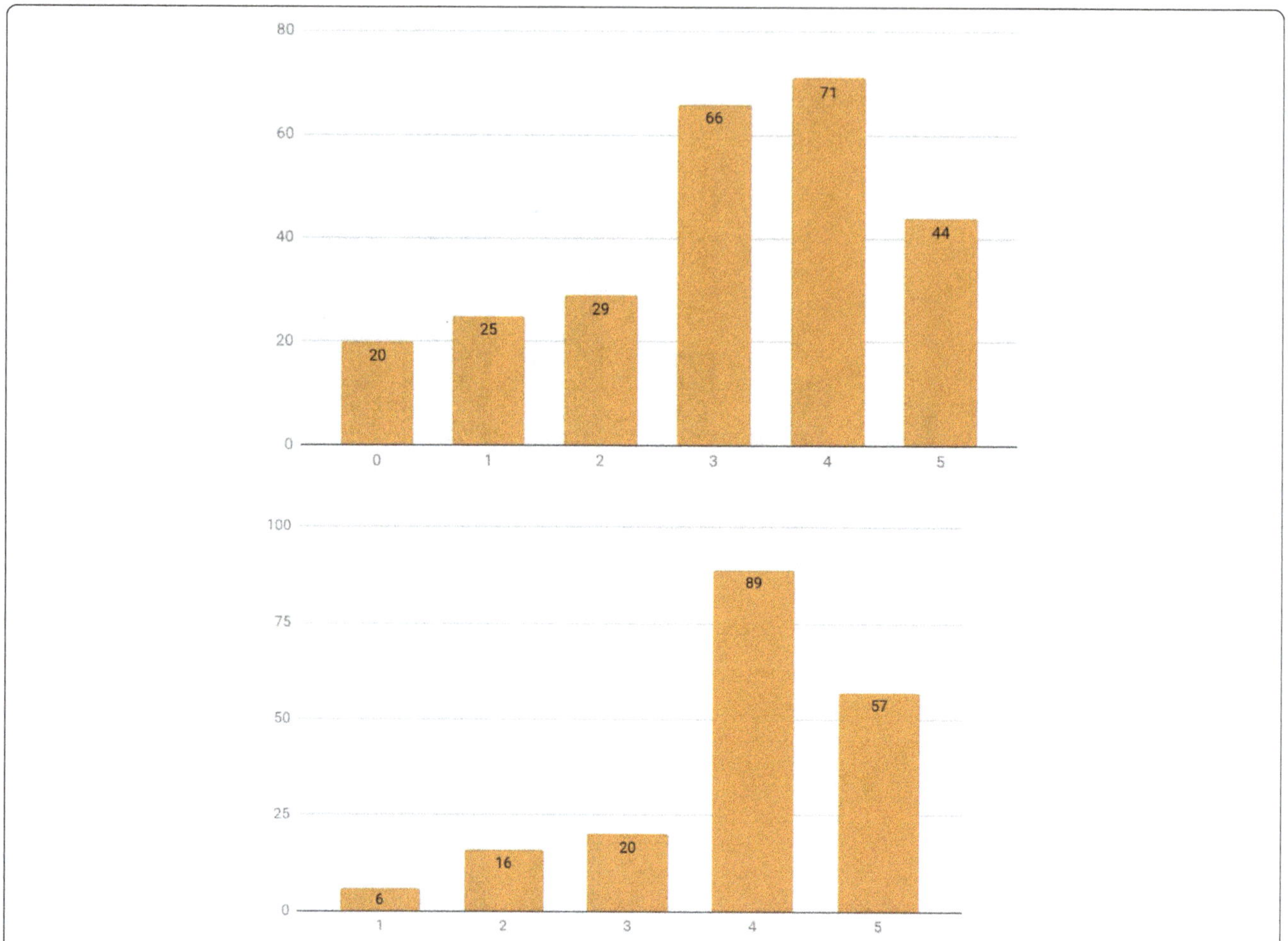

Fig. 4 Peripherals Confidence level (scale: 0 to 5): Specialists (left) vs. trainees (right). x axis – Confidence level category, y axis – absolute number of survey answers

market. This Smartphone "Confidence - Active use" gap might be explained by a yet unripe and ununiformed anesthesia app market. A perceptive phenomenon of unrealistic and consequently unfulfilled expectations by users must also be considered as possible, although formal prospective user experience assessments are needed for this purpose.

In line with the study of Green et al., dosage apps were chosen by the majority as the most useful [3]. Digital books and perioperative apps followed. Such choice pattern is not counter-intuitive considering the still limited interactivity between handheld devices and anesthesia monitoring devices, although such justification is purely speculative as formal assessments to this point are lacking. The increasing focus on portability and cross-connectivity might lead to a pattern change, and future studies would be useful to analyse a trend shift.

Table 1 Active Usage of Mobile Apps and Peripherals per subgroup

	Apps	Peripherals
Specialists	95 (37.3%)	9 (3.5%)
Trainees	63 (67.0%)	2 (1.2%)
Total	158 (45.3%)	11 (3.2%)

Cell values represent the absolute number of individuals. Within parenthesis the percentages are relative to total of individuals within the same cell line-group (i.e., relative to either specialists, trainees or total surveyees)

The observed positive disposition towards mHealth usage as well as its focus on mobile apps is apparent on indexed literature analysis. In fact, notwithstanding a possible positive publication bias, the publication of mHealth applications within all domains of healthcare has been steadily increasing [13]. Curiously, and notwithstanding the fact that representative reports on global mHealth usage patterns are lacking, analysis of an individual application's trends have shown a higher penetration of these low cost aids in low income countries [14].

Within the anesthesia domain, developed applications range from crisis management support apps, to post-operative pain assessment, but also to non-medical topics such as logistic optimisation of Operation room

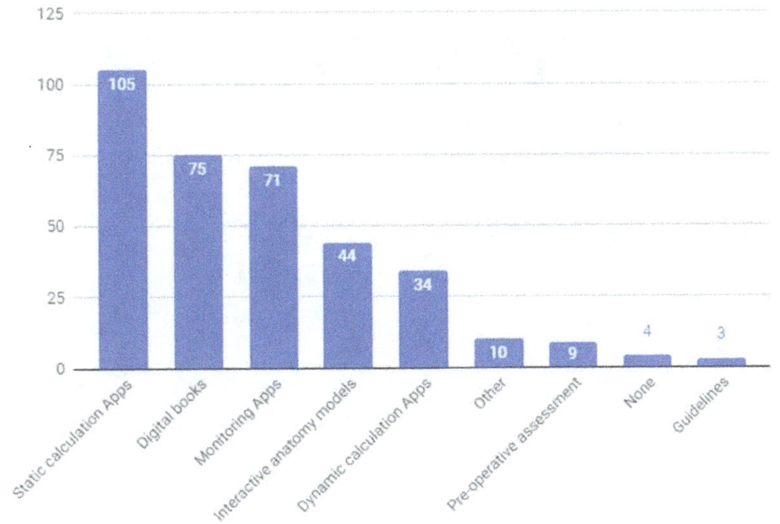

Fig. 5 Categorization of the most appealing Apps ("Which kind of Apps appeal you the most?"). x axis – App category, y axis – absolute number of survey answers

supplies [15–17]. Most of these reports are descriptive and lack usability testing to allow a direct comparison to the present study's results.

As opposed to the study of Green et al., our group found significant differences between anesthesia trainees and specialists. Although there was a global positivity trend towards mobile apps in both groups, training anesthesiologists displayed a significantly higher confidence on mobile apps than consultants (71.3% vs 51.8%, respectively, $p = 0.001$). This positivity trend was similarly true for smartphone peripherals (45.1% vs 77.7%, respectively), although this difference didn't retain statistical significant on further difference testing ($p = 0.09$). Besides the evident cultural and contextual medical practice differences between the sampled subjects (American vs. European), the collected data on both studies is insufficient to put forward a phenomenological explanation.

According to data from the Belgian National Institute for Health and Disability Insurance (RIZIV / INAMI), in the beginning of 2016, Belgium had 2441 active anesthesia specialists (certified specialists and trainees) [18]. This sets this survey's cross-sectional percentage at 14.2% of the total active Belgian anesthesiologists, 13.2% of the certified Belgian anesthesiologists, and 17.5% of the Belgian anesthesiology trainees. Concerning the accredited specialists (diploma-holding), it is however not known if all of them are dedicated in exclusivity to anesthesia-related fields such as Intensive care, Emergency or Chronic Pain. It is thus possible that the

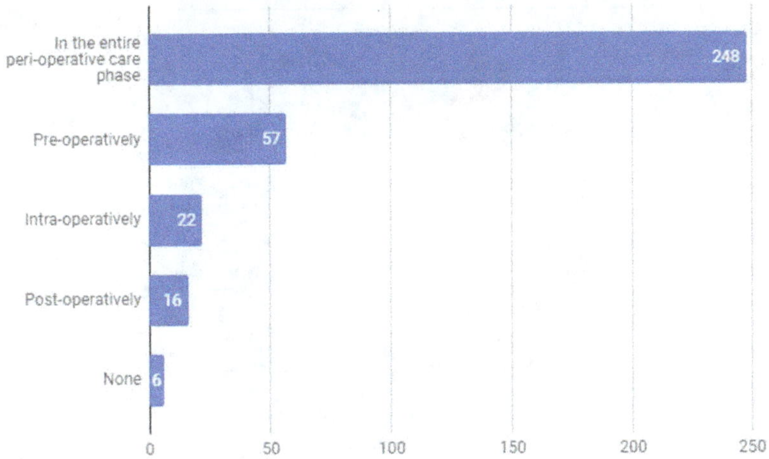

Fig. 6 Phase in which Smartphone Apps can be more useful ("In which phase of perioperative care can Smartphone Apps be more useful?"). x axis – absolute number of survey answers, y axis – Perioperative phase category

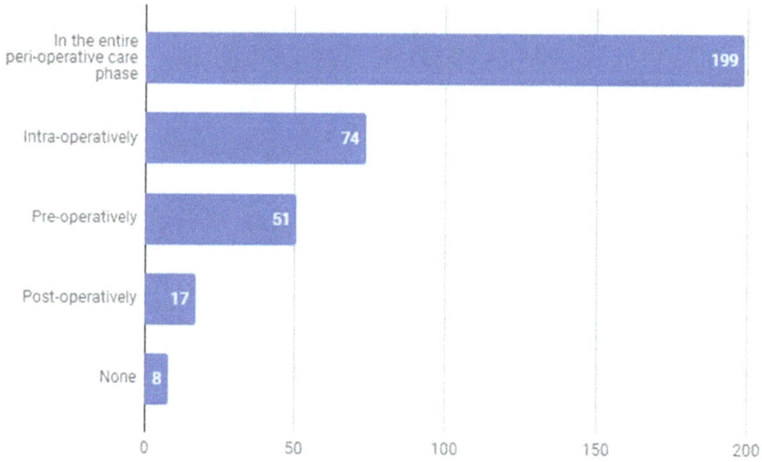

Fig. 7 Phase in which Smartphone Peripherals can be more useful ("In which phase of perioperative care can Smartphone Peripherals be more useful?"). x axis – absolute number of survey answers, y axis – Perioperative phase category

representability percentage of this survey is different than calculated, although practically very difficult to confirm.

These definitely promising technologies are increasingly being introduced in our daily practice and play an important facilitating role. However, one must not forget that these freely available tools are not always subject to formal approval procedures that scientifically validate their clinical use. Most of these are part of the off-label/ "use at own risk" category (commonly referred to as "Grey Area Apps") - applications freely available without formal evaluation of their function for their stated (medical) use [8]. Taking this into mind, the European Union (EU) has created between 2016 and 2017 a workgroup for the development of mHealth assessment guidelines [19]. However, the group was not able to endorse concrete guidelines by failure to reach a minimal intra-group consensus [20]. As of this moment, Grey Area Apps remain unregulated. There is, however, a non-binding "privacy code of conduct on mobile health apps" that outlines the core values that should guide mobile health application development [21]. It provides a theoretical competitive advantage against non-conform Applications and speeds up an eventual CE-label request. As for applications aiming for a formal regulated national market entry, compliance with the EU regulation 2017/745 (from 5 April 2017) is mandatory. Together with the EU norm 2017/746, they regulate the European market of medical devices since May 2017. European Union state members fall, thus, under these norms.

It is self-evident that mobile Applications and Peripherals are quickly permeating all phases of Healthcare, with the right steps are being taken for their scientific, national and intracontinental integration [22–33]. Peripherals still lag behind mobile applications although

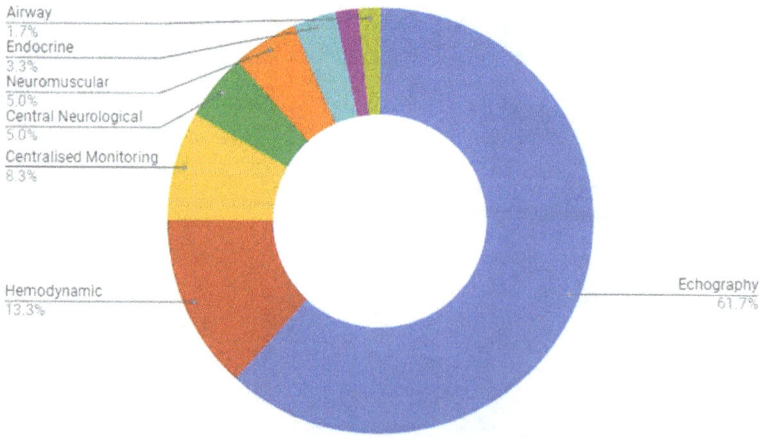

Fig. 8 Wishes for smartphone peripheral device development per monitoring category ("Which peripherals would you like to see developed in the coming future?"). Percentages represent the total number of votes per specific category relative to total number of votes

they constitute an economically and clinically important area. Care must still be taken considering the majority of available Apps fall within the unregulated category of "Grey Area Apps". Last, but not least, care is necessary in avoiding over-reliability/dependency on Apps, with the consequent side-tracking of basic clinical skills. Notwithstanding this warning note, the education potential of apps as supplement to classical learning techniques is increasingly being explored with some educational centers incorporating such solutions within anesthesia training programmes [34]. The development of applicationS should ideally use a user-centered design for and optimal and successful adoption [15].

The present study is limited in the fact that it doesn't directly address user experience. Initially designed primarily to address the acceptance of Apps and Peripherals, user experience and expectations were left out in the need for a compromise between brevity and completeness. A mixed-method experience analysis would be a relevant top-up survey that would allow this quantification as well as to potentially guide App and Peripheral development based on end user experience and expectations. Secondly, the survey is further limited in the fact that the transversal population assessment was estimated at 14.3% (349 out of 2441 active anesthesia specialists), raising the obvious concern of non-responder bias. Finally, the fact that digital books have been considered Apps might constitute a classification bias depending on surveyee interpretation. In fact, digital books might also come in non-app form (for example as *.pdf or *.chm format), which could potentially affect the perception of the respondents.

Conclusions

Belgian Anesthesia practitioners show a positive attitude towards smartphone-based solutions within Anesthesia care, mirroring international reported trends within other medical sectors. There is evidence of an international recognition of the potential of these technologies within the healthcare domain, with consequently rising regulatory efforts from medical societies and national legislative bodies.

Abbreviations

Apps: Mobile Applications; BARA: Belgian Association for Regional Anesthesia; BSAR: Belgian Society for Anesthesia and Reanimation; CE: Conformité Européenne; EU: European Union; FDA: Food and Drug Administration; mHealth: Mobile Health; RIZIV/INAMI: Belgian National Institute for Health and Disability Insurance; TAM: Technology Acceptance Model; USA: United States of America; VUB: Vrije Universiteit Brussel

Acknowledgements

We would like to thank the study nurses (Veerle Van Mossevelde, Dirk De Clippeleir, and Annelies de Cock) for their unconditional support throughout the study.

Authors' contributions

HNC and MV contributed to the design and the methods, HNC and MV acquired the data, HNC and MV analysed the data and are responsible for the integrity of the data and the analyses, all the authors contributed to the interpretation, HNC and MV redacted the first draft, reviewed and modified by PF and JP. All the authors approved the final version.

Author details

[1]Vrije Universiteit Brussel (VUB), Universitair Ziekenhuis Brussel (UZ Brussel), Brussels, Belgium. [2]Business Informatics Research Group, Universiteit Gent, Ghent, Belgium. [3]Institute of Applied Health Sciences, NHS Grampian, University of Aberdeen, Aberdeen, UK.

References

1. Boulos M, Wheeler S, Tavares C, Jones R. How smartphones are changing the face of mobile and participatory healthcare: an overview, with example from eCAALYX. Biomed Eng Online. 2011;10(1):24. https://doi.org/10.1186/1475-925X-10-24.
2. American Medical Association. Physician smartphone popularity shifts health IT focus to mobile use. In: American Medical News; 2010. http://www.amednews.com/article/20100823/business/308239976/1/. Accessed 18 Dec 2019.
3. Green MS, Mathew JJ, Gundigi A, Green P, Tariq R. Utilization of smartphone applications by anesthesia providers. Anesthesiol Res Pract. 2018;2018:8694357. https://doi.org/10.1155/2018/8694357.
4. Wood L. Mobile health (mHealth) app market industry trends, opportunities and forecasts to 2023—Research and markets. In: Business Wire; 2017. https://www.businesswire.com/news/home/20171215005299/en/Mobile-Health-mHealth-App-Market-Industry-Trends . Accessed 30 Nov 2018.
5. U.S. Food and Drug Administration. Mobile medical applications. Guidance for industry and food and drug administration staff. 2015. https://www.fda.gov/downloads/MedicalDevices/DeviceRegulationandGuidance/GuidanceDocuments/UCM263366.pdf. Accessed 22 Feb 2019.
6. Davis FD. Perceived usefulness, perceived ease of use, and user acceptance of information technology. MIS Q. 1989;13(3):319–40. https://doi.org/10.2307/249008.
7. Venkatesh V, Davis FD, Morris MG. Dead or alive? The development, trajectory and future of technology adoption research. J AIS. 2007;8(4):1. https://doi.org/10.17705/1jais.0012.
8. Davies I, Green P, Rosemann M, Indulska M, Gallo S. How do practitioners use conceptual modeling in practice? Data Knowl Eng. 2006;58(3):358–80. https://doi.org/10.1016/j.datak2005.07.007.
9. Ponce LB, Mendez JAJ, Garcia-Penalvo FJ. Analysis of certificated mobile application for medical education purposes. Proceedings of the Second International Conference on Technological Ecosystems for Enhancing Multiculturality. ACM. 2014:13–7. https://doi.org/10.1145/2669711.2669871.
10. Martínez-Pérez B, de la Torre-Díez I, Candelas-Plasencia S, López-Coronado M. Development and evaluation of tools for measuring the quality of experience (QoE) in mHealth applications. J Med Syst. 2013;37(5):9976. https://doi.org/10.1007/s10916-013-9976-x.
11. Robinson T, Cronin T, Ibrahim H, Jinks M, Molitor T, Newman J, Shapiro J. Smartphone use and acceptability among clinical medical students: a questionnaire-based study. J Med Syst. 2013;37(3):9936. https://doi.org/10.1007/s10916-013-9936-5.
12. Jensen R, Lauridsen N, Poulsen A, Tofte C, Christensen F. Analysis of subjective evaluation of user experience with headphones. Audio Engineering Society Conference: 2016 AES International Conference on Headphone Technology. Audio Engineering Society, 2016. Permalink: http://www.aes.org/e-lib/browse.cfm?elib=18345. Accessed 26 Jan 2019.
13. Meidert U, Heidrun KB, Mandy S. M-Health apps and self-quantification technologies on the rise: opportunities and risks for use in practice. Capetown: World Congress of Occupational Therapy; 2018.
14. O'Reilly-Shah VN, Kitzman J, Jabaley CS, Lynde GC. Evidence for increased use of the Society of Pediatric Anesthesia Critical Events Checklist in resource-limited environments: a retrospective observational study of app data. Pediatr Anesth. 2018;28(2):167–73. https://doi.org/10.1111/pan.13305.
15. Schild S, Sedlmayr B, Schumacher AK, Sedlmayr M, Prokosch HU, Pierre MS. German Cognitive Aid Working Group. A Digital Cognitive Aid for Anesthesia to Support Intraoperative Crisis Management: Results of the User-Centered Design Process. JMIR mHealth and uHealth. 2019;7(4):e13226. https://doi.org/10.2196/13226.

16. Highland KB, Tran J, Edwards H, Bedocs P, Suen J, Buckenmaier CC. Feasibility of App-Based Postsurgical Assessment of Pain, Pain Impact, and Regional Anesthesia Effects: A Pilot Randomized Controlled Trial. Pain Med. 2019;20(8):1592–9. https://doi.org/10.1093/pm/pny288.
17. Matava CT, Magbitang J, Choi S, Bhatia S, Tan M. A novel open-source novel app improves anesthesia operating room equipment supply. J Med Syst. 2018;42(9):167. https://doi.org/10.1007/s10916-018-1026-2.
18. Rijksinstituut voor Ziekte- en Invaliditeitsverzekering. Beroepsbeoefenaars met recht om prestaties te verrichten. 2016. https://www.inami.fgov.be/SiteCollectionDocuments/statistiek_2016_gv_proff_tabel2.pdf. Accessed 26 Jan 2019.
19. European Commission. Report of the Working Group on mHealth Assessment Guidelines. 2017. http://ec.europa.eu/newsroom/document.cfm?doc_id=45251, Accessed 26 Jan 2019.
20. European Commission. Report of the Working Group on mHealth assessment guidelines. 2017. https://ec.europa.eu/digital-single-market/en/news/report-working-group-mhealth-assessment-guidelines. Accessed 26 Jan 2019.
21. European Commission. Privacy Code of Conduct on mobile health apps. 2018. https://ec.europa.eu/digital-single-market/en/privacy-code-conduct-mobile-health-apps, Accessed 26 Jan 2019.
22. Agoria and beMedTech. mHealth Belgium platform. 2019. http://www.mhealthbelgium.be/. Accessed 26 Jan 2019.
23. Beleidscel van de minister van Sociale Zaken en Volksgezondheid. Medische apps krijgen plaats in Belgische gezondheidszorg. 2018. https://www.deblock.belgium.be/nl/medische-apps-krijgen-plaats-belgische-gezondheidszorg. Accessed 26 Jan 2019.
24. Barton AJ. Regulation of mobile health applications. BMC Med. 2012;10(1):46. https://doi.org/10.1186/1741-7015-10-46.
25. Hamilton AD, Brady RRW. Medical professional involvement in smartphone "apps" in dermatology. Br J Dermatol. 2012;167(1):220–1. https://doi.org/10.1111/j.1365-2133.2012.10844.x.
26. Rosser BA, Eccleston C. Smartphone applications for pain management. J Telemed Telecare. 2011;17(6):308–12. https://doi.org/10.1258/jtt.2011.101102.
27. Buijink AWG, Visser BJ, Marshall L. Medical apps for smartphones: lack of evidence undermines quality and safety. Evid Based Med. 2013;18(3):90–2. https://doi.org/10.1136/eb-2012-100885.
28. McCartney M. How do we know whether medical apps work? Br Med J. 2013;346:f1811. https://doi.org/10.1136/bmj.f1811.
29. Haute Autorité de santé. Good practice guidelines on health apps and smart devices (mobile health or mhealth). 2016. https://www.has-sante.fr//portail/jcms/c_2681915/en/good-practice-guidelines-on-health-apps-and-smart-devices-mobile-health-or-mhealth?cid=fc_1249702&portal=r_1455081. Accessed 26 Jan 2019.
30. IGES Institut. Health apps & co: safe digital care products. 2016. https://www.iges.com/clients/health/forschungsergebnisse/2016/health-apps-ii/index_eng.html. Accessed 22 Nov 2018.
31. UK GOV. Guidance: Medical devices: software applications (apps). 2018. https://www.gov.uk/government/publications/medical-devices-software-applications-apps. Accessed 26 Jan 2019.
32. Agencia de Calidad Sanitaria de Andalucía. Complete list of recommendations on design, use and assessment of health Apps. 2013. http://www.calidadappsalud.com/en/listado-completo-recomendaciones-app-salud/. Accessed 26 Jan 2019.
33. Fundació TicSalut. mHealth.cat Office. 2014. http://www.ticsalut.cat/observatori/mhealth/en_index/. Accessed 26 Jan 2019.
34. Monroe KS, Evans MA, Mukkamala SG, Williamson JL, Jabaley CS, Mariano ER, O'Reilly-Shah VN. Moving anesthesiology educational resources to the point of care: experience with a pediatric anesthesia mobile app. Korean J Anesthesiol. 2018;71(3):192. https://doi.org/10.4097/kja.d.18.00014.

Permissions

All chapters in this book were first published by BioMed Central; hereby published with permission under the Creative Commons Attribution License or equivalent. Every chapter published in this book has been scrutinized by our experts. Their significance has been extensively debated. The topics covered herein carry significant findings which will fuel the growth of the discipline. They may even be implemented as practical applications or may be referred to as a beginning point for another development.

The contributors of this book come from diverse backgrounds, making this book a truly international effort. This book will bring forth new frontiers with its revolutionizing research information and detailed analysis of the nascent developments around the world.

We would like to thank all the contributing authors for lending their expertise to make the book truly unique. They have played a crucial role in the development of this book. Without their invaluable contributions this book wouldn't have been possible. They have made vital efforts to compile up to date information on the varied aspects of this subject to make this book a valuable addition to the collection of many professionals and students.

This book was conceptualized with the vision of imparting up-to-date information and advanced data in this field. To ensure the same, a matchless editorial board was set up. Every individual on the board went through rigorous rounds of assessment to prove their worth. After which they invested a large part of their time researching and compiling the most relevant data for our readers.

The editorial board has been involved in producing this book since its inception. They have spent rigorous hours researching and exploring the diverse topics which have resulted in the successful publishing of this book. They have passed on their knowledge of decades through this book. To expedite this challenging task, the publisher supported the team at every step. A small team of assistant editors was also appointed to further simplify the editing procedure and attain best results for the readers.

Apart from the editorial board, the designing team has also invested a significant amount of their time in understanding the subject and creating the most relevant covers. They scrutinized every image to scout for the most suitable representation of the subject and create an appropriate cover for the book.

The publishing team has been an ardent support to the editorial, designing and production team. Their endless efforts to recruit the best for this project, has resulted in the accomplishment of this book. They are a veteran in the field of academics and their pool of knowledge is as vast as their experience in printing. Their expertise and guidance has proved useful at every step. Their uncompromising quality standards have made this book an exceptional effort. Their encouragement from time to time has been an inspiration for everyone.

The publisher and the editorial board hope that this book will prove to be a valuable piece of knowledge for researchers, students, practitioners and scholars across the globe.

List of Contributors

Gergely H. Fodor
Unit for Anesthesiological Investigations Department of Anesthesiology Pharmacology and Intensive Care, University of Geneva, Geneva, Switzerland
Department of Medical Physics and Informatics, University of Szeged, 9 Koranyi fasor, Szeged H-6720, Hungary

Federica Lovisari
Unit for Anesthesiological Investigations Department of Anesthesiology Pharmacology and Intensive Care, University of Geneva, Geneva, Switzerland
University of Milano-Bicocca, Milan, Italy

Walid Habre
Unit for Anesthesiological Investigations Department of Anesthesiology Pharmacology and Intensive Care, University of Geneva, Geneva, Switzerland
Pediatric Anesthesia Unit, Geneva Children's Hospital, Geneva, Switzerland
Unit for Anesthesiological Investigations, Department of Anesthesiology, Pharmacology and Intensive Care, University Hospitals of Geneva, University of Geneva, 1 Rue Michel Servet, CH-1205 Geneva, Switzerland

Sam Bayat
Unit for Anesthesiological Investigations Department of Anesthesiology Pharmacology and Intensive Care, University of Geneva, Geneva, Switzerland
Inserm UA7 STROBE Laboratory, University of Grenoble, Grenoble, France
Department of Clinical Physiology, Sleep and Exercise, Grenoble University Hospital, Grenoble, France

Sean Coeckelenbergh, Amélie Delaporte, Djamal Ghoundiwal, Javad Bidgoli, Denis Schmartz and Philippe Van der Linden
Department of Anesthesiology, CHU Brugmann, 4, Place Van Gehuchten, 1020 Bruxelles, Belgium
Université Libre de Bruxelles, Brussels, Belgium

Jean-François Fils
Department of Anesthesiology, CHU Brugmann, 4, Place Van Gehuchten, 1020 Bruxelles, Belgium
Ars Statistica SPRL, Nivelles, Belgium

Sergio A. Terrasa
Department of Research, Italiano de Buenos Aires Hospital, Buenos Aires, Argentina

Xiaocong Huang
Department of Anesthesiology, Guangdong Provincial Cardiovascular Institute, Guangdong Provincial People's Hospital (previously called Guangdong General Hospital), Guangdong Academy of Medical Sciences, Guangzhou 510630, China

Lei Chen and Xuemei Peng
Department of Anesthesiology, the First Affiliated Hospital of Jinan University, Guangzhou 510632, China

Yujing Cai
Department of Anesthesiology, Guangdong Provincial People's Hospital (previously called Guangdong General Hospital), Guangdong Academy of Medical Sciences, Guangzhou 510630, China

Jinfeng Wei
Department of Anesthesiology, Guangdong Provincial People's Hospital (previously called Guangdong General Hospital), Guangzhou 510630, China

Lina Lin and Jie Sun
College of Pharmacy, Jinan University, Guangzhou 510632, China

Sheng Wang
Department of Anesthesiology, Guangdong Provincial Cardiovascular Institute, Guangdong Provincial People's Hospital (previously called Guangdong General Hospital), Guangdong Academy of Medical Sciences, Guangzhou 510630, China
Department of Anesthesiology, Linzhi People's Hospital, Xizang 860000, China

Gonzalo Domenech, Matías A. Kampel, María E. García Guzzo, Delfina Sánchez Novas and Gustavo Garcia Fornari
Department of Anesthesiology, Italiano de Buenos Aires Hospital, Presidente Teniente General Juan Domingo Perón 4190, Postal Code, 1199 Buenos Aires, Argentina

Heleen J. Blussé van Oud-Alblas
Department of Anesthesiology, Erasmus Medical Center, Rotterdam, The Netherlands
Department of Anesthesiology, St. Antonius Hospital, Nieuwegein, The Netherlands

Meindert Danhof
Division of Pharmacology, Leiden Academic Center for Drug Research, Leiden University, Leiden, The Netherlands

Margreke J. E. Brill and Catherijne A. J. Knibbe
Division of Pharmacology, Leiden Academic Center for Drug Research, Leiden University, Leiden, The Netherlands
Department of Clinical Pharmacy, St. Antonius Hospital, 3430 EM Nieuwegein, The Netherlands

Mariska Y. M. Peeters
Department of Clinical Pharmacy, St. Antonius Hospital, 3430 EM Nieuwegein, The Netherlands

Dick Tibboel
Department of Pediatric Intensive Care, Erasmus Medical Center - Sophia Children's Hospital, Rotterdam, The Netherlands

Tadashi Tanioku, Akari Yoshida, Yuichi Aratani, Keisuke Fujii and Tomoyuki Kawamata
Department of Anesthesiology, Wakayama Medical University School of Medicine, Kimiidera 811-1, Wakayama 641-8509, Japan

Jonathan V. Roth
Department of Anesthesiology, Albert Einstein Medical Center, 5501 Old York Road, Philadelphia, PA, USA
Albert Einstein Healthcare Network, Philadelphia, PA, USA
Sidney Kimmel Medical School of Thomas Jefferson University, Philadelphia, PA, USA

Leonard E. Braitman and Lacy H. Hunt
Office for Research and Technology Development, Albert Einstein Medical Center, 5501 Old York Road, Philadelphia, PA, USA

Ferenc Peták
Department of Medical Physics and Informatics, University of Szeged, 9 Koranyi fasor, Szeged H-6720, Hungary

Adam L. Balogh, Roberta Südy and Barna Babik
Department of Anesthesiology and Intensive Therapy, University of Szeged, 8 Semmelweis str, Szeged H-6725, Hungary

Ulrick Sidney Kanmounye
Department of Research, Association of Future African Neurosurgeons, Kinshasa, Democratic Republic of Congo
Department of Neurosurgery, Faculty of Medicine, Bel Campus University of Technology, Kinshasa, Democratic Republic of Congo

Cynthia Kévine Wafo and Daniel Cheryl Eyaman
Department of Anesthesiology and Critical Care Medicine, Faculty of Medicine and Biomedical Sciences, University of Yaounde I, Yaounde, Cameroon

Joel Noutakdie Tochie
Department of Anesthesiology and Critical Care Medicine, Faculty of Medicine and Biomedical Sciences, University of Yaounde I, Yaounde, Cameroon
Human Research Education and Networking, Yaounde, Cameroon

Aimé Mbonda
Faculty of Medicine and Biomedical Sciences, University of Yaounde I, Yaounde, Cameroon
Surgery Unit, District Hospital of Batouri, Batouri, Cameroon
Department of Research, International Student Surgical Network, Yaounde, Cameroon

Leonid Daya
Department of Anesthesiology and Critical Care Medicine, Faculty of Medicine and Biomedical Sciences, University of Yaounde I, Yaounde, Cameroon
Department of Research, International Student Surgical Network, Yaounde, Cameroon

Thompson Hope Atem
Department of Internal Medicine, Faculty of Medicine, Bel Campus University of Technology, Kinshasa, Democratic Republic of Congo

Arsène Daniel Nyalundja
Department of Research, Association of Future African Neurosurgeons, Kinshasa, Democratic Republic of Congo
Faculty of Medicine, Catholic University of Bukavu, Bukavu, Democratic Republic of Congo

Tarig Osman
Centre for Population Health Sciences, Lee Kong Chian School of Medicine, Nanyang Technological University (Singapore), Singapore, Singapore

Eileen Lew, Rajive Dabas and Ban Leong Sng
Department of Women's Anaesthesia, KK Women's and Children's Hospital (Singapore), 100 Bukit Timah Road, Singapore 229899, Singapore

Elaine Pooi-Ming Lum
Centre for Population Health Sciences, Lee Kong Chian School of Medicine, Nanyang Technological University (Singapore), Singapore, Singapore
Duke-NUS Medical School, 8, College Road, Singapore 169857, Singapore

Louise van Galen
Centre for Population Health Sciences, Lee Kong Chian School of Medicine, Nanyang Technological University (Singapore), Singapore, Singapore
Department of Internal Medicine, VU University Medical Center, De Boelelaan 1117, Room ZH 4A58, 1081 HV Amsterdam, Netherlands

Josip Car
Centre for Population Health Sciences, Lee Kong Chian School of Medicine, Nanyang Technological University (Singapore), Singapore, Singapore
Global eHealth Unit, Department of Primary Care and Public Health, School of Public Health, Imperial College London (United Kingdom), London, UK

Yu Cui, Rong Cao, Lingmei Deng and Jia Li
Department of Anesthesiology, The Affiliated Hospital, School of Medicine, UESTC Chengdu Women's & Children's Central Hospital, No.1617, Riyue Avenue, Qingyang District, Chengdu 610091, PR China

Yu Wang
Department of Anesthesilogy, No.363 hospital, Chengdu 610041, China

Gen Li
Department of Anesthesiology, Vanderbilt University Medical Center, Nashville, TN 37232, USA

Yan Xing, Nan Lin, Ruquan Han, Yuming Peng, Jiaxin Li, Xiaoyuan Liu, Yan Li, Jia Dong, Min Zeng, Manyu Zhang and Lanyi Nie
Department of Anesthesiology, Beijing Tiantan Hospital, Capital Medical University, No.119, West Road 4th ring South, Fengtai District, Beijing 100070, China

John F. Bebawy
Departments of Anesthesiology & Neurological Surgery, Northwestern University Feinberg School of Medicine, 251 E. Huron St., F5-704, Chicago, IL 60611, USA

Jingli Chen, Caihua Liu, Chang Liu, Quanyuan Fu, Dingwei Pei, Linyun Ren and Hong Yan
Department of Anaesthesia, The Central Hospital of Wuhan, Tongji Medical College, Huazhong University of Science and Technology, Wuhan 430014, Hubei, China

Marieke Poterman, Pieter L. Buisman, Michel M. R. F. Struys and Thomas W. L. Scheeren
Department of Anaesthesiology, University Medical Center Groningen, Hanzeplein 1, 9700, RB, Groningen, The Netherlands

Alain F. Kalmar
Department of Anaesthesiology, University Medical Center Groningen, Hanzeplein 1, 9700, RB, Groningen, The Netherlands
Department of Anaesthesiology, AZ Maria Middelares Gent Buitenring Sint-Denijs 30, 9000 Ghent, Belgium

Hong Yin, Guangyi Zhao, Yingjie Du and Ping Zhao
Department of Anesthesiology, Shengjing Hospital of China Medical University, Shenyang 110004, China

Kore Menjie Benwu and Hagos Gebregziabher Gebremedhin
Mekelle University College of Health Science Department of Anesthesia, Mekelle, Ethiopia

Jennifer Herzog-Niescery, Martin Bellgardt, Andreas Breuer-Kaiser, Philipp Gude, Heike Vogelsang and Thomas Peter Weber
Department of Anesthesiology, Katholisches Klinikum Bochum, Ruhr-University Bochum, St. Josef Hospital, Gudrunstraße 56, 44791 Bochum, Germany

Thomas Steffens and Hans-Martin Seipp
Department of Life Science Engineering, University of Applied Sciences, Giessen, Germany

Ling Lan, Penghao Liu, Yuan Tian, Bo Zhu, Le Shen and Yuguang Huang
Department of Anaesthesiology, Peking Union Medical College Hospital, Peking Union Medical College and Chinese Academy of Medical Sciences, 100730 Beijing, P.R. China

Hong-Qian Wang
Department of Anesthesiology, Eastern Hepatobiliary Surgery Hospital, the Second Military Medical University, 225 Changhai Road, Shanghai, China

Xiao-Yan Meng and Wei-Feng Yu
Department of Anesthesiology, Ren Ji Hospital, School of Medicine, Shanghai Jiao Tong University, 160 Pudian Road, Shanghai, China

Xiu-Ping Zhang and Zhe Sun
Department of Hepatic Surgery, Eastern Hepatobiliary Surgery Hospital, the Second Military Medical University, 225 Changhai Road, Shanghai, China

Penghui Wei, Dong Yan, Lili Dong, Ying Zhao, Fei Rong, Jing Li, Wenxi Tang and Jianjun Li
Department of Anesthesiology, Qilu Hospital of Shandong University (Qingdao), No.758 Hefei Road, Qingdao, People's Republic of China

Jiapeng Huang
Department of Anesthesiology & Perioperative Medicine, University of Louisville, Louisville, KY, USA

Sangbin Han
Department of Emergency medicine, Cheongyang Health Center County Hospital, Chungcheongnam-do, Republic of Korea

Jaesik Park, Sang Hyun Hong, Soojin Lim and Min Suk Chae
Department of anesthesiology and Pain medicine, Seoul St. Mary's Hospital, College of Medicine, The Catholic University of Korea, 222, Banpo-daero, Seocho-gu, Seoul 06591, Republic of Korea

Yong Hyun Park
Department of Urology, Seoul St. Mary's Hospital, College of Medicine, The Catholic University of Korea, Seoul, Republic of Korea

Chiara Robba
Anaesthesia and Intensive Care, IRCCS for Oncology and Neurosciences, San Martino Policlinico Hospital, Genoa, Italy

Denise Battaglini, Paolo Pelosi and Lorenzo Ball
Anaesthesia and Intensive Care, IRCCS for Oncology and Neurosciences, San Martino Policlinico Hospital, Genoa, Italy
Department of Surgical Sciences and Integrated Diagnostics, University of Genoa, Genoa, Italy

Patricia Rieken Macêdo Rocco
Laboratory of Pulmonary Investigation, Carlos Chagas Filho Institute of Biophysics, Federal University of Rio de Janeiro, Rio de Janeiro, Brazil

Marcelo Gama De Abreu
Department of Anaesthesiology and Intensive Care Medicine, Pulmonary Engineering Group, University Hospital Carl Gustav Carus, Technische Universität Dresden, Dresden, Germany

Xia Yuan, Tingjie Liu, Chunbo Hu and Xia Shen
Department of Anesthesiology, The Eye, Ear, Nose and Throat Hospital, Fudan University, 83 fenyang road, Shanghai 200031, China

Kohei Fukuta, Asuka Kasai, Noriko Niki, Yuki Ishikawa, Ryosuke Kawanishi, Nami Kakuta, Yoko Sakai and Katsuya Tanaka
Department of Anesthesiology, Graduate School of Biomedical Sciences, Tokushima University, 3-18-15 Kuramoto, Tokushima 770-8503, Japan

Yasuo M. Tsutsumi
Department of Anesthesiology and Critical Care, Graduate School of Biomedical and Health Sciences, Hiroshima University, 1-2-3 Kasumi Minami, Hiroshima 774-8551, Japan

James Harvey Jones and Robin Aldwinckle
UC Davis Department of Anesthesiology and Pain Medicine, University of California Davis Medical Center, 4150 V Street, PSSB Suite 1200, Sacramento, CA 95817, USA

Hugo Carvalho and Jan Poelaert
Vrije Universiteit Brussel (VUB), Universitair Ziekenhuis Brussel (UZ Brussel), Brussels, Belgium

Michael Verdonck
Vrije Universiteit Brussel (VUB), Universitair Ziekenhuis Brussel (UZ Brussel), Brussels, Belgium
Business Informatics Research Group, Universiteit Gent, Ghent, Belgium

Patrice Forget
Institute of Applied Health Sciences, NHS Grampian, University of Aberdeen, Aberdeen, UK

Index

www.ingramcontent.com/pod-product-compliance
Lightning Source LLC
LaVergne TN
LVHW060518210926
848485LV00005B/1104
9781646465804